# Dry Mouth

Guy Carpenter
Editor

# Dry Mouth

## A Clinical Guide on Causes, Effects and Treatments

Springer

*Editor*
Guy Carpenter
Department of Salivary Research
Kings College London Dental Institute
London
UK

ISBN 978-3-642-55153-6 ISBN 978-3-642-55154-3 (eBook)
DOI 10.1007/978-3-642-55154-3
Springer Heidelberg New York Dordrecht London

Library of Congress Control Number: 2014953246



Printed on acid-free paper

Springer is part of Springer Science+Business Media (www.springer.com)

# Contents

**Part I Background Topics**

1 **Introduction** . . . . . . . . . . . . . . . . . . . . . . . . . . . . . . . . . . . . 3
Guy Carpenter

**Part II Causes**

2 **Diseases Causing Oral Dryness** . . . . . . . . . . . . . . . . . . . . . . . . . . . . . 7
Anne Marie Lynge Pedersen

3 **Medication-Induced Dry Mouth** . . . . . . . . . . . . . . . . . . . . . . . . . . . . 33
Gordon B. Proctor

4 **Cancer-/Cancer Treatment-Related Salivary Gland Dysfunction** . . . . . . . . . . . . . . . . . . . . . . . . . . . . . . . . . . . . 51
Andrew N. Davies

**Part III Effects**

5 **Oral Dryness, Dietary Intake, and Alterations in Taste** . . . . . . . . . . . 69
Anja Weirsøe Dynesen

6 **Xerostomia and the Oral Microflora** . . . . . . . . . . . . . . . . . . . . . . . . . 81
Antoon J.M. Ligtenberg and Annica Almståhl

7 **Subjective Aspects of Dry Mouth** . . . . . . . . . . . . . . . . . . . . . . . . . . . 103
W. Murray Thomson

**Part IV Diagnosis**

8 **Clinical Scoring Scales for Assessment of Dry Mouth** . . . . . . . . . . . . 119
Stephen J. Challacombe, Samira M. Osailan, and Gordon B. Proctor

9 **Imaging of Salivary Glands** . . . . . . . . . . . . . . . . . . . . . . . . . . . . . . . 133
Bethan Louise Thomas

**Part V Treatment**

**10 New Radiotherapy Techniques for the Prevention of Radiotherapy-Induced Xerostomia** . . . . . 147
Thomas M. Richards and Christopher M. Nutting

**11 Artificial Salivas: Why Are They Not More Useful?** . . . . . 165
Guy Carpenter

**12 The Beneficial Effects of Regular Chewing** . . . . . 175
Taichi Inui

**13 Future Prevention and Treatment of Radiation-Induced Hyposalivation** . . . . . 195
Robert P. Coppes and Tara A. van de Water

**Index** . . . . . 213

# Contributors

**Annica Almståhl, PhD, Dental Hygenist** Department of Oral Microbiology and Immunology, Sahlgrenska Academy, University of Gothenburg, Gothenburg, Sweden

**Guy Carpenter** Salivary Research, King's College London Dental Institute, London, UK

**Stephen J. Challacombe, PhD, FRC(Path), FDSRCS, FMedSci** Department of Oral Medicine, King's College London, Guys and St Thomas' Hospital, London, UK

**Robert P. Coppes, PhD** Department of Radiation Oncology and Cell Biology, University Medical Center Groningen, Groningen, The Netherlands

**Andrew N. Davies, FRCP** Palliative Medicine, Palliative Care, Royal Surrey County Hospital, Guildford, Surrey, UK

**Anja Weirsøe Dynesen, DDS, MSc. Human Nutrition, PhD** Department of Odontology, Faculty of Health and Medical Sciences, University of Copenhagen, Copenhagen Nørrebro, Denmark

**Taichi Inui, PhD** Department of R&D, Wm. Wrigley Jr. Company, Chicago, IL, USA

**Antoon J. M. Ligtenberg, PhD** Department of Oral Biochemistry, Academic Centre for Dentistry Amsterdam, Amsterdam, The Netherlands

**Christopher M. Nutting, MBBS, BSc, MD, PhD, MRCP, FRCR** Head and Neck Unit, The Royal Marsden Hospital, London, UK

**Samira M. Osailan, BDS, PhD** Department of Oral Surgery, King Abdulaziz University, Jeddah, Saudi Arabia

**Anne Marie Lynge Pedersen, PhD, DDS** Section of Oral Medicine, Clinical Oral Physiology, Oral Pathology and Anatomy, Department of Odontology, Faculty of Health and Medical Sciences, University of Copenhagen, Copenhagen, Denmark

**Gordon B. Proctor, BSc, PhD** Mucosal and Salivary Biology Division, King's College London Dental Institute, London, UK

**Thomas M. Richards, BSc, MBBS, MRCP, FRCR** Head and Neck Unit, The Royal Marsden Hospital, London, UK

**Bethan Louise Thomas, BDS, BSc (Hons), PhD, DDMFR RCR** Dental and Maxillofacial Radiology, Guy's Hospital, Guy's and St Thomas' NHS Foundation Trust, London, UK

Dental RadiologyThe Eastman Dental Hospital, University College London Hospitals NHS Foundation Trust, London, UK

**W. Murray Thomson, BSc, BDS, MA, MComDent, PhD** Dental Epidemiology and Public Health, Oral Sciences, Faculty of Dentistry, Sir John Walsh Research Institute, The University of Otago, Dunedin, Otago, New Zealand

**Tara A. van de Water, PhD** Department of Radiation Oncology, University Medical Center Groningen, Groningen, The Netherlands

# Part I

# Background Topics

# Introduction

# 1

Guy Carpenter

**Abstract**

This book has come about following a symposium organized by the editor to encourage further research into dry mouth and its causes. The symposium was held at the Pan-European meeting of the IADR, and as a consequence, this book is largely based on contributions from Europeans. This may lead to variations compared to US-based books as there are differences in drug prescribing, irradiation protocols, and even diagnostic criteria that may influence the healthcare professional. Using even the most conservative of estimates, this book will still be relevant to the 30 million dry mouth sufferers in the European region. In trying to stimulate research in this field, a more scientific than clinical approach has been taken although, of course, the two go hand in hand.

Dry mouth is surprisingly a common symptom. For the entire population, it is estimated that 10–30 % may experience a troublesome dry mouth with a smaller percentage suffering serious impact on their quality of life. Salivary secretion is an autonomic reflex stimulated mainly by taste and chewing. The resting flow rate that maintains a hydrated mouth between meals is driven mostly by cortical activity. It is often the decline in the resting rate of salivary secretion that causes most people most problems – particularly at night when cortical activity will be at its lowest. As we discover in the initial chapters, dry mouth can develop from three main causes: by specific diseases of the salivary glands (Chap. 2 – Dr Pedersen), as a side effect of head and neck irradiation treatment for cancer (Chap. 4 – Dr Davies), or most commonly as a side effect of prescribed drugs (Chap. 3 – Prof Proctor). One

G. Carpenter
Salivary Research, King's College London Dental Institute,
Floor 17, Tower wing, London SE1 9RT, UK
e-mail: guy.carpenter@kcl.ac.uk

 
G. Carpenter (ed.), *Dry Mouth: A Clinical Guide on Causes, Effects and Treatments*, DOI 10.1007/978-3-642-55154-3_1

of the problems with dry mouth is that because it is subjectively reported, it is harder to diagnose than an objective measure, such as salivary flow rate. It should follow that dry mouth is caused by decreased saliva production, but this is not always the case. Due to a wide variation in flow rates of a normal population, there is little to separate a hyposalivator from an individual with a normal range of salivation. A recent development has been a clinical scoring system to aid general practitioners and healthcare workers to determine the severity of the dry mouth. The Challacombe scale is fully explained by its originator (Chap. 8 – Prof Challacombe) and set within the background of other scoring systems which are notoriously complicated and variable. Within the hospital setting, (Chap. 9 – Dr Thomas) explores some different imaging modalities and recent advances that can be used to identify glandular changes that would cause hyposecretion and therefore dry mouth.

The rate of change from normal salivation to dry mouth often makes a difference as to when subjects report dry mouth to a clinician. For example, subjects on medication that have xerostomia as a side effect (around 50 % of all drugs have this property) develop dry mouth relatively quickly and are more likely to report dry mouth than subjects with a slow change, perhaps caused by an autoimmune condition such as Sjögren's syndrome. To emphasize the point, children born with a lack of salivary glands (aplasia) often do not report dry mouth as a problem probably because they have never known what a normally hydrated mouth feels like. Dry mouth is widely perceived as a minor symptom except by those that suffer from it. This seemingly unjust situation probably occurs because it is not life threatening. Yet the impact on quality of life (Chap. 7 – Dr Thompson) is considerable often leaving patients socially isolated. This is because saliva affects all functions of the mouth and thus a lack of saliva will have an impact on eating, chewing and swallowing leading to a poorer diet (Chap. 5 – Dr Dynesen). Furthermore, the oral health of dry mouth patients is challenged by a change in the oral flora. Saliva has many antibacterial proteins, but it also has pro-microbial factors that help to maintain a normal healthy flora commensal to the host. The changes and impacts of an altered oral flora with dry mouth are fully described by Prof Ligtenberg (Chap. 6). Overall the impact of a dry mouth is considerable, leading to subjects losing weight and becoming dehydrated which also impacts on their quality of life.

The final section of the book addresses recent research in treating or even remedying dry mouth. Of immediate availability are artificial salivas (Dr Carpenter – Chap. 11), and the benefits of chewing gum in improving oral health are further discussed (Dr Inui – Chap. 12). For those patients who have to undergo head and neck irradiation for the treatment of cancer, improvements in the irradiation protocol and equipment are outlined in Chap. 10 by Dr Richards and Prof Nutting. The field of stem cells and their beneficial healing properties as well as regenerating properties offers great hope for future treatments (Chap. 13 – Prof Coppes).

# Part II

# Causes

# Diseases Causing Oral Dryness

# 2

Anne Marie Lynge Pedersen

**Abstract**

Saliva is important for the maintenance of oral health and also plays an essential role in a number of oral and gastrointestinal functions. Consequently, patients with reduced salivary secretion and changes in their saliva composition are more susceptible to dental caries, oral infections and mucosal lesions and often have symptoms of a dry and sore mouth, burning and itching oral mucosa, difficulties in chewing and swallowing dry foods, impaired sense of taste, difficulty in speaking and problems with acid reflux. These distressing consequences of salivary hypofunction also have a significant negative impact on quality of life and general health status. Several diseases and medical conditions as well as the medications used for treating them are associated with salivary gland hypofunction (objective evidence of diminished salivary output) and xerostomia (subjective sensation of dry mouth). In autoimmune diseases like Sjögren's syndrome, salivary gland dysfunction is largely related to structural changes in the salivary glands and in endocrine and metabolic disorders mainly related to pathophysiological changes that affect the formation of saliva. Other diseases affect the autonomic outflow pathway involving the salivary gland innervation, the central nervous system and the salivation centre. This chapter reviews systemic diseases and medical conditions associated with salivary gland hypofunction and xerostomia.

A.M.L. Pedersen, PhD, DDS
Section of Oral Medicine, Clinical Oral Physiology, Oral Pathology and Anatomy,
Department of Odontology, Faculty of Health and Medical Sciences,
University of Copenhagen, Noerre Allé 20, Copenhagen 2200, Denmark
e-mail: amlp@sund.ku.dk



G. Carpenter (ed.), *Dry Mouth: A Clinical Guide on Causes, Effects and Treatments*, DOI 10.1007/978-3-642-55154-3_2

## Xerostomia and Salivary Gland Hypofunction

Inadequate salivary function is often associated with the sensation of dry mouth referred to as xerostomia. Xerostomia usually occurs when the unstimulated whole saliva flow rate is reduced with about 50 % of its normal value in any given individual [1]. However, xerostomia also occurs in the presence of normal salivary secretion [2] indicating that also the quality of saliva may be of importance to oral comfort.

Xerostomia is a common complaint, estimated to daily and persistently affect at least 10 % of an adult population [3, 4] and about 30 % of the elderly people [4]. The increase in prevalence of xerostomia with age is primarily ascribed to a higher incidence of systemic diseases and intake of medications among the elderly [4–6]. Although age-related changes in the structure of the salivary glands might suggest hypofunction, there is no clinically significant reduction in the overall gland output with aging in healthy, non-medicated adults [7].

The term hyposalivation is based on objective measures of the salivary secretion (sialometry) and refers to the condition where the unstimulated whole saliva flow rate is ≤0.1 ml/min and/or the chewing-stimulated whole saliva flow rate is ≤0.7 ml/min [8, 9]. The normal unstimulated whole saliva flow rate ranges between 0.3 and 0.5 ml/min and the normal stimulated whole saliva flow rate between 1.0 and 1.5 ml/min [8, 9]. The most commonly used method for measuring the whole saliva flow rate is the so-called draining method. This method is highly reproducible and simple to use in the dental office [10]. Evaluation of salivary gland function should be a routine part of any oral examination in order to manage and prevent the serious consequences of salivary gland dysfunction (Fig. 2.1). Despite comprehensive and systematic evaluation, it may in some cases be difficult to determine whether the symptoms of oral dryness and the salivary gland hypofunction are caused by the systemic disease itself or by the pharmacological treatment.

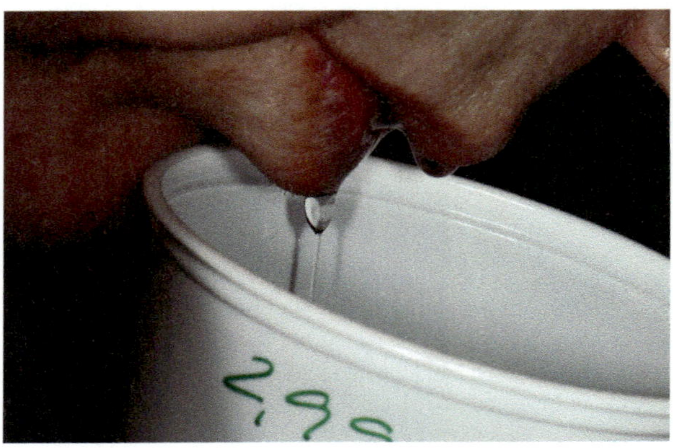


**Fig. 2.1** Measurement of the unstimulated whole saliva flow rate using the drooling method

## Autoimmune Diseases

Autoimmune diseases include a large number of chronic inflammatory connective tissue diseases like Sjögren's syndrome, rheumatoid arthritis, systemic lupus erythematosus and scleroderma, but also sarcoidosis, inflammatory bowel diseases and endocrine diseases. Overlap between the various autoimmune diseases is common.

## Chronic Inflammatory Connective Tissue Diseases

### Sjögren's Syndrome

Sjögren's syndrome (SS) is a chronic, systemic autoimmune inflammatory disorder that affects the exocrine glands and particularly the salivary and lacrimal glands [11]. The most prominent disease manifestations include hyposalivation and keratoconjunctivitis sicca, which result in symptoms of oral and ocular dryness. Although characterised as an exocrinopathy, non-exocrine organs may also be affected [11, 12]. The aetiology remains unknown, but most likely includes an interaction between immunological, genetic, hormonal and environmental factors. SS can occur at all ages, but the median age of presentation is around 50 years. A female preponderance is seen with a female to male ratio of 9:1 [11, 12]. Diagnosis is often delayed which reflects the fact that the onset of disease is often insidious, and patients often present various and non-specific symptoms like fatigue, myalgia, arthralgia and intermittent fever [11–13]. SS can occur alone as primary SS or in conjunction with another chronic inflammatory connective tissue disease such as rheumatoid arthritis, systemic lupus erythematosus, scleroderma or mixed connective tissue disease, designated as secondary SS [14]. The prevalence of primary SS is about 0.6 %, but the prevalence varies depending on the population sampled and the diagnostic criteria used [15]. At present, there are no specific diagnostic tests for SS. The diagnosis is based on a combination of questions regarding oral and ocular symptoms and clinical tests for evaluation of the salivary and lacrimal gland function as well as labial salivary gland biopsy and serological analysis for presence of serum autoantibodies (anti-Ro/SSA and anti-La/SSB) [16]. The classification criteria for SS currently used by clinicians and researchers around the world are the American-European Consensus Classification Criteria [16] (Table 2.1). The diagnosis of SS requires presence of focal lymphocytic infiltrates in the labial salivary glands and/or presence of serum autoantibodies as indicators of autoimmune activity [16]. Recently, a new set of classification criteria was proposed that are based entirely on objective measures [17]. At present, there is no curative therapy for SS, and current management is mainly symptomatic. Patients with SS are at risk of developing diseases of the oral hard and soft tissues due to hyposalivation and therefore require special attention by the dentist.

The histological findings of the labial salivary glands that have been given diagnostic significance are characterised by focal, periductal infiltration of lymphocytes, comprising about 80 % T lymphocytes and 20 % B lymphocytes [18, 19]

**Table 2.1** American-European classification criteria for Sjögren's syndrome [16]

| |
|---|
| I. Ocular symptoms, positive response for at least one of the following questions |
| 1. Have you felt your eyes dry for the past 3 months? |
| 2. Do you have a recurrent feeling of sand in your eyes? |
| 3. Do you use tear substitutes more than 3 times a day? |
| II. Oral symptoms, positive response for at least one of the following questions |
| 1. Have you felt your mouth dry for the past 3 months? |
| 2. Have you had persistent or recurrent swollen salivary glands in your adult life? |
| 3. Do you normally drink liquids to help you swallow dry foods? |
| III. Ocular impairment signs, positive results in one of the two following tests |
| 1. Schirmer I test (≤5 mm/5 min) |
| 2. Rose bengal staining (≥4 according to van Bijsterveld's scoring system) |
| IV. Histopathology: presence of focal lymphocytic infiltration with focus score ≥1 in minor salivary gland biopsy |
| V. Salivary gland involvement, positive results in one of the two following tests |
| 1. Whole saliva sialometry ≤1.5 ml/15 min |
| 2. Parotid sialography (presence of diffuse punctate sialectasia) |
| 3. Salivary scintigraphy (delayed uptake, reduced concentration and/or decreased excretion of tracer) |
| VI. Presence of serum autoantibodies |
| 1. Antibodies to Ro(SSA) or La(SSB) antigens or both |

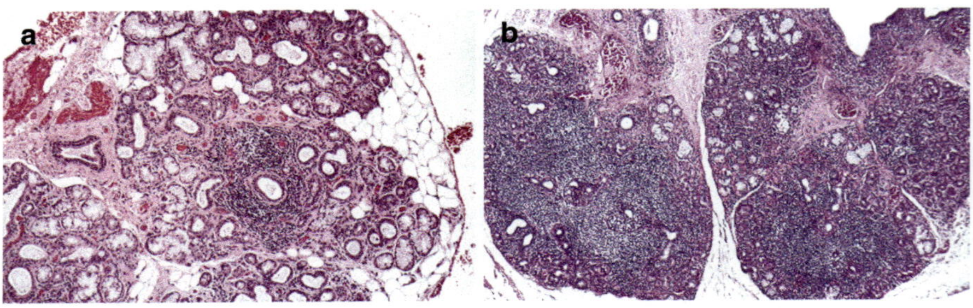


**Fig. 2.2** Labial salivary gland specimens from patients with Sjögren's syndrome. (**a**) Presence of focal periductal lymphocytic infiltrates. Note the normal-appearing acinar cells adjacent to the infiltrate. (**b**) Confluent foci of lymphocytes in labial salivary gland tissue

(Fig. 2.2). The lymphocytic infiltrates may in severe cases replace the acinar tissue. The degree of lymphocytic infiltration is evaluated semi-quantitatively by means of a focus scoring system in which a focus is defined as an aggregate of more than 50 lymphocytes per 4 $mm^2$ of glandular tissue [18]. A focus score is derived by calculating the number of foci per 4 $mm^2$ of the total salivary gland tissue in the specimen [18]. A focus score ≥1 is considered consistent with the diagnosis of SS, provided that other criteria are fulfilled [16, 17].

However, focal lymphocytic infiltrates in labial salivary glands are not specific for SS, but may be seen in other disorders such as type 1 diabetes mellitus [20, 21], myasthenia gravis [22], primary biliary cirrhosis [23] and SOX syndrome [24].

Acute and chronic graft-versus-host disease [25], HIV infection [26], leukaemia or lymphoid malignancies [27] and sarcoidosis [28] display symptoms and salivary gland histopathology that resembles SS, and they are also among the exclusion criteria in the American-European Consensus Classification Criteria for SS [16].

The impaired salivary gland function and xerostomia are considered to be consequences of progressive lymphocyte-mediated destruction of the gland tissue [29, 30]. However, the extent of focal lymphocytic infiltration in labial salivary glands is not always associated with the functional capacity of the salivary glands [31, 32]. Thus, some patients with markedly diminished salivary secretion may lack significant focal lymphocytic infiltration in their labial salivary glands indicating an earlier involvement of the major salivary glands than of the minor ones. On the other hand, a recent study indicates that the diagnostic value of labial and parotid biopsies is comparable, and the advantage of taking a parotid biopsy is that it allows comparison of flow rate with histopathological findings from the same gland [33].

It has been suggested that the exocrine gland hypofunction is not merely a result of immune-mediated inflammation, but could be the result of a neurogenic, autonomic dysfunction. It has been shown that stimulation of labial salivary gland cells of isolated patients with primary SS produces an almost identical rise in the intracellular calcium concentration as that of healthy controls, which indicate that patients with SS possess functional receptor systems on their salivary gland cells, despite severely impaired salivary flow [34]. Along this it has been reported that the M3 muscarinic receptors are up-regulated in labial salivary gland acinar cells of patients with primary SS [35] and that these cells have a lowered sensitivity to acetylcholine [36]. These findings suggest that the receptors on the salivary gland cell membranes are not activated either due to inactivation or increased breakdown of the neurotransmitters (most likely acetylcholine) in the synaptic cleft or inhibition of the receptor systems by autoantibodies or cytokines or defect in the intracellular second messenger systems required for stimulus-secretion coupling in acinar cells [12, 34]. Experimental studies in animals suggest that SS-autoantibodies and cytokines play a role in the pathogenesis of exocrine hypofunction by interacting with the muscarinic receptors [37, 38] and that antibodies inhibit the function of the salivary and lacrimal glands [39, 40]. The potential involvement of autoantibodies in SS is further substantiated by the demonstration of Ro/SSA and La/SSB autoantibody-producing cells in labial salivary glands of patients with SS having circulating serum autoantibodies [41]. In addition, interaction of the salivary gland cells with infiltrating lymphocytes seems to lead to increased secretion of cytokines such as IL-6 and TNF-α than can interfere with the binding of neurotransmitters to the receptor system and thereby contribute to salivary gland dysfunction in SS. Moreover, it has recently been shown that autonomic symptoms are common in SS and are associated with the disease activity and symptom burden [42].

Other salivary measures that have been used diagnostically include sialometry with measurement of unstimulated whole saliva flow rate. It has been reported that in primary SS patients with the lowest unstimulated whole salivary flow rates, i.e. <0.05 ml/min, the sensation of oral dryness had the most significant negative impact on general health. These patients were also more severely affected by non-exocrine disease involvement and serological hyperactivity and had more extensive focal lymphocytic infiltrates than patients with flow rates >0.05 ml/min [43]. Measurement of the paraffin chewing-stimulated whole saliva flow rate with a pathological cut-off value of ≤3.5 ml/5 min has a relatively low diagnostic sensitivity (66 %) and specificity (56 %) and is not included in the classification criteria [16]. On the other hand, it provides information regarding the residual secretory capacity of the salivary glands and is useful in monitoring disease progression and efficacy of therapeutic intervention. Selective measurement of the parotid, submandibular and sublingual and the minor salivary gland flow provides important information concerning the function of each of these glands and the composition of the saliva that is produced in these glands, but are not included in the classification criteria. Nevertheless, measurements from these glands indicate that mucous glands/acini are affected earlier than the serous ones [44].

Sialochemical analyses have demonstrated elevated concentrations of sodium and chloride in whole saliva and parotid and submandibular/sublingual saliva despite markedly diminished flow rates, which indicate an impairment of ductal reabsorption of sodium and chloride [44, 45].

Cytokines are assumed to play an essential role in the pathogenesis and B-cell development in SS. It has been reported that serum levels of members of the tumour necrosis factor (TNF) superfamily and levels of the B-cell-activating factor (BAFF) are increased in SS compared to controls and are found correlated with the focal lymphocytic infiltrates in the labial salivary glands [46, 47]. More recent analyses of salivary changes in SS using proteomics, genomics and systems biology assays have opened new possibilities for easier and earlier detection of SS as well as for monitoring the effects occurring in salivary gland physiology induced by treatment with biological agents [48, 49].

Intermittent or persistent enlargement of the salivary glands, particularly the parotid glands, occurs in 20–30 % of patients with SS [50]. It may be unilateral or bilateral. The swelling is usually related to benign lymphoepithelial lesions in the gland tissue. A persistent, unilateral salivary gland enlargement should give suspicion of lymphoma development, since patients with SS have an increased risk of developing non-Hodgkin's lymphomas, typically the mucosa-associated lymphoid tissue (MALT) type that is about 18 times greater than in the general population [51]. Risk factors for the development of lymphoma include low complement C4 levels, presence of cryoglobulins and palpable purpura [52].

## Rheumatoid Arthritis

Rheumatoid arthritis (RA) is a chronic systemic inflammatory disease which affects multiple joints of the body. The inflammatory process primarily affects the lining of the joints (synovial membrane), but can also affect other organs. The inflamed synovium leads to erosions of the cartilage and bone, which may result in joint deformity and disability. It affects 0.5–1.0 % of the population with a female to male ratio of 3:1 [53]. The onset of RA is usually 25–45 years of age, but it may occur in all age groups. The aetiology is unknown, but probably involves interplay between genetic and environmental factors (smoking, viral infections, vitamin D deficiency) that triggers a specific autoimmune response. RA primarily affects the small joints in the hands, wrists and feet. It may also in rare cases affect the temporomandibular joint. The symptoms include malaise, fatigue, weakness, muscle soreness, fever and weight loss which often precede the symptoms of the joints (pain, stiffness, redness and swelling). RA is classified according to the 2010 American College of Rheumatology (ACR) and European League Against Rheumatism (EULAR) classification criteria for rheumatoid arthritis.

A study of 636 patients with RA found that 50 % had symptoms of dry mouth and 17 % diminished unstimulated whole saliva flow rates [54]. It has also been shown that patients with RA have significantly lower saliva secretion from the submandibular gland compared to healthy controls, while the parotid saliva flow rate was in the normal range [55]. The concentrations of acidic proline-rich proteins and statherin in saliva from the submandibular gland were lower in the RA patients with xerostomia than in RA patients without xerostomia and healthy controls [55]. Other studies have also reported an increased frequency of xerostomia and hyposalivation in RA [56–58]. Enlargement of the major salivary glands is relatively seldom, and the risk of lymphoma is low. On the other hand, the labial salivary glands may display inflammatory changes like those seen in patients with SS [59, 60]. About 30 % of patients with RA also have SS (secondary SS), but xerostomia and the salivary hypofunction and histopathology may be present, independent of SS [61, 62].

## Systemic Lupus Erythematosus

Systemic lupus erythematosus (SLE) is a chronic, autoimmune, inflammatory disease which affects the joints, skin, kidneys, membranes such as the pleura and pericardium, central nervous system and blood-forming system. The overall prevalence is approx. 50 per 100,000. The onset of SLE is usually in the age of 20–30 years, and the female to male ratio is 10:1. Apart from symptoms like fatigue, weight loss and intermittent fever, SLE is characterised by a facial exanthema (butterfly-like rash), photophobia, vasculitis, hair loss, arthritis, Raynaud's phenomenon, pleuritis, pericarditis, glomerulonephritis, seizure and psychosis. It has been reported that 75 % of patients with SLE have oral symptoms including mucosal soreness and xerostomia [63]. It has also been shown that the unstimulated whole saliva flow rate in some cases is decreased and that the concentration of statherin in saliva from the parotid gland is lower, whereas the concentration of acidic proline-rich proteins from parotid and submandibular gland saliva is higher than in controls [64]. The stimulated whole saliva flow rate has also been found decreased in SLE in addition to increased salivary concentrations of sodium, calcium, protein and carbohydrates and decreased concentration of phosphate [65]. About 30 % of patients with SLE also have SS [66]. Inflammatory changes have been demonstrated in labial salivary glands in 49 % of patients with SLE of whom 25 % had SS [67].

## Scleroderma

Scleroderma is a chronic disease characterised by excessive deposits of collagen especially in the skin, but also in other organs. The generalised type of the disease is designated systemic sclerosis, which can be lethal due to damage to the heart, kidneys or lungs. It is four times more common in women than in men. Symptoms predominantly occur at the age of 40. The characteristic disease manifestations include fibrotic changes of the skin of the fingers, hands, arms and face, sclerodactyly (localised thickening and tightness of the skin of the fingers or toes), telangiectasia, Raynaud's phenomenon, oesophageal changes, microstomia, arthralgia, myalgia, lung fibrosis, nephropathy and hypertension. SS presents in approx. 20 % of the patients. It has been found that up to 70 % of the patients with scleroderma complain of xerostomia, and about 50 % display diminished whole saliva flow rates. A large variety of inflammatory changes including glandular fibrosis may be seen in the labial salivary glands [68, 69].

## Mixed Connective Tissue Disease

Mixed connective tissue disease (MCTD) is a chronic disease characterised by swollen fingers, Raynaud's phenomenon and non-erosive polyarthritis. MCTD has overlapping features of SLE, scleroderma and polymyositis, and consequently the diagnosis is often delayed. MCTD mostly affects women (90 %), and the onset is often at the age of 30. Xerostomia and salivary hypofunction as well as histopathological changes in terms of focal lymphocytic infiltrates are common conditions in MCTD [70].

## Sarcoidosis

Sarcoidosis is a chronic granulomatous disease of unknown aetiology. It is usually seen in the age of 20–40 years and affects women more often than men. The prevalence is about 10:100,000. The tissue of any organ may be affected by the progressive non-caseating granulomatous inflammation, but the lungs, lymph nodes, skin, eyes and salivary glands are most commonly affected. Sarcoidosis may be asymptomatic and may resolve spontaneously within 2 years [71]. However, the symptoms and clinical signs including enlargement of the major salivary glands, symptoms of oral and ocular dryness and salivary hypofunction may resemble those of SS [72]. Histopathologically, the salivary gland tissue is characterised by the presence of epithelioid cell granulomas and not focal lymphocytic infiltration. Sarcoidosis can lead to loss of acinar cell which may explain the reduction in salivary flow seen in some of the patients [73].

# Chronic Inflammatory Bowel Diseases

## Crohn's Disease

Crohn's disease (CD) is a chronic, inflammatory, granulomatous disease which mainly affects the lowest portion of the small intestine known as the terminal ileum, but it may affect any part of the gastrointestinal tract, from the mouth to the anus. The cause is unknown. The inflammation often leads to erosions, ulcers, intestinal obstruction and formation of fistulas and abscesses. The onset of CD most commonly occurs between ages of 15 and 30. Symptoms include chronic diarrhoea, abdominal pain, fever, weight loss, arthritis and ocular infections. More than 30 % of children with CD display mucosal tags, lip swelling, gingivitis, aphthous ulcerations and pyostomatitis vegetans. Also the salivary gland tissue may display non-caseating granulomatous inflammation [74]. About 30 % of patients with CD complain of xerostomia, but whole saliva flow rates and buffer capacity appear to be unaffected [75]. In addition there appear to be no changes in salivary levels of antimicrobial proteins [75].

## Ulcerative Colitis

Ulcerative colitis (UC) is a chronic inflammation of the large intestine (colon). The inflammation affects the mucosa and submucosa, leading to ulcers. The symptoms include abdominal pain, diarrhoea, rectal bleeding, painful spasms, fever, fatigue, arthritis and inflammation of the eyes. The cause of UC remains elusive. The onset of UC usually occurs between the ages of 15 and 30. It has been shown that the levels of IgA and IgG in parotid and whole saliva are elevated compared to healthy controls [76]. Salivary levels of nitric oxide and transforming growth factor-beta are also elevated, although not found correlated to the severity of UC [77].

## Coeliac Disease

Coeliac disease is an autoimmune disease with small intestine (duodenum and jejunum) inflammation caused by intolerance to gluten, which is found in wheat, oats, barley and rye. Ingestion of gluten is assumed to initiate an abnormal activation of the immune system leading to inflammation in genetically predisposed persons. Symptoms include diarrhoea, dyspepsia, abdominal pain, weight loss, fatigue, anaemia, infertility, depression, osteoporosis, muscle weakness and neuropathy. Oral symptoms include aphthous ulcers, sore tongue, glossitis and stomatitis. Coeliac disease is also related to an increased frequency of dental enamel defects. The mean age of diagnosis is 40 years, but it can occur at any age. It has been shown that patients following a strict gluten-free diet have lower levels of amylase, IgA and IgM in stimulated whole saliva than healthy controls [78]. The whole and parotid saliva flow rates appear to be unaffected. As expected, oral symptoms such as itching and burning mouth, dry mouth and altered taste sensations as well as history of RAS were more prevalent among the patients than the healthy controls, and these results support previous observations [79].

## Autoimmune Liver Diseases

In chronic autoimmune inflammatory liver diseases, the hepatocytes, small bile ducts or the entire biliary system are target for an immune-mediated attack. The cause is unknown. The most prevalent of them include autoimmune hepatitis (AIH), primary biliary cirrhosis (PBC) and primary sclerosing cholangitis (PSC). AIH and PBC are most often seen in young women, while PSC mainly affects young men, of whom 75 % also have an inflammatory bowel disease. The symptoms include fatigue, fever, jaundice, polymyalgia, arthralgia and symptoms of progressive hepatic dysfunction. Autoimmune liver diseases often present in association with other autoimmune diseases like SS, RA, type 1 diabetes, autoimmune thyroiditis and ulcerative colitis. Both xerostomia and decreased salivary flow have been reported in autoimmune liver diseases [80]. About 90 % of PBC patients have focal lymphocytic infiltrates in their labial salivary glands [81]. Antimitochondrial autoantibodies to 2-oxo-acid dehydrogenase enzymes have been detected in saliva from patients with PBC suggesting that the salivary glands may participate in the pathogenesis [82, 83].

## Amyloidosis

Amyloidosis covers various conditions in which amyloid, an abnormal protein polysaccharide substance with starchlike characteristics, is deposited in tissues and organs and thereby affects their function. Primary amyloidosis occurs independently of other diseases and often affects the skin, tongue, thyroid gland, intestines, liver, heart, lung, spleen and kidneys. Secondary amyloidosis is the most prevalent type, and it usually occurs with other chronic diseases such as rheumatoid arthritis, Crohn's disease, multiple myeloma, osteomyelitis or tuberculosis, and it often affects the vascular system, lymph nodes, kidneys, liver and spleen. Disease manifestations include cardiomyopathy, nephropathy, purpura, neuropathy, carpal tunnel syndrome, arthritis, bursitis, macroglossia, diarrhoea, constipation and malabsorption. Amyloidosis is typically diagnosed at the age of 40–60 years. Most patients are men. Salivary hypofunction and changes in saliva composition have been demonstrated in patients with familial amyloidotic polyneuropathy [84]. Labial salivary gland biopsy is a highly sensitive method for the diagnosis of primary and secondary amyloidosis [85].

## Endocrine Diseases

### Diabetes Mellitus

The term diabetes mellitus (DM) refers to a group of metabolic diseases characterised by hyperglycaemia, which develops as a result of insufficient insulin secretion and/or reduced insulin sensitivity. The two most prominent forms are type 1 and type 2 diabetes. Type 1 diabetes is characterised by a progressive immune-mediated destruction of the insulin-producing β-cells in the pancreas. Exogenous supply of insulin is vitally necessary, and if left untreated, it will lead to diabetic coma and death. Type 1 diabetes mainly affects children and adolescents, but it may occur at any age. The initial classical symptoms include fatigue, weakness, weight loss, irritability, polydipsia, polyphagia, polyuria and pruritus. Type 2 diabetes is caused by a combination of insufficient insulin secretion in the pancreatic β-cells and insulin resistance in mainly the skeletal muscles and hepatic cells. Type 2 diabetes typically develops in middle-aged and older people. It is well known that both type 1 and type 2 diabetes are associated with an increased susceptibility to periodontitis and fungal infections. However, xerostomia and salivary hypofunction also appear to be prominent conditions, particularly in inadequately controlled diabetics. It has been shown that 16 % of patients with type 1 with a disease duration of 10 years have symptoms of dry mouth [86] and 54 % of type 2 diabetics with similar duration [87]. The difference in prevalence can be explained by the fact that type 2 diabetics often are older, display more late-diabetic complications, have other medical diseases and take more medications that may cause hyposalivation and xerostomia than type 1 diabetics [88]. In both type 1 and type 2 diabetes, xerostomia has been found related to diminished unstimulated and stimulated whole saliva flow [89–94]. However, other studies found no differences between diabetic patients and healthy controls [88, 95]. Saliva composition in terms of electrolytes, pH, buffer capacity, antimicrobial proteins and total protein has also been studied, but the results are conflicting [for review 96]. Dehydration, occurring as the result of prolonged hyperglycaemia and consequently polyuria, is considered an important cause of xerostomia and salivary gland hypofunction in diabetics [92]. However, structural changes have also been observed in the salivary glands. Thus, 10–25 % of type 1 or type 2 diabetics may develop sialosis, a bilateral asymptomatic enlargement of the major salivary glands, particularly the parotid glands [97–100]. The salivary gland tissue of these enlarged glands is characterised by enlargement of acinar cells, reduction in the acinar tissue, fatty infiltration, fibrosis and no signs of inflammation [99]. It is likely that the neuropathy and microangiopathy associated with diabetes affect the autonomic innervation and microcirculation of the glandular tissue and thereby contribute to salivary hypofunction. Lymphocytic infiltrates have been found in labial salivary glands of children with type 1 diabetes [20], indicating that the salivary gland tissue may be a target for the same autoimmune process as the pancreas.

## Thyroiditis

Thyroiditis is a group of diseases that cause inflammation in the thyroid gland and destruction of the thyroid cells. Some of the most common types include Hashimoto's thyroiditis, postpartum thyroiditis, acute and subacute thyroiditis, drug-induced thyroiditis and radiation-induced thyroiditis. Hashimoto's thyroiditis, an autoimmune inflammatory disorder, is the most prevalent cause of hypothyroidism, i.e. reduced activity of the thyroid gland. Diseases causing thyroiditis occur three to five times more often in women than in men. The average age of onset is between 30 and 50 years of age. The symptoms are related to thyroid gland hypofunction and include fatigue, weight gain, dry skin, myalgia, constipation and depression. Thyroiditis is common in SS (30–60 %) [101], but autoimmune thyroiditis itself has been found associated with xerostomia (30 %) and inflammatory changes in the salivary glands [102]. Moreover, it has been shown that both unstimulated and stimulated salivary flow are decreased in patients with autoimmune thyroiditis and xerostomia [103].

## Neurological Disorders

### CNS Trauma

A number of head and brain trauma including, among others, craniofacial fractures, neural disruption by surgical trauma, cerebrovascular accidents including stroke, cerebral ischaemia or haemorrhage and brain stem injury may result in sequelae comprising xerostomia and salivary dysfunction.

### Cerebral Palsy

Cerebral palsy syndromes occur in 0.1–0.2 % of children. The prevalence is higher in babies born prematurely. The term covers a group of conditions affecting body movement, balance and posture caused by abnormal development or damage of the part(s) of the brain that controls muscle tone and motor activity. Thus, this CNS damage is characterised by lack of muscle coordination when performing voluntary movements (ataxia), and also stiff muscles and exaggerated reflexes (spasticity) are common. It has been shown that patients with cerebral palsy have diminished whole saliva flow rates and changes in the composition of saliva including increased total protein concentration, decreased amylase and peroxidase activity, decreased sodium and increased potassium concentrations and impaired buffer capacity [104, 105]. Dysphagia and sialorrhoea are common conditions in cerebral palsy. Drooling is often related to swallowing difficulties rather than hypersialorrhoea.

## Bell's Palsy

Bell's palsy is an idiopathic unilateral facial nerve paralysis. The condition usually has a rapid onset of partial or total facial paralysis. It is generally self-limiting, and in about 70 % of the patients, there is a spontaneous recovery within weeks or few months. However, in some cases it persists, and in rare cases (<1 %) it occurs bilaterally causing total facial paralysis. Several conditions are associated with facial paralysis including pregnancy, diabetes, autoimmune diseases like SS, ear infections and herpes simplex virus infection. The underlying mechanism is assumed to involve swelling and thereby pressure on the facial nerve in the narrow bone canal it passes through in the temporal bone. The facial nerve comprises parasympathetic nerve fibres that supply the salivary glands and travel with the facial nerve, and consequently, Bell's palsy is characterised by salivary gland hypofunction due to compromised innervation of the gland. Impaired sensation of taste is also common.

## Parkinson's Disease

Parkinson's disease (PD) is a progressive neurodegenerative cerebral disease of unknown aetiology. It is predominantly diagnosed in persons above 50 years of age.

Degeneration of dopamine neurons results in motor dysfunction, and the four cardinal features of PD are tremor, rigidity, bradykinesia and postural instability and gait disorder. It has been reported that unstimulated and stimulated whole saliva flow rates are reduced in untreated patients with PD indicating that salivary hypofunction is an early manifestation of PD and also a sign of autonomic dysfunction [106]. Furthermore, it has been shown that the salivary concentrations of amylase, sodium and chloride are increased [107]. Xerostomia is also a common symptom in PD, increasing with the progression of the disease. This can be ascribed to the adverse effects of the medication, especially anticholinergic agents, taken by PD patients. However, selective administration of levodopa has been shown to increase saliva flow rates [107]. Drooling and dysphagia are prevalent conditions in PD. Drooling is assumed to be related to reduced swallowing activity rather than hypersialorrhoea.

## Alzheimer's Disease

Alzheimer's disease (AD) is a progressive neurodegenerative disorder and the most common cause of dementia among elderly people. It is mostly diagnosed in persons above the age of 60. Dementia is characterised by loss of cognitive functioning like memory, reasoning and judgement, as well as loss of behavioural abilities that affect the person's daily life and activities. It has been shown that untreated patients with AD have salivary hypofunction [108] which may be related to an autonomic dysfunction. Patients with AD are often treated with "xerogenic" medication that can further aggravate salivary gland hypofunction leading to further impairment of the oral health.

### Burning Mouth Syndrome

Burning mouth syndrome (BMS) is an orofacial pain condition of unknown aetiology, characterised by a persistent burning sensation in a clinically normal-appearing oral mucosa. There is increasing evidence supporting that BMS is a form of neuropathic pain condition. The average age of onset is usually 50 years. Xerostomia is a common complaint in patients with BMS (30–70 %), but overall both whole and parotid saliva flow rates are within the normal range [109, 110]. Results are conflicting with regard to changes in saliva composition [110]. It has been shown that the salivary concentrations of chloride, phosphate and potassium are elevated [111]. Total protein concentrations appear to be reduced in patients with BMS [111, 112] and also the expression of low molecular weight proteins [111]. A study, comparing the expression levels of MUC1 and Toll-like receptor-2 between patients with BMS, patients with oral lichen planus and healthy women, showed increases in MUC1 transcripts in BMS patients, indicating a role of salivary mucins in BMS [113].

A number of other neurological conditions and disease that can cause xerostomia and hyposalivation include anxiety and depression [114], narcolepsia [115] and autonomic disorders like Holmes-Adie syndrome [for review 116].

## Infectious Diseases

### Human Immunodeficiency Virus

Human immunodeficiency virus (HIV) is a retrovirus, which is transmitted via blood. Infection with HIV is chronic and leads to a significant drop in the number of CD4+ T cells and consequently immunodeficiency. HIV infection may affect the salivary glands leading to enlargement of one or more of the major salivary glands due to lymphocytic infiltration. Clinical and histopathological manifestations of HIV-associated salivary gland disease are similar to those of Sjögren's syndrome with xerostomia, salivary gland hypofunction and lymphocytic infiltration. However, in patients with HIV, the focal lymphocytic infiltrations in the salivary gland tissue are less pronounced and mainly comprise CD8+ T cells [117]. HIV-associated lymphoma may involve parotid lymphoid tissue leading to a rapid enlargement of the glands [117]. It has been shown that patients with HIV have various changes in their saliva composition with decreased protein concentration and increased secretory IgA, lysozyme and albumin [118], but results are conflicting as to whether various components are unchanged, increased or decreased due to HIV infection. HIV is present at low concentrations in saliva of infected persons, but the virus does not spread by contact with saliva. Low whole salivary flow rates have been associated with low CD4+ cell counts and highly active antiretroviral therapy (HAART) reflecting disease progression and adverse effects of the treatment.

## Hepatitis C Virus

Hepatitis C virus (HCV) is primarily transmitted via blood in relation to transfusions and intravenous drug use and insufficient sterilised medical equipment. Chronic HCV infection is associated with an increased risk of liver cirrhosis and liver cancer. It has been reported that about 50 % of patients with HCV infection have salivary gland hypofunction [119] and also histological signs of inflammation including lymphocytic infiltrations of the salivary gland tissue. These may resemble signs of SS, but there is no female predominance and no SS-autoantibodies, and the infiltrates in the salivary glands mainly comprise CD8+ T cells [120, 121]. HCV is not the cause of SS and is among the exclusion criteria in the classification criteria set [16].

### Epstein-Barr Virus and Cytomegalovirus

Epstein-Barr virus (EBV) and cytomegalovirus (CMV) as well as other herpes viruses have been associated with xerostomia and salivary gland hypofunction. EBV infection generally occurs during childhood and is asymptomatic, but in adolescents and adults it causes mononucleosis with sore throat, fever, malaise, cervical lymphadenopathy and in some cases hepatosplenomegaly. EBV is primarily transmitted through saliva. EBV infection may in rare cases present as parotitis. EBV is associated with various lymphoid and epithelial malignancies, and EBV-associated oral tumours can involve the parotid gland. EBV has been related to the development of lymphomas, particularly in immunosuppressed patients. In patients with Sjögren's syndrome, increased levels of antibodies against EBV have been found in salivary gland tissue and blood serum. It has been reported that HIV-positive patients with CMV in their saliva suffer more from xerostomia than the HIV-positive patients without CMV in their saliva [122].

### Epidemic Parotitis (Mumps)

Epidemic parotitis is a contagious disease caused by a paramyxovirus. It is the most prevalent salivary gland disease. The virus is transmitted by droplet infection carried in the saliva. The incubation period is about 3 weeks. Mumps is predominantly a childhood disease, but in parts of the world where the MMR (measles, mumps and rubella) vaccine is routinely used, the prevalence of the disease is declining. Mumps is characterised by a painful swelling of one or both parotid glands that persists for 1–2 weeks, fever and malaise.

## Genetic and Developmental Diseases

### Cystic Fibrosis

Cystic fibrosis (CF) is an autosomal recessive genetic disease that primarily affects the lungs, pancreas, liver and intestine. CF is caused by a mutation in the gene for the protein cystic fibrosis transmembrane conductance regulator (CFTR). Since CFT plays an important role in the regulation of chloride and sodium ions across epithelial membranes and the protein secretion in exocrine glands, CF is characterised by abnormal transport of chloride and sodium across the epithelial membranes leading to secretion of highly viscous fluids. The clinical manifestations include salty tasting skin and accumulation of sticky mucus leading to frequent and often severe pulmonary infections. The salt concentrations (sodium and chloride) are elevated in sweat, pancreatic and lacrimal fluids and pancreatic insufficiency may occur due to mucous obstruction. CF has been found associated with quantitative and qualitative changes of saliva from the submandibular gland. Thus, it has been shown that the submandibular saliva flow rate is decreased, and the saliva has a high viscosity with elevated concentrations of total calcium and total phosphate as well as of elevated levels of lipids [123–125]. Furthermore, xerostomia and salivary gland hypofunction in CF patients may be further aggravated by the fact that many of them have a daily intake of "xerogenic" medications. Histopathological manifestations in the submandibular and sublingual gland tissue can be mucous plugs causing obstruction and chronic inflammation [126].

### Ectodermal Dysplasia

Ectodermal dysplasia (ED) is an inherited disorder, which affects the ectoderm. X-linked recessive hypohidrotic ED is the most prevalent type. The ectoderm contributes to the formation of the skin, hair, nails, teeth and salivary, lacrimal and sweat glands. The clinical characteristics are reduced hair growth and (hypotrichosis) reduced or absent sweat secretion (hypohidrosis) and hypodontia or anodontia (congenital missing number of teeth or absence of all teeth). Hypoplasia and aplasia of the major salivary glands have been demonstrated [127, 128]. It has also been shown that both unstimulated and stimulated whole saliva as well as submandibular saliva flow rates are diminished, whereas parotid flow rate is not [129]. Furthermore, saliva composition may be changed with higher concentrations of sodium, chloride, potassium, calcium and phosphate [130].

### Prader-Willi Syndrome

Prader-Willi syndrome (PWS) is associated with genetic abnormalities of chromosome 15. Manifestations of PWS are abnormal growth (short stature, small hands and feet, prominent forehead), abnormally low muscle tone, hypogonadism, increased appetite leading to obesity, strabismus and various degree of mental retardation. Tooth eruption may be delayed and the teeth may be hypoplastic. Salivary secretion is markedly reduced and the saliva is highly viscous [131]. Changes in saliva composition have also been reported including higher concentrations of sodium, chloride, calcium, phosphate, fluoride as well as proteins [132].

## Dehydration

Dehydration is a common cause of xerostomia and hyposalivation, especially in elderly people with an insufficient intake of fluids. It may also occur as a consequence of intensive exercise combined with limited intake of water or due to disease- or medication-induced changes in the water and salt balance [100, 133].

It has been shown that dehydration is associated with decreased parotid saliva flow rates and that these changes are age independent in healthy adults [133]. An insufficiently regulated diabetes can lead to polyuria and consequently dehydration. Dehydration and imbalances in the body's salt and water homeostasis may also be seen in patients with renal diseases and diarrhoea and in abusers of alcohol. Medications which affect the regulation of the body's salt and water balance such as diuretics may cause xerostomia and in some cases lead to reduced salivary flow rates and changes in the saliva composition [100, 133]. It has recently been shown that dehydration not only reduces whole saliva flow rates but also decreases the secretion rates of α-amylase and lysozyme, which are antimicrobial proteins playing an important role for mucosal immunity [134]. These findings indicate that dehydration may compromise host defence.

## Eating Disorders

### Anorexia Nervosa

Anorexia nervosa is an eating disorder mostly seen in young women. It is characterised by an irrational fear of gaining weight, an immoderate food restriction as well as a distorted body self-perception. The restriction of food intake causes metabolic and hormonal disturbances. Consequently, young postmenarcheal females often suffer from amenorrhoea. The purging type of anorexia nervosa is usually characterised by self-induced vomiting and misuse of laxatives and diuretics, whereas the restricted type displays no history of vomiting. Xerostomia and salivary gland dysfunction often occur as consequences of various factors including nutritional deficiencies and consequent metabolic disturbances, "xerogenic" medications as well as psychological disturbances [135]. There are no reports on specific changes of saliva composition, apart from increased salivary amylase activity in patients with the purging type of anorexia nervosa [136].

## Bulimia Nervosa

Bulimia nervosa is an eating disorder which primarily affects young women. It is characterised by recurrent episodes of binge eating and self-induced vomiting as well as misuse of medication such as diuretics and laxatives to prevent weight gain. Also excessive exercise and fasting are characteristic behaviours. Clinical manifestations often include intermittent, asymptomatic bilateral enlargement of the major salivary glands, particularly the parotids [137], and dental erosions due to vomiting. Complaints of oral dryness are common, and the saliva flow rates and composition may be also affected due to dehydration, nutritional imbalance by binge eating, self-induced vomiting, misuse of diuretics and laxatives, excessive exercise and intake of antidepressants, which influence saliva formation [137, 138]. Histological examination of enlarged salivary gland tissue reveals acinar hyperplasia but no signs of inflammation [137]. Elevated serum amylase levels have been found associated with salivary gland enlargements and self-induced vomiting [139]. It has also been shown that the salivary alpha-amylase activity is increased in patients with bulimia nervosa [140]. Recently, it was demonstrated that the enzymatic activities of proteases, collagenase and pepsin were increased in unstimulated whole saliva and proteases increased in stimulated whole saliva in bulimics with erosion compared with controls [141]. Proteolytic enzymes are considered relevant for the initiation and progression of dental erosion directly after vomiting, and the results may explain the high prevalence of dental erosion in bulimics.

In summary, a large number of medical conditions and systemic diseases may cause or be associated with xerostomia and salivary gland dysfunction. A comprehensive diagnostic examination is imperative in order to determine the cause of the patient's dry mouth complaints and/or observed clinical signs of salivary gland hypofunction and consequently initiate proper treatment and prevention. Establishing collaboration between the patient's physician and specialists is also essential for optimal diagnosis and patient care.

## References

1. Dawes C. Physiological factors affecting salivary flow rate, oral sugar clearance, and the sensation of dry mouth in man. J Dent Res. 1987;66:648–53.
2. Ship JA, Fox PC, Baum BJ. How much saliva is enough? 'Normal' function defined. J Am Dent Assoc. 1991;122:63–9.
3. Thomson WM, Poulton R, Broadbent JM, Al-Kubaisy S. Xerostomia and medications among 32-year-olds. Acta Odont Scand. 2006;64:249–54.
4. Sreebny LM. The enigma of dry mouth. In: Sreebny LM, Vissink A, editors. Dry mouth. The malevolent symptom: a clinical guide. London: Wiley-Blackwell Publishing; 2010. p. 3–9.
5. Thomson WM, Chalmers JM, Spencer AJ, Slade GD. Medication and dry mouth: findings from a cohort study of older people. J Public Health Dent. 2000;60(1):12–20.
6. Smidt D, Torpet LA, Nauntofte B, Heegaard KM, Pedersen AML. Associations between oral and ocular dryness, salivary flow rates, systemic diseases, medication in a sample of older people. Community Dent Oral Epidemiol. 2011;39(3):276–88.
7. Turner MD, Ship JA. Dry mouth and its effects on the oral health of elderly people. J Am Dent Assoc. 2007;138:15–20.

8. Heintze U, Birkhed D, Bjorn H. Secretion rate and buffer effect of resting and stimulated whole saliva as a function of age and sex. Swed Dent J. 1983;7(6):227–38.
9. Sreebny LM. Dry mouth: a multifaceted diagnostic dilemma. In: Sreebny LM, Vissink A, editors. Dry mouth. The malevolent symptom: a clinical guide. London: Wiley-Blackwell Publishing; 2010. p. 33–51.
10. Navazesh M, Christensen CM. A comparison of whole mouth resting and stimulated salivary measurement procedures. J Dent Res. 1982;61:1158–62.
11. Fox RI. Sjögren's syndrome. Lancet. 2005;366(9482):321–31.
12. Pedersen AM, Nauntofte B. Primary Sjögren's syndrome: oral aspects on pathogenesis, diagnostic criteria, clinical features and approaches for therapy. Expert Opin Pharmacother. 2001;2:1415–36.
13. Haga HJ, Jonsson R. The influence of age on disease manifestations and serological characteristics in primary Sjögren's syndrome. Scand J Rheumatol. 1999;28:227–32.
14. Manthorpe R, Oxholm P, Prause JU, Schøidt M. Copenhagen criteria for Sjögren's syndrome. Scand J Rheumatol. 1986;61(Suppl):19–21.
15. Haugen AJ, Peen E, Hultén, Johannessen AC, Brun JG, Halse AK, Haga HJ. Estimation of the prevalence of primary Sjögren's syndrome in two age-different community-based populations using two sets of classification criteria: the Hordaland Health Study. Scan J Rheumatol. 2008;37(1):30–4.
16. Vitali C, Bombardieri S, Jonsson R, Moutsopoulos HM, Alexander EL, Carsons SE, Daniels TE, Fox PC, Fox RI, Kassan SS, Pillemer SR, Talal N, Weisman MH, European Study Group on Classification Criteria for Sjögren's Syndrome. Classification criteria for Sjögren's syndrome: a revised version of the European criteria proposed by the American-European Consensus Group. Ann Rheum Dis. 2002;61:554–8.
17. Shiboski SC, Shiboski CH, Criswell LA, Baer AN, Challacombe S, Lanfranchi H, Schiødt M, et al. American College of Rheumatology classification criteria for Sjögren's syndrome: a data-driven, expert consensus approach in the Sjögren's International Collaborative Clinical Alliance Cohort. Arthritis Care Res. 2012;64(4):475–87.
18. Daniels TE. Labial salivary gland biopsy in Sjögren's syndrome. Assessment and a diagnostic criterion in 362 suspected cases. Arthritis Rheum. 1984;27:147–56.
19. Adamson FV. Immunohistologic analysis of lymphoid infiltrates in primary Sjögren's syndrome using monoclonal antibodies. J Immunol. 1983;130:203–8.
20. Markopoulos AK, Belazi M. Histopathological and immunohistochemical features of the labial salivary glands in children with type I diabetes. J Diabetes Complications. 1998;12:39–42.
21. Groule V, Reibel J, Bendtson Falch I, Pedersen AML. Labial salivary gland inflammation and function in type 1-diabetic children. In preparation.
22. Lindhahl G, Hedfors E. Lymphocytic infiltrates and epithelial HLA-DR expression in lip salivary glands in connective tissue disease patient lacking sicca: a prospective study. Br J Rheumatol. 1989;28:293–8.
23. Hansen BU, Lindgren S, Erikson S, Henricsson V, Larsson A, Manthorpe R, Warfvinge G. Clinical and immunological features of Sjögren's syndrome in patients with primary biliary cirrhosis with emphasis on focal sialadenitis. Acta Med Scand. 1988;224: 611–9.
24. Kassimos DG, Shirlaw PJ, Choy EH, Hockey K, Morgan PR, Challacombe SJ, Panayi GS. Chronic sialadenitis in patients with nodal osteoarthritis. Br J Rheumatol. 1997;36:1312–7.
25. Nakhleh RE, Miller W, Snover DC. Significance of mucosal vs salivary gland changes in lip biopsies in the diagnosis of chronic graft-vs-host disease. Arch Pathol Lab Med. 1989;113:932–4.
26. Haddad J, Deny P, Munz-Gotheil C, Ambrosini JC, Trinchet JC, Pateron D, Mal F, Callard P, Beaugrand M. Lymphocytic sialoadenitis of Sjögren's syndrome associated with chronic hepatitis C virus liver disease. Lancet. 1992;339(8789):321–3.
27. Itescu S. Diffuse infiltrative lymphocytosis syndrome in human deficiency virus infection – Sjögren's like disease. Rheum Dis Clin North Am. 1991;17:99–115.

28. Melsom RD, Speight PM, Ryan J, Perry JD. Sarcoidosis in a patient presenting with clinical and histopathological features in primary Sjögren's syndrome. Ann Rheum Dis. 1988;14:77–103.
29. Talal N. Recent developments in the immunology of Sjögren's syndrome (autoimmune exocrinopathy). Scand J Rheumatol. 1986;61(Suppl):76–82.
30. Moutsopoulos HM, Talal N. Immunological abnormalities in Sjögren's syndrome. In: Talal N, Moutsopoulos HM, Kassan SS, editors. Sjögren's syndrome. Clinical and immunological aspects. Heidelberg: Springer; 1987. p. 258–65.
31. Jonsson R, Kroneld U, Bäckman K, Magnusson B, Tarkowski A. Progression of sialadenitis in Sjögren's syndrome. Br J Rheumatol. 1993;32:578–81.
32. Atkinson JC, Travis WD, Slocum L, Ebbs WL, Fox PC. Serum anti-SS-B/La and IgA rheumatoid factor are markers of salivary gland disease activity in primary Sjögren's syndrome. Arthritis Rheum. 1992;35:1368–72.
33. Pijpe J, Kalk WW, van der Wal JE, Vissink A, Kluin PM, Roodenburg JL, Bootsma H, Kallenberg CG, Spijkervet FK. Parotid gland biopsy compared with labial biopsy in the diagnosis of patients with primary Sjögren's syndrome. Rheumatology (Oxford). 2007;46(2):335–41.
34. Pedersen AM, Dissing S, Fahrenkrug J, Hannibal J, Reibel J, Nauntofte B. Innervation pattern and Ca2+ signalling in labial salivary glands of healthy individuals and patients with primary Sjögren's syndrome. J Oral Pathol Med. 2000;29:97–109.
35. Beroukas D, Goodfellow R, Hiscock J, Jonsson R, Gordon TP, Waterman SA. Up-regulation of M3 receptors in labial salivary gland acini in primary Sjögren's syndrome. Lab Invest. 2002;82(2):203–10.
36. Dawson LJ, Field A, Harmer AR, Smith PM. Acetylcholine-evoked calcium mobilization and ion channel activation in labial gland acinar cells from patients with primary Sjögren's syndrome. Clin Exp Immunol. 2001;124:480–5.
37. Waterman SA, Gordon TP, Rischmueller M. Inhibitory effects of muscarinic receptor autoantibodies on parasympathetic neurotransmission in Sjögren's syndrome. Arthritis Rheum. 2000;43(7):1647–54.
38. Cha S, Singson E, Cornelius J, Yagna JP, Knot HJ, Peck AB. Muscarinic acetylcholine type-3 receptor desensitization due to chronic exposure to Sjögren's syndrome-associated autoantibodies. J Rheumatol. 2006;33(2):296–306.
39. Bacman S, Sterin-Borda L, Camusso JJ, Arana R, Hubscher O, Borda E. Circulating antibodies against rat parotid M3 muscarinic receptors in primary Sjögren's syndrome. Clin Exp Immunol. 1996;104:454–9.
40. Robinson CP, Brayer J, Yamachika S, Esch TR, Peck AB, Stewart CA, Peen E, Jonsson R, Humphreys-Beher MG. Transfer of human serum IgG to nonobese diabetic $Ig\mu^{null}$ mice reveals a role for autoantibodies in the loss of secretory function of exocrine tissues in Sjögren's syndrome. Proc Natl Acad Sci U S A. 1998;95:7538–43.
41. Tengner P, Halse AK, Haga HJ, Jonsson R, Wahren-Herlenius M. Detection of anti-Ro/SSA and anti-La/SSB autoantibody-producing cells in salivary glands from patients with Sjögren's syndrome. Arthritis Rheum. 1998;41:2238–48.
42. Newton JL, Frith J, Powell D, Hackett K, Wilton K, Bowman S, Price E, Pease C, Andrews J, Emery P, Hunter J, Gupta M, Vadivelu S, Giles I, Isenberg D, Lanyon P, Jones A, Regan M, Cooper A, Moots R, Sutcliffe N, Bombardieri M, Pitzalis C, McLaren J, Young-Min S, Dasgupta B, Griffiths B, Lendrem D, Mitchell S, Ng WF, UK primary Sjögren's syndrome registry. Autonomic symptoms are common and are associated with overall symptom burden and disease activity in primary Sjogren's syndrome. Ann Rheum Dis. 2012;71(12):1973–9.
43. Pedersen AM, Reibel J, Nauntofte B. Primary Sjögren's syndrome: subjective symptoms and salivary findings. J Oral Pathol Med. 1999;28:303–11.
44. Kalk WW, Vissink A, Stegenga B, Bootsma H, Nieuw Amerongen AV, Kallenberg CG. Sialometry and sialochemistry: a non-invasive approach for diagnosing Sjögren's syndrome. Ann Rheum Dis. 2002;61(2):137–44.
45. Pedersen AM, Bardow A, Nauntofte B. Salivary changes and dental caries as potential oral markers of autoimmune salivary gland dysfunction in primary Sjögren's syndrome. BMC Clin Pathol. 2005;5(1):4.

46. Jonsson MV, Szodoray P, Jellestad S, Jonsson R, Skarstein K. Association between circulating levels of the novel TNF family members APRIL and BAFF and lymphoid organization in primary Sjögren's syndrome. J Clin Immunol. 2005;34:49–55.
47. Szodoray P, Alex P, Jonsson MV, Knowlton N, Dozmorov I, Nakken B, Delaleu N, Jonsson R, Centola M. Distinct profiles of Sjögren's syndrome patients with ectopic salivary gland germinal centers revealed by serum cytokines and BAFF. Clin Immunol. 2005;117:168–76.
48. Hu S, Wang J, Meijer JM, Ieong S, Xie Y, Yu T, Zhou H, Henry S, Vissink A, Pijpe J, Kallenberg CG, Elashoff D, Loo JA, Wong DT. Salivary proteomic and genomic biomarkers for primary Sjögren's syndrome. Arthritis Rheum. 2007;56(11):3588–600.
49. Hu S, Zhou M, Jiang J, Wang J, Elashoff D, Gorr S, Michie SA, Spijkervet FK, Bootsma H, Kallenberg CG, Vissink A, Horvath S, Wong DT. Systems biology analysis of Sjögren's syndrome and mucosa-associated lymphoid tissue lymphoma in parotid glands. Arthritis Rheum. 2009;60(1):81–92.
50. Garcia-Carrasco M, Ramos-Casals M, Rosas J, Pallares L, Calvo-Alen J, Cervera R, Font J, Ingelmo M. Primary Sjögren's syndrome: clinical and immunologic disease patterns in a cohort of 400 patients. Medicine (Baltimore). 2002;81:270–80.
51. Zintzaras E, Voulgarelis M, Moutsopoulos HM. The risk of lymphoma development in autoimmune diseases: a meta-analysis. Arch Intern Med. 2005;165(20):2337–44.
52. Voulgarelis M, Skopouli FN. Clinical, immunologic, and molecular factors predicting lymphoma development in Sjögren's syndrome patients. Clin Rev Allergy Immunol. 2007;32:265–74.
53. Silman AJ, Hochberg MC. Epidemiology of the rheumatic diseases. 2nd ed. New York: Oxford University Press; 2001.
54. Uhlig T, Kvien TK, Jensen JL, Axell T. Sicca symptoms, saliva and tear production, and disease variables in 636 patients with rheumatoid arthritis. Ann Rheum Dis. 1999;58:415–22.
55. Jensen JL, Uhlig T, Kvien TK, Axell T. Characteristics of rheumatoid arthritis patients with self-reported sicca symptoms: evaluation of medical, salivary and oral parameters. Oral Dis. 1997;3:254–61.
56. Moen K, Bertelsen LT, Hellem S, Jonsson R, Brun JG. Salivary gland and temporomandibular joint involvement in rheumatoid arthritis: relation to disease activity. Oral Dis. 2005;11(1):27–34.
57. Nederfors T, Holmström G, Paulsson G, Sahlberg D. The relation between xerostomia and hyposalivation in subjects with rheumatoid arthritis or fibromyalgia. Swed Dent J. 2002;26(1):1–7.
58. Nagler RM, Salameh F, Reznick AZ, Livshits V, Nahir AM. Salivary gland involvement in rheumatoid arthritis and its relationship to induced oxidative stress. Rheumatology (Oxford). 2003;42(10):1234–41.
59. Markkanen SO, Syrjanen SM, Lappalainen R, Markkanen H. Assessment of labial salivary gland changes in patients with rheumatoid arthritis by subjective and quantitative methods. Appl Pathol. 1989;7:233–40.
60. Cimmino MA, Salvarani C, Macchioni P, Montecucco C, Fossaluzza V, Mascia MT, Punzi L, Davoli C, Filippini D, Numo R. Extra-articular manifestations in 587 Italian patients with rheumatoid arthritis. Rheumatol Int. 2000;19(6):213–7.
61. Helenius LM, Meurman JH, Helenius I, Kari K, Hietanen J, Suuronen R, Hallikainen D, Kautiainen H, Leirisalo-Repo M, Lindqvist C. Oral and salivary parameters in patients with rheumatic diseases. Acta Odontol Scand. 2005;63(5):284–93.
62. Brun JG, Madland TM, Jonsson R. A prospective study of sicca symptoms in patients with rheumatoid arthritis. Arthritis Rheum. 2003;49(2):187–92.
63. Rhodus NL, Johnson DK. The prevalence of oral manifestations of systemic lupus erythematosus. Quintessence Int. 1990;21:461–5.
64. Jensen JL, Bergen HO, Gilboe I-M, Husby G, Axell T. Oral and ocular sicca symptoms and findings are prevalent in systemic lupus erythematosus. J Oral Pathol Med. 1999;28:317–22.
65. Jonsson R, Bratthall D, Nyberg G. Histologic and sialochemical findings indicating sicca syndrome in patients with systemic lupus erythematosus. Oral Surg Oral Med Oral Pathol. 1982;54(6):635–9.

66. Grennan DM, Ferguson M, Williamson J, Mavrikakis M, Dick WC, Buchanan WW. Sjögren's syndrome in SLE: part I. The frequency of the clinical and subclinical features of Sjogren's syndrome in patients with SLE. N Z Med J. 1977;86(598):374–6.
67. Skopouli F, Siouna-Fatourou H, Dimou GS, Galanopoulou D, Papadimitriou CS, Moutsopoulos HM. Histologic lesion in labial salivary glands of patients with systemic lupus erythematosus. Oral Surg Oral Med Oral Pathol. 1991;72:208–12.
68. Wood RE, Lee P. Analysis of the oral manifestations of systemic sclerosis (scleroderma). Oral Surg Oral Med Oral Pathol. 1988;65:172–8.
69. Nagy G, Kovacs J, Zeher M, Czirjak L. Analysis of the oral manifestations of systemic sclerosis. Oral Surg Oral Med Oral Pathol. 1994;77:141–6.
70. Konttinen YT, Tuominen TS, Piirainen HI, Könönen MH, Wolf JE, Hietanen JH, Malmström MJ. Signs and symptoms in the masticatory system in ten patients with mixed connective tissue disease. Scand J Rheumatol. 1990;19:363–73.
71. Vasil'ev VI, Logvinenko OA, Simonova MV, Safonova TN, Radenska-Lopovok SG, Bozh'eva LA, Shornikova NS, Andrianov SG. Sicca syndrome in sarcoidosis and involvement of the salivary and lacrymal glands. Ter Arkh. 2005;77(1):52–7.
72. Sack KE, Carteron NL, Whitcher JP, Greenspan JS, Daniels TE. Sarcoidosis mimicking Sjögren's syndrome: histopathologic observations. J Clin Rheumatol. 1998;4(1):13–6.
73. Nitzan DW, Shteyer A. Sarcoidosis of the parotid salivary glands. J Oral Maxillofac Surg. 1982;40:443–6.
74. van der Walt JD, Leake J. Granulomatous sialadenitis of the major salivary glands. A clinicopathological study of 57 cases. Histopathology. 1987;11:131–44.
75. Sundh B, Emilson CG. Salivary and microbial conditions and dental health in patients with Crohn's disease: a 3-year study. Oral Surg Oral Med Oral Pathol. 1989;67(3):286–90.
76. Crama-Bohbouth G, Pena AS, Verspaget HW, et al. Immunological findings in whole and parotid saliva of patients with ulcerative colitis and healthy controls. Hepatogastroenterology. 1989;36:185–7.
77. Rezaie A, Khalaj S, Shabihkhani M, Nikfar S, Zamani MJ, Mohammaddirad A, Daryani NE, Abdollahi M. Study on the correlations among disease activity index and salivary transforming growth factor-β1 and nitric oxide in ulcerative colitis patients. Signal transduction pathways, part C: cell signaling in health and disease. Ann N Y Acad Sci. 2007;1095:305–14.
78. Lenander-Lumikari M, Ihalin R, Lahteenoja H. Changes in whole saliva in patients with coeliac disease. Arch Oral Biol. 2000;45(5):347–54.
79. Lähteenoja Lahteenoja H, Toivanen A, Viander M, Maki M, Irjala K, Raiha I, Syrjänen S. Oral mucosal changes in coeliac patients on a gluten-free diet. Eur J Oral Sci. 1998;106(5):899–906.
80. Mang FW, Michieletti P, O'Rourke K, Cauch-Dudek K, Diamant N, Bookman A, Heathcote J. Primary biliary cirrhosis, sicca complex, and dysphagia. Dysphagia. 1997;12(3):167–70.
81. Tsuneyama K, Van De Water J, Yamazaki K, Suzuki K, Sato S, Takeda Y, Ruebner B, Yost BA, Nakanuma Y, Coppel RL, Gershwin ME. Primary biliary cirrhosis an epithelitis: evidence of abnormal salivary gland immunohistochemistry. Autoimmunity. 1997;26(1):23–31.
82. Ikuno N, Mackay IR, Jois J, Omagari K, Rowley MJ. Antimitochondrial autoantibodies in saliva and sera from patients with primary biliary cirrhosis. J Gastroenterol Hepatol. 2001;16(12):1390–4.
83. Reynoso-Paz S, Leung PS, Van De Water J, Tanaka A, Munoz S, Bass N, Lindor K, Donald PJ, Coppel RL, Ansari AA, Gershwin ME. Evidence for a locally driven mucosal response and the presence of mitochondrial antigens in saliva in primary biliary cirrhosis. Hepatology. 2000;31(1):24–9.
84. Johansson I, Ryberg M, Steen L, Wigren L. Salivary hypofunction in patients with familial amyloidotic polyneuropathy. Oral Surg Oral Med Oral Pathol. 1992;74(6):742–8.
85. Sacsaquispe SJ, Antúnez-de Mayolo EA, Vicetti R, Delgado WA. Detection of AA-type amyloid protein in labial salivary glands. Med Oral Patol Oral Cir Bucal. 2011; 16(2):149–52.

86. Moore PA, Guggenheimer J, Etzel KR, Weyant RJ, Orchard T. Type 1 diabetes mellitus, xerostomia and salivary flow rates. Oral Surg Oral Med Oral Pathol Oral Radiol Endod. 2001;92:281–91.
87. Sandberg GE, Sundberg HE, Fjellström CA, Wikblad KF. Type 2 diabetes and oral health. A comparison between diabetic and non-diabetic subjects. Diabetes Res Clin Pract. 2000;50:27–34.
88. Meurman JH, Collin H-L, Niskanen L, Töyry J, Alakuijala P, Keinänen S, Uusitupa M. Saliva in non-insulin-dependent diabetic patients and control subjects. Oral Surg Oral Med Oral Pathol Oral Radiol Endod. 1998;86:69–76.
89. Ben-Aryeh H, Cohen M, Kanter Y, Szargel R, Laufer D. Salivary composition in diabetic patients. J Diabet Complications. 1988;2:96–9.
90. Thorstensson H, Falk H, Hugoson A, Olsson J. Some salivary factors in insulin-dependent diabetics. Acta Odontol Scand. 1989;47:175–83.
91. Newrick PG, Bowman C, Green D, O'Brien IA, Porter SR, Scully C, Corrall RJ. Parotid salivary secretion in diabetic autonomic neuropathy. J Diabet Complications. 1991;5:35–7.
92. Sreebny LM, Yu A, Green A, Valdini A. Xerostomia in diabetes mellitus. Diabetes Care. 1992;15:900–4.
93. Lamey PJ, Darwazeh AM, Frier BM. Oral disorders associated with diabetes mellitus. Diabet Med. 1992;9:410–6.
94. Dodds MW, Dodds AP. Effects of glycemic control on saliva flow rates and protein composition in non-insulin-dependent diabetes mellitus. Oral Surg Oral Med Oral Pathol Oral Radiol Endod. 1997;83:465–70.
95. Chávez EM, Borrell LN, Taylor GW, Ship JA. A longitudinal analysis of salivary flow in control subjects and older adults with type 2 diabetes. Oral Surg Oral Med Oral Pathol Oral Radiol Endod. 2001;91(2):166–73.
96. Pedersen AML. Diabetes mellitus and related oral manifestations. Oral BioSci Med. 2004;1(4):229–48.
97. Russotto SB. Asymptomatic parotid gland enlargement in diabetes mellitus. Oral Surg. 1981;52:594–8.
98. Murrah VA. Diabetes mellitus and associated oral manifestations: a review. J Oral Pathol. 1985;14:271–81.
99. Lindeberg A, Andersen L. Size and composition of the submandibular glands in late onset diabetes. Arch Otorhinolaryngol. 1987;244:100–3.
100. Greenspan D. Xerostomia: diagnosis and management. Oncology (Huntingt). 1996;10:7–11.
101. D'Arbonneau F, Ansart S, Le Berre R, Dueymes M, Youinou P, Pennec YL. Thyroid function in primary Sjögren's syndrome: a long-term follow-up study. Arthritis Rheum. 2003;49(6):804–9.
102. Soy M, Guldiken S, Arikan E, Altun BU, Tugrul A. Frequency of rheumatic diseases in patients with autoimmune thyroid disease. Rheumatol Int. 2007;27(6):575–7.
103. Changlai SP, Chen WK, Chung C, Chiou SM. Objective evidence of decreased salivary function in patients with autoimmune thyroiditis (chronic thyroiditis, Hashimoto's thyroiditis). Nucl Med Commun. 2002;23(10):1029–33.
104. Ferreira MC, Pastore C, Imada R, Guaré R, Leite M, Poyares D, Santos MT. Autonomic nervous system in individuals with cerebral palsy: a controlled study. J Oral Pathol Med. 2011;40(7):576–81.
105. Santos MT, Ferreira MC, Leite MF, Guaré RO. Salivary parameters in Brazilian individuals with cerebral palsy who drool. Child Care Health Dev. 2011;37(3):404–9.
106. Cersósimo MG, Tumilasci OR, Raina GB, Benarroch EE, Cardoso EM, Micheli F, Pazo JH. Hyposialorrhea as an early manifestation of Parkinson disease. Auton Neurosci. 2009;150(1–2):150–1.
107. Tumilasci OR, Cersósimo MG, Belforte JE, Micheli FE, Benarroch EE, Pazo JH. Quantitative study of salivary secretion in Parkinson's disease. Mov Disord. 2006;21(5):660–7.
108. Ship JA, Puckett SA. Longitudinal study on oral health in subjects with Alzheimer's disease. J Am Geriatr Soc. 1994;42(1):57–63.

109. Gorsky M, Silverman Jr S, Chinn H. Clinical characteristics and management outcome in the burning mouth syndrome. An open study of 130 patients. Oral Surg Oral Med Oral Pathol. 1991;72(2):192–5.
110. Pedersen AML, Smidt D, Nauntofte B, Christiani CJ, Jerlang BB. Burning mouth syndrome: etiopathogenic mechanisms, symptomatology, diagnosis and therapeutic approaches. Oral BioSci Med. 2004;1(1):3–19.
111. de Moura SA, de Sousa JM, Lima DF, Negreiros AN, Silva Fde V, da Costa LJ. Burning mouth syndrome (BMS): sialometric and sialochemical analysis and salivary protein profile. Gerodontology. 2007;24(3):173–6.
112. Tammiala-Salonen T, Söderling E. Protein composition, adhesion, and agglutination properties of saliva in burning mouth syndrome. Scand J Dent Res. 1993;101:215–8.
113. Kho HS, Chang JY, Kim YY, Kim Y. MUC1 and toll-like receptor-2 expression in burning mouth syndrome and oral lichen planus. Arch Oral Biol. 2013;58(7):837–42.
114. Anttila SS, Knuuttila ML, Sakki TK. Depressive symptoms as an underlying factor of the sensation of dry mouth. Psychosom Med. 1998;60:215–8.
115. Nordgarden H, Lamkin M, Oppenheim FG, Storhaug K, Jensen JL. Salivary secretions: narcolepsy and central nervous system stimulants. J Dent Res. 1998;77:1817–22.
116. Jensen SB, Nauntofte B, Pedersen AML. The causes of dry mouth. In: Sreebny LM, Vissink A, editors. Dry mouth. The malevolent symptom: a clinical guide. London: Wiley-Blackwell Publishing; 2010. p. 158–81.
117. Schiødt M, Greenspan D, Daniels TE, Nelson J, Leggott PJ, Wara DW, Greenspan JS. Parotid gland enlargement and xerostomia associated with labial sialadenitis in HIV-infected patients. J Autoimmun. 1989;2(4):415–25.
118. Schiødt M, Dodd CL, Greenspan D, Daniels TE, Chernoff D, Hollander H, Wara D, Greenspan JS. Natural history of HIV-associated salivary gland disease. Oral Surg Oral Med Oral Pathol. 1992;74(3):326–31.
119. Coates EA, Brennan D, Logan RM, Goss AN, Scopacasa B, Spencer AJ, Gorkic E. Hepatitis C infection and associated oral health problems. Aust Dent J. 2000;45(2):108–14.
120. Pirisi M, Scott C, Fabris C, Ferraccioli G, Soardo G, Ricci R, Toniutto P, Avellini C, Vitulli D, Miotti AM, et al. Mild sialoadenitis: a common finding in patients with hepatitis C virus infection. Scand J Gastroenterol. 1994;29(10):940–2.
121. Scott CA, Avellini C, Desinan L, Pirisi M, Ferraccioli GF, Bardus P, Fabris C, Casatta L, Bartoli E, Beltrami CA. Chronic lymphocytic sialoadenitis in HCV-related chronic liver disease: comparison of Sjögren's syndrome. Histopathology. 1997;30(1):41–8.
122. Greenberg MS, Glick M, Nghiem L, Stewart JC, Hodinka R, Dubin G. Relationship of cytomegalovirus to salivary gland dysfunction in HIV-infected patients. Oral Surg Oral Med Oral Pathol Oral Radiol Endod. 1997;83(3):334–9.
123. Davies H, Bagg J, Goodchild MC, McPherson MA. Examination of submandibular fluid in cystic fibrosis. Acta Univ Carol Med (Praha). 1990;36(1–4):84–5.
124. Aps JK, Delanghe J, Martens LC. Salivary electrolyte concentrations are associated with cystic fibrosis transmembrane regulator genotypes. Clin Chem Lab Med. 2002;40(4):345–50.
125. Slomiany BL, Aono M, Murty VL, Slomiany A, Levine MJ, Tabak LA. Lipid composition of submandibular saliva from normal and cystic fibrosis individuals. J Dent Res. 1982;61(10):1163–6.
126. Durie PR, Kent G, Phillips MJ, Ackerley CA. Characteristic multiorgan pathology of cystic fibrosis in a long-living cystic fibrosis transmembrane regulator knockout murine model. Am J Pathol. 2004;164(4):1481–93.
127. McDonald FG, Mantas J, McEwen CG, Ferguson MM. Salivary gland aplasia: an ectodermal disorder? J Oral Pathol. 1986;15(2):115–7.
128. Singh P, Warnakulasuriya S. Aplasia of submandibular salivary glands associated with ectodermal dysplasia. J Oral Pathol Med. 2004;33(10):634–6.
129. Nordgarden H, Storhaug K, Lyngstadaas SP, Jensen JL. Salivary gland function in persons with ectodermal dysplasias. Eur J Oral Sci. 2003;111(5):371–6.

130. Lexner MO, Bardow A, Hertz JM, Almer L, Nauntofte B, Kreiborg S. Whole saliva in X-linked hypohidrotic ectodermal dysplasia. Int J Paediatr Dent. 2007;17(3):155–62.
131. Hart PS. Salivary abnormalities in Prader-Willi syndrome. Ann N Y Acad Sci. 1998;15(842):125–31.
132. Saeves R, Reseland JE, Kvam BM, Sandvik L, Nordgarden H. Saliva in Prader-Willi syndrome: quantitative and qualitative characteristics. Arch Oral Biol. 2012;57(10):1335–41.
133. Ship JA, Fischer DJ. The relationship between dehydration and parotid salivary gland function in young and older healthy adults. J Gerontol A Biol Sci Med Sci. 1997;52:310–9.
134. Fortes MB, Diment BC, Di Felice U, Walsh NP. Dehydration decreases saliva antimicrobial proteins important for mucosal immunity. Appl Physiol Nutr Metab. 2012;37(5):850–9.
135. Montecchi PP, Custureri V, Polimeni A, Cordaro M, Costa L, Marinucci S, Montecchi F. Oral manifestations in a group of young patients with anorexia nervosa. Eat Weight Disord. 2003;8(2):164–7.
136. Scheutzel P, Gerlach U. Alpha-amylase isoenzymes in serum and saliva of patients with anorexia and bulimia nervosa. Z Gastroenterol. 1991;29(7):339–45. Article in German.
137. Coleman H, Altini M, Nayler S, Richards A. Sialadenosis: a presenting sign in bulimia. Head Neck. 1998;20(8):758–62.
138. Dynesen AW, Bardow A, Petersson B, Nielsen LR, Nauntofte B. Salivary changes and dental erosion in bulimia nervosa. Oral Surg Oral Med Oral Pathol Oral Radiol Endod. 2008;106(5):696–707.
139. Wolfe BE, Jimerson DC, Smith A, Keel PK. Serum amylase in bulimia nervosa and purging disorder: differentiating the association with binge eating versus purging behavior. Physiol Behav. 2011;104(5):684–6.
140. Kronvall P, Fahy TA, Isaksson A, Theander S, Russell GF. The clinical relevance of salivary amylase monitoring in bulimia nervosa. Biol Psychiatry. 1992;32(2):156–63.
141. Schlueter N, Ganss C, Pötschke S, Klimek J, Hannig C. Enzyme activities in the oral fluids of patients suffering from bulimia: a controlled clinical trial. Caries Res. 2012;46(2):130–9.

# Medication-Induced Dry Mouth

# 3

Gordon B. Proctor

**Abstract**

A wide range of medications have been found to be associated with xerostomia, the subjective symptom of dry mouth. The assessment of medication-induced xerostomia (MIX) is usually made through a subject's responses to relevant questions or the use of visual analogue scales whereby the subject is asked to rate the severity of their oral dryness. It is uncertain how much MIX is accompanied or can be ascribed to medication-induced salivary gland hypofunction and reduced secretion of saliva. MIX in older age groups is associated with the number of medications being taken and is higher than seen in the younger subjects. Many medications cause xerostomia as a side effect, but some of these, for example, selective serotonin reuptake inhibitors, do not appear to cause salivary gland hypofunction. However, there have been relatively few studies assessing objective changes in salivary flow in response to medications. The salivary reflex has peripheral and central components which can be the targets of medications, leading to interruption of the reflex and medication-induced salivary gland dysfunction (MISGD) characterized by reduced production of saliva. The principal peripheral target is the cholinergic muscarinic (M3) receptor of salivary gland acinar cells which is blocked by antimuscarinic drugs used in the treatment of, for example, irritable bladder and chronic obstructive pulmonary disease. Tricyclic antidepressants not only have targets in the central nervous system but interact with and block muscarinic receptors in the periphery. Sympathetic nerve-mediated stimuli enhance salivary secretion, and there is no peripheral inhibition. Although adrenergic antagonists cause MIX, there is no evidence that they reduce salivary secretion. However, antihypertensive β-adrenoceptor blockers

G.B. Proctor, BSc, PhD
Mucosal and Salivary Biology Division, King's College London Dental Institute,
Floor 17 Guy's Tower Strand, London SE1 9RT, UK
e-mail: gordon.proctor@kcl.ac.uk



G. Carpenter (ed.), *Dry Mouth: A Clinical Guide on Causes, Effects and Treatments*, DOI 10.1007/978-3-642-55154-3_3

such as propranolol reduce the protein concentration of saliva which may impact on 'mouthfeel'. The main target for the central action of drugs causing MISGD is α2 adrenoceptors, and antihypertensive drugs that stimulate these receptors such as clonidine cause MIX and MISGD. Mixed serotonin and noradrenaline reuptake inhibitors (SNRIs) used in the treatment of depression, such as venlafaxine, cause significant MIX and MISGD. It may be that the mechanism of action involves activation of α2 adrenoceptors due to central accumulation of noradrenaline. Opioids such as tramadol that cause MIX and MISGD may have a similar mechanism of action. Gum chewing has been demonstrated to be effective for increasing salivary secretion in subjects with dry mouth and has been used to alleviate MIX. Parasympathomimetics might be appropriate for relieving xerostomia and salivary hypofunction resulting from non-anticholinergic xerogenic medications. Saliva substitutes with lubricative properties may also be appropriate.

## Introduction

In considering medication-induced dry mouth alongside other forms of dry mouth, it might be concluded that it occupies an area roughly in the middle of a pyramid of dry mouth severity. Dry mouth due to irradiation therapy for head and neck cancer is severe and affects relatively small numbers of subjects, whilst medication-induced dry mouth affects a larger number of subjects with a range of severity. Intuitively, this seems correct, given the high percentages of the population taking prescribed medications, up to 80 % in the over 60 age group [1], and the rates of reported xerostomia, 20–30 % of all age groups taking one prescribed medication [2, 3]. However, published studies of patients attending dry mouth clinics do not always support the higher prevalence of medication-induced dryness compared to disease-induced dryness [4–6]. Most likely this can be attributed to dry mouth clinics not being an accurate reflection of oral dryness in the general population.

A wide range of medications have been identified as xerogenic, that is, they have been found to be associated with xerostomia, the subjective symptom of dry mouth. A visit to the website www.drymouth.info indicates that medication-induced dry mouth is associated with an extensive list of over 1,500 drugs in a variety of drug groups including: analgesics, anorectics, antiarrhythmics, anticholinergics, anticonvulsants, antidepressants, antidiarrhoeals, anti-emetics, antihistamines/decongestants, antihypertensives, antiparkinsonians, antipsychotics, antispasmodics and diuretics [7]. Given the variety of mechanisms of action of these xerogenic drugs, it is to be expected that medication-induced dry mouth will encompass a wide range of severity with perhaps the most severe medication-related dryness being associated with anticholinergics. Many medicated individuals take more than one drug, and this adds to the complexity and a potential for enhanced dry mouth.

## What Is Medication-Induced Dry Mouth?

A wide range of drugs have been identified as xerogenic, that is, they have been found to be associated with xerostomia, the subjective symptom of dry mouth. Drug- or medication-induced xerostomia (MIX) is a drug-induced sensation of dry mouth. However, it is uncertain how much MIX is accompanied or can be ascribed to medication-induced salivary gland hypofunction (MISGD) which is defined as a reduced production of saliva which may also have an altered composition. Depending upon the degree of reduction in saliva production, MISGD tends to be accompanied by objective, observed signs of oral dryness including dry, sticky mucosal surfaces, lobulated anterior surface of the tongue and cervical caries (see Challacombe, Chap. 8 of this volume; [8]) and is usually accompanied by xerostomia. The observed signs of dryness result from a reduction of salivary function presumably due to either decreased volume or altered composition and retention of saliva on surfaces.

## Medication-Induced Xerostomia

Most published studies concerning medication-induced oral dryness are based on reported perception of dryness, and relatively few studies have objectively assessed aspects of saliva production. Apart from reduced production of saliva or retention on oral surfaces, it may also be that medication-induced xerostomia results from altered orosensory perception due to the action of medications on the peripheral or central nervous system.

Medication-induced dryness is usually reported as the subjective complaint of dry mouth, and relatively few studies undertake measurement of salivary flow rate or clinical assessment of dryness. The assessment of MIX is often made through subjects responses to relevant questions or the use of visual analogue scales whereby the subject is asked to rate the severity of their oral dryness. Nederfors et al. [9] asked over 4,000 subjects aged from 20 to 89 years old the question, 'Does your mouth usually feel dry?' and the results suggested a prevalence of 21 and 27 % in men and women, respectively [9]. There was a trend of increasing prevalence in subjects in their sixth, seventh and eighth decades which was evident in those on medications. Other studies on smaller sample sizes have derived prevalence figures of between 10 and 80 % most likely due to differences in the study populations. It is generally considered that age per se causes insignificant increases in the prevalence of dry mouth [10], and this conclusion is supported by the Nederfors study.

## Dose, Duration and Number of Medications

MIX in older age groups is associated with the number of medications being taken [9, 11–14]. The relationship is seen regardless of whether each medication has been found to be xerogenic alone. Nederfors et al. [9] and Sreebny et al. [15] found xerostomia rates of around 40 % in those taking three medications daily. Smidt et al. included the question, 'Have you had a daily sensation of dry mouth for more than 3 months?' in their assessment of xerostomia in a study of 668 community dwelling elderly (over 65 years) subjects [12]. The rates of xerostomia were lower than the above studies, 12.3 % overall and rising to 16.6 % in those taking two to three medications. It appears that elderly subjects exhibit higher rates of xerostomia with polypharmacy compared to younger subjects; for example, in subjects taking two or more medications, a rate of 15 % was found in subjects in their 30s [16] compared to a rate of 60 % in elderly subjects [17].

For some drugs, the dose and duration of medication have been associated with severity of xerostomia. Selective serotonin reuptake inhibitors (SSRIs) used as anorexiants (sibutramine) or as antidepressants (desvenlafaxine) were found to cause dose-dependent increases in xerostomia [18, 19]. Anticholinergics used to treat chronic obstructive pulmonary disease (tiotropium) and irritable bladder (tolterodine) caused increased xerostomia with increased dose [20]. Similarly, the antihypertensive alpha-2 adrenoceptor agonist guanfacine was found to cause dry mouth in higher percentages of treated subjects as the dose increased (Chap. 3, [1]).

It may be thought that a longer duration of medication would cause increased xerostomia, but recently published studies of specific drugs do not support this view. In a trial of tolterodine, a higher percentage of subjects experienced xerostomia during the period of up to 12 weeks compared to longer periods of 6 or 12 months [21]. Guanfacine was found to cause dry mouth in 60 % of subjects in the first year of treatment compared to 15 % after 1 year [1]. The latter pattern might be due to subjects becoming accustomed to or familiarized with 'their xerostomia'.

The severity of xerostomia is likely to be dependent upon the type of medication; although there are relatively few published studies examining severity and drug class or formulation, many of these have compared different antimuscarinic receptor drugs used in the treatment of overactive bladder, a condition characterized by an urgent and frequent need to urinate [22]. Results from a number of studies suggest that slow (osmotic system) release formulations of anticholinergic agents appear to be better tolerated, as indicated by rates of discontinuation due to dry mouth, than immediate release formulations [23–26], although other studies have found high discontinuation rates even with extended release formulations [27, 28]. The alpha-2 adrenoceptor agonist clonidine caused less dry mouth when administered as a transdermal patch compared to a tablet formulation [29, 30].

In the treatment of depression, tricyclic antidepressants (TCAs) are poorly tolerated compared to more modern SSRIs or mixed serotonin and noradrenaline reuptake inhibitors (SNRIs), as indicated by the reported rates of dry mouth – the most frequently reported adverse drug reaction (ADR) [22]. Thus the SSRI paroxetine was reported to cause less dry mouth than seen with TCAs [31]. A comparison of different

SNRIs indicates that many produced rates of reported xerostomia comparable to the placebo; however, in these patient groups, reported xerostomia is often high in the placebo group, presumably due to xerostomia associated with depression itself [1].

## Medication-Induced Salivary Gland Dysfunction (MISGD)

Salivary gland dysfunction is frequently reported as an ADR in response to prescribed medications (see [3]). MISGD can be defined as a medication-induced reduction in saliva production by salivary glands or an altered composition of secreted saliva. Intuitively we would consider that hyposalivation is the main cause of oral dryness and that medication-induced xerostomia is due to the effects of drugs on salivary flow rates. Wolff and Kleinberg [32] utilized paper-strip (Sialopaper) sampling of residual mucosal saliva and demonstrated reduced oral mucosal wetness in hyposalivators versus normosalivators [32]. Osailan et al. used the same method to demonstrate reduced mucosal wetness in subjects with reduced UWMS flow rate (see Challacombe, this volume) [33]. In order to determine the correlation of MIX with MISGD, we must define what we mean by MISGD (see later). Using a cut-off of 0.1 ml/min for UWMS flow rate, Smidt et al. [34] found a significant increase in salivary gland hypofunction in subjects experiencing xerostomia compared to those without xerostomia. Dawes [35] found that a group of subjects with normal salivary flow rates perceived oral dryness when their salivary flow rate decreased below 50 % [35]. So, we might conclude that subjects experience drug-induced dryness regardless of the 0.1 ml/min cut-off when salivary flow rate is substantially reduced.

Many medications cause xerostomia as a side effect, but very few have been tested for objective changes in salivary flow [36]. Salivary gland hypofunction is usually assessed by measuring salivary flow rates which are dependent upon nerve-mediated stimulation (see Fig. 3.1). During the 24-h day, salivary secretion is stimulated by overt taste or chewing stimulation for only short periods (total approx. 4 h). Therefore salivary flow during the waking period (approx. 15 h) in the absence of stimulation might be considered to be the most relevant to dry mouth. Unstimulated whole mouth saliva (UWMS) flow rate is therefore usually measured in order to assess salivary hypofunction, ideally for a period of not less than 5 min in order to reduce variation [37]. However, hyposalivation is difficult to define since salivary flow rates show a wide range in the normal population (see Challacombe, this volume). Sreebny and Vissink [1] presented UWMS flow rates from a number of studies, and it can be concluded that normal mean flow rate for all ages is approximately 0.35 ml/min, but standard deviations tend to be high (approximately 0.3 ml/min). When studies comparing males and females of all age groups are compared, it has been found that overall female UWMS flow rate is 70 % of male flow rates (see summary data in [1]). In addition a 12-h circadian variation in UWMS flow has been shown in which measured flows might differ by up to 70 % depending upon the time of day of collection [38]. Against this backdrop of variation, a generally accepted figure for very low UWMS flow rate is 0.1 ml/min, whilst 0.15 ml/min or

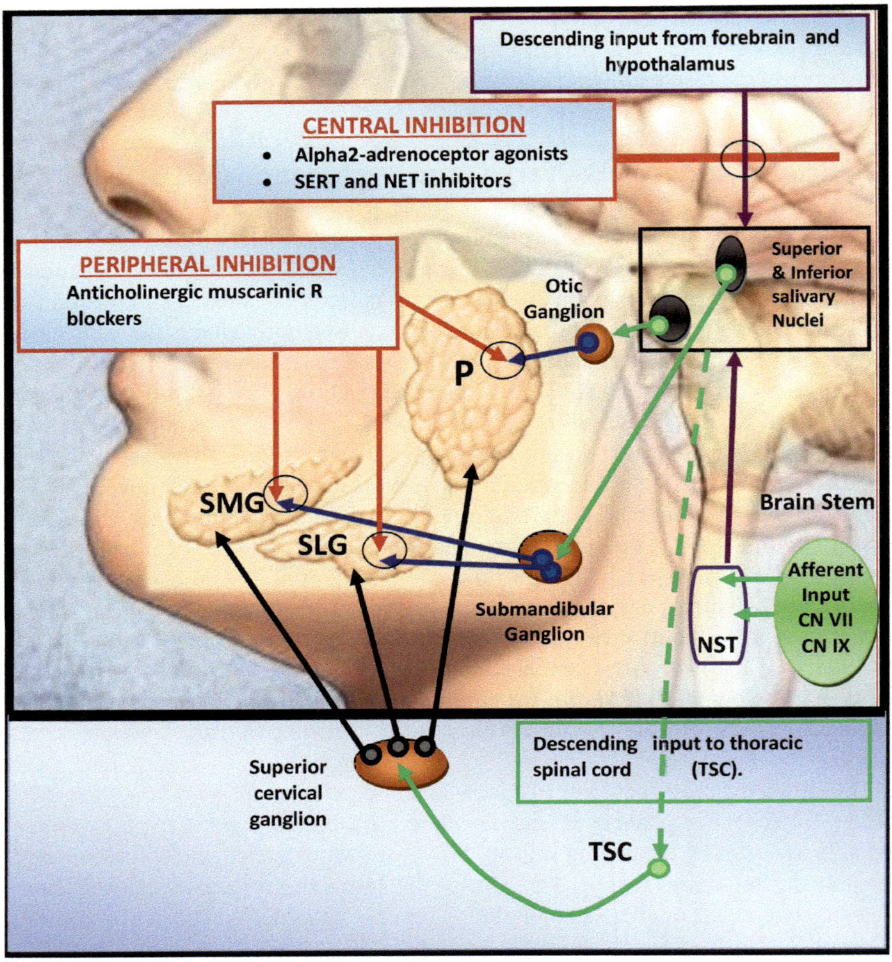


**Fig. 3.1** Peripheral and central targets of medications inhibiting nerve signalling in the salivary reflex. The illustration of the salivary reflex shows afferent stimuli arriving via cranial nerves VII and IX at the nucleus of the solitary tract (*NST*) in the brainstem. Central neural tracts connect to the salivary nuclei, and parasympathetic nerves from the superior salivary nucleus innervate the submandibular (*SMG*)/sublingual (*SLG*) glands via the submandibular ganglion, whilst parasympathetic nerves from the inferior salivary nucleus innervated the parotid (*P*) gland. Not shown is central integration of afferent (chewing, chemical) stimuli from cranial nerve V. Descending tracts from the cortex via the lateral hypothalamus modulate transmission of stimuli in the salivary nuclei and alpha-2 adrenoceptor agonists (e.g. antihypertensives) produce an inhibitory effect on transmission and cause MISGD. Inhibitors of SERT and NET, serotonin and noradrenaline transporters responsible for reuptake, appear to cause MISGD through activation of alpha-2 adrenoceptors by elevating endogenous levels of noradrenaline. The main peripheral target of drugs causing MISGD is cholinergic muscarinic receptors (M3 an M1) on salivary gland acinar cells. Central connections and sympathetic outflow are also shown. Antihypertensive (and maybe also nasal decongestant) drugs may alter saliva protein content by acting on peripheral beta-1 adrenoceptors, but there is little evidence that substantial MISGD is caused through receptors in this pathway

less can be regarded as low. Looking at individual published studies, the figure might be adjusted slightly; for example, a study of over 1,000 subjects by Dodds & Johnson [39] suggests a figure of 0.14 ml/min for the lowest 10 %, and a similar figure can be deduced from a study by Heintze et al. [40].

The ages of study subjects have been found to influence salivary flow rates with older age groups showing reduced flow. However, the extent of this reduction appears to be mostly influenced by the increased consumption of medications in the older age groups. The effects of age per se, in a non-medicated population, have been less frequently studied with some researchers finding an effect of age [39, 41] and others suggesting that such an effect is not significant [10] since there is little evidence of age-related (per se) xerostomia. The observed differences between the sexes referred to above need also to be considered in the light of medication. For example [12], a study of older (over 65 years) subjects found that UWMS flow rate in female subjects was 63 % of males. However, this difference was not seen when non-medicated subjects were considered as a separate group.

How is it that subjects might experience MIX in the absence of reduced saliva production? One possibility is that altered salivary composition and properties may affect salivary function including coating and retention on soft tissue surfaces. Osailan et al. studied a group of dry mouth patients with mixed diagnoses including drug-induced dryness, and a substantial proportion (20 %) had signs (scored using a clinical scale) and symptoms (scored using relevant questions and a VAS) of dryness even though their unstimulated salivary flow rate was greater than 0.2 ml/min, well above the accepted figure for hypofunction of 0.1 (or 0.15) ml/min [33]. Analysis of the composition of saliva from patients did not reveal decreased levels of high-molecular-weight mucin (MUC5B), an important glycoprotein in determining the viscoelastic properties of saliva [42]. More recent studies suggest reduced extensional rheology in these ‘higher salivary flow’ dry mouth patients which may be linked with a reduced function on mucosal surfaces (Chaudhury et al. 2014, unpublished findings).

## What Are the Mechanisms of MISGD?

### Interruption of Reflex Signalling at the Periphery: Afferent Signalling

Secretion of fluid from salivary glands is a nerve-mediated reflex (Fig. 3.1). Secretion from the major salivary glands is evoked by tastants with citric acid and other strong sour tastes evoking high flows of saliva, whilst salt, bitter and sweet evoke less saliva. High salivary flow rates are also produced following activation of mechanoreceptors in the periodontal ligament and mucosae [43]. Minor salivary glands may also increase secretion in response to taste stimulation [44], but perhaps mechanoreceptors responding to movement and tactile stimulation of the mucosa play a more important role in evoking secretion from submucosal labial and palatine minor salivary glands [45, 46]. Interference with afferent signalling does not appear to play a primary role in MISGD although it might be speculated that dietary consumption of softer foods, as a result of insufficient saliva to moisten/process harder foods, may exacerbate a dry mouth condition due to reduced chewing reflex stimulation of salivary glands. Reduced reflex stimulation can result in salivary gland atrophy [47].

## Interruption of Reflex Signalling at the Periphery: Efferent Signalling

Salivary secretion is dependent upon autonomic nerve-mediated signals. Under anaesthesia, most salivary glands do not secrete fluid, and there are only a few examples of spontaneously secreting salivary glands, and even in these glands secretion ceases when the autonomic nerve supply to salivary glands is severed [48]. When the parasympathetic nerve supply is stimulated electrically under anaesthesia, large volumes of saliva are evoked, whilst similar stimulation of sympathetic nerves evoked only a small volume of fluid. Dual parasympathetic and sympathetic nerve stimulation experiments under anaesthesia have demonstrated that the individual actions of the nerves, particularly protein secretion evoked by the sympathetic nerve, are augmented, whilst the volume of secretion is maintained in rat parotid [47]. Such dual stimulation experiments are thought to better reflect the events leading to reflex secretion of saliva, since it is expected that both parasympathetic and sympathetic impulses are acting on secretory cells simultaneously. The concept of peripheral sympathetic inhibition of salivary secretion, which later became widely accepted, was appreciated as an experimental artefact over a century ago. Experimental electrical stimulation of the sympathetic nerve supply to salivary glands or use of alpha-1 adrenoceptor agonists in anaesthetized animals leads to a vasoconstriction of glandular blood vessels in addition to activation of parenchymal cells. In contrast under reflex conditions, only sympathetic secretomotor nerve fibres and not vasoactive nerve fibres to salivary glands are activated. Thus vasoconstriction is not part of the salivary reflex.

Denervation studies in the rat have demonstrated that sympathetic impulses make a contribution to the amount of protein secreted under reflex taste stimulation [49]. The importance of an intact parasympathetic innervation is clear when one considers the dryness caused by blockade of the effects of acetylcholine by atropine and its analogues. Blockade of the effects of sympathetically mediated stimuli by the beta-blocker propranolol and its analogues causes reductions in protein concentration of saliva.

Although adrenergic signalling from sympathetic nerves leads to an augmentation of protein secretion by parotid and submandibular glands, mucin secretion from mucous glands such as the rat sublingual gland and human minor glands is dependent upon parasympathetic stimulation and peptidergic stimulation [50]. Thus, although parasympathetic nerve-mediated stimuli appear to universally cause fluid secretion from salivary glands, the role of the sympathetic innervation in evoking protein secretion is variable.

## Efferent Signalling and Muscarinic Receptor Antagonists

Salivary secretion is largely dependent upon the activation of muscarinic acetylcholine receptors (mAchRs) on salivary acinar cells by acetylcholine released from parasympathetic nerves [47]. Pharmacological studies suggest that secretion is almost entirely dependent upon signalling through m3AchRs in the rat parotid gland whilst submandibular gland secretion in rat and rabbit is dependent on both m3AchRs and m1AchRs. Selective knockout of muscarinic receptor subtypes in mice indicates that m1AchRs play a role in whole mouth saliva secretion in response to stimulation with cholinergic agonists, including pilocarpine [51, 52]. The m1AchRs are not expressed on all submandibular cells, and activation appears to require higher doses of agonist compared to activation of m3AchR, and studies of calcium signalling in submandibular acinar cells in vitro indicate, unlike m3 receptors, that m1 receptors are not ubiquitously expressed [51].

Given the paramount importance of cholinergic signalling in salivary secretion, it is clear that xerostomia associated with anticholinergic medications (see earlier) is most likely due to medication-induced salivary gland hypofunction (Table 3.1; Fig. 3.1). Oxybutynin, tolterodine, trospium, solifenacin, darifenacin and fesoterodine are muscarinic receptor antagonists commonly used in the treatment of overactive bladder, and each of these drugs blocks M3 and/or M2 receptors, which are the intended targets since the latter mediate smooth muscle relaxation in the bladder. Dry mouth is an ADR of varying severity depending on the drug; for example, tolterodine appears to produces less dry mouth than fesoterodine although each drug interacts with a number of muscarinic receptors including M3 ([53], [54], [55], [56]). Studies on the mouse have compared some prescribed anticholinergics used in the treatment of overactive bladders – oxybutynin, solifenacin and tolterodine. Submandibular gland secretion was less affected by solifenacin and tolterodine compared to oxybutynin, and solifenacin dissociated from muscarinic receptors more easily than oxybutynin [57].

Dry mouth may be offset to a degree through controlled drug-release formulations compared to immediate release [58] as described above. Tiotropium is an inhaled bronchodilator used in the treatment of chronic obstructive pulmonary disease which interacts with muscarinic receptors including M3 and was found to cause dry mouth as an ADR in 9.3–16 % of the subjects compared to 1.6–2.7 % of the subjects in a placebo group [59, 60]. Tiotropium results in more dry mouth symptoms than new LAMA (glycopyrronium bromide). The efficacy of this drug in

**Table 3.1** Pharmacological mechanisms of peripherally acting xerogenic drugs

| Drug type | Intended action | Decreased salivation | Mechanism of MISGD |
|---|---|---|---|
| Overactive bladder | Anticholinergic (M3) | Y | Anticholinergic (M3) |
| Anti-emetics | Anticholinergic | Y | Anticholinergic (M3) |
| Tricyclic antidepressants | SNRI | Y | Anticholinergic (M3) |
| Antihistamines | Anti-H1 receptor | Y | Anticholinergic (M3) |
| Antihypertensives | β-Adr antagonist | N (reduced protein secretion) | β-Adr antagonist |

controlling COPD still needs confirmation by a phase III study [61]. Orphenadrine, procyclidine and trihexyphenidyl are anticholinergics that antagonize muscarinic receptors and can cause dry mouth as a side effect, presumably due to blockade of M3 and M1 receptors.

### Medications with an Unintended Antimuscarinic Effect

Tricyclic antidepressants (TCAs) used in the treatment of depression not only inhibit reuptake of serotonin and noradrenaline by transporters in the CNS but interact with muscarinic receptors as demonstrated by competitive radioligand binding assays [62]. TCAs cause dry mouth in a substantial (27 %) percentage of treated subjects [63], and the TCAs amitriptyline and nortriptyline have been demonstrated to reduce stimulated salivary secretion [64–66] whilst amitriptyline and the TCA dothiepin also significantly reduced (58 %) stimulated parotid salivary flow rate.

Early formulated antihistamines such as clemastine, diphenhydramine and brompheniramine used in the treatment of allergy, nausea and vomiting cause varying degrees of dry mouth in subjects, and this appears to be due to an interaction with muscarinic receptors. More specific histamine H1 receptor blockers are less associated with dry mouth as an ADR [1, 22]. Some anti-emetic medications such as scopolamine used in the control of motion sickness have an anticholinergic action and cause hyposalivation and dry mouth through this mechanism.

## Central Interruption of Reflex Signalling

Taste, mechanical or pungency signals generate afferent signals in fibres of the facial (CN VII), glossopharyngeal (CN IX) and trigeminal (CN V) nerves. The nucleus of the solitary tract is innervated by the CN VII and CN IX and sends interneurons to the salivary centres, respectively, the superior and inferior salivary nuclei in the medulla oblongata. Interneurons presumably supply the primary sympathetic salivary centres which are located in the upper thoracic segments of the spinal cord although it remains unclear precisely where in this region [67]. Efferent nerve fibres from the salivary nuclei conduct efferent signals via the chorda lingual nerve to the submandibular ganglion and thence to the submandibular and sublingual glands. The parotid gland is supplied by efferent fibres in the glossopharyngeal (tympanic branch) nerve to the otic ganglion and postganglionic fibres in the auriculotemporal nerve (see Fig. 3.1).

The salivary reflex is profoundly influenced by central nerves from other nuclei in the brain supplying the salivary nuclei in the medulla oblongata. The salivary nuclei have various inputs from the frontal cortical areas as demonstrated by nerve-tracing experiments [68]. This central neural activity appears to contribute towards the resting rate of salivary secretion into the mouth since salivary flow rates are lower during sleep and virtually absent during anaesthesia. Retrograde labelling of neurons has demonstrated that the primary parasympathetic salivary centres form connections with the lateral hypothalamus where the regulation of feeding, drinking and body temperature occurs. Both excitatory (gamma-aminobutyric acid containing) and inhibitory (glycine containing) nerves synapse with the salivary centres [67].

Suppression of impulse traffic from the salivary nuclei to salivary glands leading to reduced salivation and dry mouth is most obviously demonstrated during fear and anxiety and, like other autonomic regulations, involves a complex interaction with higher (limbic and cortical) centres in the brain. Different sensory modalities, including auditory, visual and somatosensory, are associated with fear and may potentially impact on salivary secretion through pathways in the amygdala, the hypothalamus and the brainstem.

Previous neuroanatomical studies have shown that there are also cholinergic inputs to the salivary centres from other nuclei including the substantia innominata, pedunculopontine nucleus (PPN) and lateral dorsal tegmental nucleus (LDT). It has recently been demonstrated that neurons in the SSN express M3 and other muscarinic acetylcholine receptors [69].

Since cholinergic neurons from the PPN and LDT are associated with the maintenance of wakefulness and show increasing impulses during wakefulness, it may be that these inputs enhance activity of superior salivary nucleus neurons and increase salivation during wakefulness, whilst reduced impulse input from the PPN and LDT suppresses salivation during sleep and may account for the circadian pattern of resting or unstimulated salivation observed in man [38]. The presence of muscarinic receptors on neurons of the salivary nuclei may also partly explain the observed effects of enhanced salivary secretion evoked by intracerebroventricular injection of pilocarpine or atropine which was found to, respectively, stimulate and inhibit salivation [70, 71].

## Central Signalling and Alpha-2 Adrenoceptor Agonists

Clonidine, guanabenz, guanfacine, methyldopa and moxonidine are α2Ad agonists used in the treatment of hypertension and have been found to cause dry mouth in high percentages of treated subjects (see Chap. 3 in [1]). Alpha-2 adrenoceptor (α2Ad) agonists (e.g. clonidine) have been demonstrated to reduce salivary secretion in human subjects (Table 3.2; Fig. 3.1). Studies in animal models indicate that the mechanism of hyposalivation involves central α2Ads which are distributed throughout the central nervous system, and high levels of specific α2Ad binding sites are found in the nuclei of the hypothalamus and amygdala. The lateral hypothalamus projects to the parasympathetic salivary nuclei in the brainstem, and lesions of the lateral hypothalamus produce a typical pattern of degeneration secretion with immediate, transient hypersalivation due to neurotransmitter release being superceded by prolonged impairment of basal salivation and reduction of pilocarpine-induced salivation [72]. Alpha-2 adrenoceptor blockade can increase salivary secretion, whilst α2Ad agonists inhibit secretion [73, 74]. Injection of moxonidine (an α2Ad and imidazoline agonist) reduced salivation induced by pilocarpine (i.p.) in rats, and prior injection of the RX 821002, an α2Ad antagonist, abolished the inhibitory effect of moxonidine [72]. It appears that under physiological conditions,

**Table 3.2** Pharmacological mechanisms of centrally acting xerogenic drugs

| Drug type | Intended action | Hyposalivation | Mechanism of MISGD |
|---|---|---|---|
| Antihypertensives | $\alpha_2$-Adr agonist | Y | $\alpha_2$-Adr agonist |
| Tricyclic antidepressants | SNRI | Y | Uncertain – $\alpha_2$-Adr agonist? |
| Antidepressants (non-TCA) | SNRI | Y | Uncertain – $\alpha_2$-Adr agonist? |
| | SSRI | N | N |
| Appetite suppressant | SNRI | Y | Uncertain – $\alpha_2$-Adr agonist? |
| | SSRI | N | N |
| Opioid analgesics | Mu-opioid receptor | N | Uncertain – $\alpha_2$-Adr agonist? |
| | SNRI | Y | N |
| Decongestant (pseudoephedrine) | $\alpha_1$-Adr agonist | Uncertain | Uncertain – $\alpha_2$-Adr agonist? |
| | β-Adr agonist | N (increased protein secretion?) | β-Adr agonist |

α2Ad signalling is part of a central inhibitory circuit related to the control of salivary gland secretion involving projections running from the rat hypothalamus to the midbrain and hindbrain autonomic centres, including the salivary nuclei. In addition, direct efferent connections exist between the forebrain and the salivary glands. The α2Ad mechanisms on salivary secretion probably involve descending pathways passing through the LH before reaching the brainstem or more caudal autonomic centres related to the control of salivary gland function. Binding studies have shown the existence of high levels of α2Ad in the LH, and moxonidine acting on α2Ad may produce inhibitory effects as a consequence of presynaptic inhibition of noradrenaline or glutamate release or postsynaptic hyperpolarization, both mechanisms consistent with the pre- and postsynaptic location of the α2Ad in the brain. Therefore, moxonidine acting on α2Ad probably located postsynaptically in the LH may inhibit the excitatory mechanisms of the LH activated by pilocarpine to induce salivation [72, 75].

## Medications with an Unintended Activation of α2 Adrenoceptors

Amphetamine is a xerogenic drug which acts on the central serotonin and noradrenaline transporters (SERT and NET) leading to increased levels of noradrenaline, dopamine and serotonin at nerve terminals [5]. Amphetamine exerts an inhibitory effect on the flow of saliva through release of noradrenaline from nerves in the medulla causing activation of inhibitory α2Ad [76]. These central effects of amphetamine that cause a dry mouth contrast with its action in the periphery leading to increased secretion of protein by salivary cells and increased salivary protein concentration.

Mixed serotonin and noradrenaline reuptake inhibitors (SNRIs) such as venlafaxine, nefazodone, duloxetine and trazodone can cause a substantial percentage of treated subjects to experience dry mouth (Table 3.2). The xerogenic mechanism is not understood but may involve elevated levels of catecholamines in central synapses leading to activation of α2Ads by a similar mechanism to that of amphetamine. Venlafaxine was found to significantly decrease salivary output measured using a cotton wool roll by 30 and 32 % at doses of 75 and 150 mg, respectively

[77]. In the same study, the TCA desipramine reduced salivary output almost 50 %, whilst the SSRI paroxetine (20 mg) had no effect on salivary output in agreement with a previous report that paroxetine (30 mg) did not affect salivation [78]. Dry mouth is one of the self-reported side effects of venlafaxine in clinical trials, and it seems that the reduction in salivation produced by venlafaxine may be due to the reduced activity of parasympathetic salivary neurons in the brainstem resulting from accumulation of noradrenergics due to the inhibition of noradrenaline reuptake blockade. It is of interest that the selective noradrenaline uptake blocker reboxetine also reduces salivation, probably via the same mechanism [77] and it might be that TCAs like desipramine owe some of their xerogenic effect to this mechanism in addition to the anticholinergic effect described earlier.

SSRIs such as citalopram, paroxetine, fluoxetine, fluvoxamine and sertraline used in treatment of depression can cause dry mouth although to a lesser extent than seen with the SNRIs [1]. However, unlike TCAs, these drugs were found not to reduce stimulated parotid saliva secretion [66]. Smidt et al. [12] found that SSRIs (ATC N06AB) did reduce UWMS flow rate ($p=0.049$) compared to subjects not taking the medications, but the degree of reduction (34 %) was less than seen for the subgroup of psychoanaleptics (ATC N06) as a whole which showed a 44 % reduction ($p=0.001$).

Tramadol, morphine and other opioids exert an antinociceptive effect through inhibition of central reuptake of noradrenaline by NET transporters as well as binding to mu-opioid receptors [79]. A randomized double-blind placebo-controlled study using tramadol confirmed that dry mouth was associated with decreased salivary flow rates in 75 % of subjects [80]. The mechanism of action of tramadol was investigated in a rat model in which the secretion in response to the application of citric acid on the tongue was assessed and found to be reduced by 38 % and by 64 %, respectively, at 5 and 10 mg/kg (i.v.) of tramadol. There was no anticholinergic effect on salivary gland secretion, and tramadol exerted its principal xerogenic effect by activating inhibitory pathways in the central nervous system. It is likely that the reduced salivation on reflex stimulation was due to raised levels of noradrenaline in central synapses and interaction with central $\alpha 2$ adrenoceptors.

## Treatment of Medication-Induced Xerostomia and Salivary Gland Dysfunction

There are few studies that address treatment of MIX specifically, but clearly interventions that can relieve xerostomia should be of use in those experiencing xerostomia due to medications.

### Drug Substitution

Different formulations of drugs – slow release using osmotic systems, for example – may cause less severe xerostomia as described above [22]. It may be a therapeutic option to substitute a drug treatment with a different class of drug in order to relieve xerostomia as an ADR. An example is seen in the treatment of depression using

TCAs, which have been shown to cause a high incidence of xerostomia and MISGD; SSRIs, which cause a much lower incidence of xerostomia and have not been demonstrated to cause MISGD, might be substituted for TCAs. Similarly, SNRIs which also cause MIX and MISGD might be replaced by SSRIs.

## Pharmacological Stimulation

Parasympathomimetics such as pilocarpine (Salagen) and cevimeline are used to treat xerostomia associated with Sjögren syndrome and following radiotherapy for head and neck cancer [81, 82]. A more recent study by Götrick et al. indicates that oral pilocarpine is of use for the treatment of opioid (tramadol)-induced xerostomia. The randomized, double-blind, placebo-controlled trial of 65 individuals found that both xerostomia and hyposalivation induced by tramadol were reversed by oral pilocarpine [83]. Although the study was conducted on healthy volunteers, it may be of significance for patients in palliative care who frequently experience xerostomia as a symptom due to treatment with opioids. Clearly, parasympathomimetics are not an option for the treatment of xerostomia caused by anticholinergic drugs used in the treatment of an overactive bladder since both drug classes target cholinergic muscarinic receptors.

## Gum Chewing and Saliva Substitutes

Xerostomia may be experienced during the day, at night or both. For those subjects experiencing daytime xerostomia, it appears to manifest as a need to moisten dry food when eating, and questions relating to eating have proved to be useful in detecting and assessing xerostomia; such questions are a major part of the Summated Xerostomia Inventory-Dutch Version [84]. Since xerostomia is particularly manifested during consumption of food, it might be concluded that stimulation of secretion by gum chewing would not represent an effective means of relief from xerostomia. However, xerostomia is also likely to be a symptom related to the condition/feel of the mouth during periods of unstimulated secretion which occupy most of the waking day between periods of consumption of food or drink. Secretion from the submandibular/sublingual glands contributes a greater proportion of unstimulated whole mouth salivary secretion, and a study by Wolff et al. [85] concluded that users of many common medication categories – cardiovascular drugs, antihistamines, tranquillizers/sedatives and antidepressants – display greater reductions in salivary flow rate from submandibular/sublingual glands than parotid glands. Since parotid secretion forms a greater proportion of chewing than stimulated salivary secretion, it would seem that gum chewing should be an effective means of increasing saliva secretion in those with MISGD and alleviating dryness xerostomia [85].

The Cochrane review on 'Interventions for the management of dry mouth: topical therapies' [86] concluded that gum chewing was neither more nor less effective than available saliva substitutes in relieving dry mouth. For example, Bots et al. [87] studied alleviation of thirst in haemodialysis patients and found that both saliva substitute and gum chewing significantly relieved dryness [87]. However, 20 % preferred the Xialine spray, and 80 % preferred the chewing gum. A more relevant study to MISGD is that of Davies (2000) who studied patients in palliative care. The results indicated that gum chewing and the mucin-based saliva substitute Saliva Orthana relieved xerostomia and that subjects preferred gum chewing [88]. The Cochrane review concluded that water/electrolyte-based topical sprays were less effective than formulations such as oxygenated glycerol triester which have lubricative/surface active properties. As an alternative to gum chewing, a recent study found that the use of a 1 % malic acid spray mixed with xylitol and fluoride produced relief in subjects with dry mouth induced by antidepressant medication [89]. However, previously the Cochrane review concluded that the use of acidic saliva stimulation by those with dry mouth should be avoided owing to the likelihood of tooth erosive demineralization [86].

**Acknowledgement** The author thanks Dr. Abeer Shaalan, King's College London - Dental Institute, for the preparation of Fig. 3.1 and for help in preparing the manuscript.

## References

1. Sreebny LM, Vissink A. Dry mouth. The malevolent symptom: a clinical guide. Ames: Wiley-Blackwell; 2010.
2. Sreebny LM, Valdini A. Xerostomia. 1. Relationship to other oral symptoms and salivary-gland hypofunction. Oral Surg Oral Med Oral Pathol Oral Radiol Endod. 1988;66(4):451–8.
3. Nederfors T. Xerostomia and hyposalivation. Adv Dent Res. 2000;14:48–56.
4. Longman LP, et al. Salivary gland hypofunction in elderly patients attending a xerostomia clinic. Gerodontology. 1995;12(12):67–72.
5. Field EA, et al. The establishment of a xerostomia clinic: a prospective study. Br J Oral Maxillofac Surg. 1997;35(2):96–103.
6. Kaplan I, Zuk-Paz L, Wolff A. Association between salivary flow rates, oral symptoms, and oral mucosal status. Oral Surg Oral Med Oral Pathol Oral Radiol Endod. 2008;106(2):235–41.
7. Sreebny LM, Schwartz SS. A reference guide to drugs and dry mouth–2nd edition. Gerodontology. 1997;14(1):33–47.
8. Osailan S, et al. A validated clinical oral dryness score. Oral Dis. 2010;16(6):538.
9. Nederfors T, et al. Prevalence of perceived symptoms of dry mouth in an adult Swedish population – relation to age, sex and pharmacotherapy. Community Dent Oral Epidemiol. 1997; 25(3):211–6.
10. Ship JA, Baum BJ. Old age in health and disease. Lessons from the oral cavity. Oral Surg Oral Med Oral Pathol. 1993;76(1):40–4.
11. Narhi TO, et al. Association between salivary flow rate and the use of systemic medication among 76-, 81-, and 86-year-old inhabitants in Helsinki, Finland. J Dent Res. 1992;71(12): 1875–80.
12. Smidt D, et al. Associations between labial and whole salivary flow rates, systemic diseases and medications in a sample of older people. Community Dent Oral Epidemiol. 2010;38(5): 422–35.
13. Sreebny LM. Salivary flow in health and disease. Compend Suppl. 1989;13:S461–9.
14. Wu AJ, Ship JA. A characterization of major salivary gland flow rates in the presence of medications and systemic diseases. Oral Surg Oral Med Oral Pathol. 1993;76(3):301–6.

15. Sreebny LM, Valdini A, Yu A. Xerostomia. Part II. Relationship to nonoral symptoms, drugs, and diseases. Oral Surg Oral Med Oral Pathol. 1989;68(4):419–27.
16. Thomson WM, et al. The occurrence of xerostomia and salivary gland hypofunction in a population-based sample of older South Australians. Spec Care Dentist. 1999;19(1):20–3.
17. Ikebe K, et al. Perception of dry mouth in a sample of community-dwelling older adults in Japan. Spec Care Dentist. 2001;21(2):52–9.
18. Gallagher JC, et al. The effect of dose titration and dose tapering on the tolerability of desvenlafaxine in women with vasomotor symptoms associated with menopause. J Womens Health (Larchmt). 2012;21(2):188–98.
19. Deecher DC, et al. Desvenlafaxine succinate: a new serotonin and norepinephrine reuptake inhibitor. J Pharmacol Exp Ther. 2006;318(2):657–65.
20. Malone-Lee JG, Walsh JB, Maugourd MF. Tolterodine: a safe and effective treatment for older patients with overactive bladder. J Am Geriatr Soc. 2001;49(6):700–5.
21. Takei M, Homma Y. Long-term safety, tolerability and efficacy of extended- release tolterodine in the treatment of overactive bladder in Japanese patients. Int J Urol. 2005;12(5):456–64.
22. Scully C. Drug effects on salivary glands: dry mouth. Oral Dis. 2003;9(4):165–76.
23. Appell RA, et al. Prospective randomized controlled trial of extended-release oxybutynin chloride and tolterodine tartrate in the treatment of overactive bladder: results of the OBJECT Study. Mayo Clin Proc. 2001;76(4):358–63.
24. Diokno AC, et al. Prospective, randomized, double-blind study of the efficacy and tolerability of the extended-release formulations of oxybutynin and tolterodine for overactive bladder: results of the OPERA trial. Mayo Clin Proc. 2003;78(6):687–95.
25. Elinoff V, et al. Symptom-specific efficacy of tolterodine extended release in patients with overactive bladder: the IMPACT trial. Int J Clin Pract. 2006;60(6):745–51.
26. Gupta SK, Sathyan G. Pharmacokinetics of an oral once-a-day controlled- release oxybutynin formulation compared with immediate-release oxybutynin. J Clin Pharmacol. 1999;39(3):289–96.
27. Chung SD, et al. The efficacy of additive tolterodine extended release for 1-year in older men with storage symptoms and clinical benign prostatic hyperplasia. Neurourol Urodyn. 2011;30(4):568–71.
28. Kaplan SA, Walmsley K, Te AE. Tolterodine extended release attenuates lower urinary tract symptoms in men with benign prostatic hyperplasia. J Urol. 2005;174(6):2273–5; discussion 2275–6.
29. Breidthardt J, Schumacher H, Mehlburger L. Long-term (5 year) experience with transdermal clonidine in the treatment of mild to moderate hypertension. Clin Auton Res. 1993;3(6): 385–90.
30. Burris JF, Mroczek WJ. Transdermal administration of clonidine: a new approach to antihypertensive therapy. Pharmacotherapy. 1986;6(1):30–4.
31. Ravindran AV, et al. A double-blind, multicenter study in primary care comparing paroxetine and clomipramine in patients with depression and associated anxiety. Paroxetine Study Group. J Clin Psychiatry. 1997;58(3):112–8.
32. Wolff M, Kleinberg I. Oral mucosal wetness in hypo- and normosalivators. Arch Oral Biol. 1998;43(6):455–62.
33. Osailan S, et al. Investigating the relationship between hyposalivation and mucosal wetness. Oral Dis. 2011;17(1):109–14.
34. Smidt D, Torpet LA, Nauntofte B, et al. Associations between oral and ocular dryness, labial and whole salivary flow rates, systemic diseases and medications in a sample of older people. Community Dent Oral Epidemiol. 2011;39(3):276–88.
35. Dawes C. Physiological factors affecting salivary flow rate, oral sugar clearance, and the sensation of dry mouth in man. J Dent Res. 1987;66(Spec):648–53.
36. Napenas JJ, Brennan MT, Fox PC. Diagnosis and treatment of xerostomia (dry mouth). Odontology. 2009;97(2):76–83.
37. Navazesh M, Kumar SK. Measuring salivary flow: challenges and opportunities. J Am Dent Assoc. 2008;139(Suppl):35S–40.
38. Dawes C. Circadian rhythms in human salivary flow rate and composition. J Physiol. 1972;220(3):529–45.
39. Dodds MW, Johnson DA, Yeh CK. Health benefits of saliva: a review. J Dent. 2005;33(3):223–33.

40. Heintze U, Birkhed D, Bjorn H. Secretion rate and buffer effect of resting and stimulated whole saliva as a function of age and sex. Swed Dent J. 1983;7(6):227–38.
41. Percival RS, Challacombe SJ, Marsh PD. Flow rates of resting whole and stimulated parotid saliva in relation to age and gender. J Dent Res. 1994;73(8):1416–20.
42. Pramanik R, et al. Protein and mucin retention on oral mucosal surfaces in dry mouth patients. Eur J Oral Sci. 2010;118(3):245–53.
43. Hector MP, Linden RW. Reflexes of salivary secretion. In: Garrett JR, Ekstrom J, Anderson LC, editors. Neural mechanisms of salivary secretion. Basel: Karger; 1999. p. 196–217.
44. Speirs RL. Secretion of saliva by human lip mucous glands and parotid glands in response to gustatory stimuli and chewing. Arch Oral Biol. 1984;29(11):945–8.
45. Boros I, Keszler P, Zelles T. Study of saliva secretion and the salivary fluoride concentration of the human minor labial glands by a new method. Arch Oral Biol. 1999;44 Suppl 1:S59–62.
46. Veerman ECI, et al. Human glandular salivas: their separate collection and analysis. Eur J Oral Sci. 1996;104(4):346–52.
47. Proctor GB, Carpenter GH. Regulation of salivary gland function by autonomic nerves. Auton Neurosci. 2007;133(1):3–18.
48. Emmelin N. Nervous control of mammalian salivary-glands. Phil Trans Roy Soc London Ser B Biol Sci. 1981;296(1080):27–35.
49. Matsuo R, et al. Reflex secretion of proteins into submandibular saliva in conscious rats, before and after preganglionic sympathectomy. J Physiol. 2000;527(Pt 1):175–84.
50. Culp DJ, et al. Rat sublingual gland as a model to study glandular mucous cell secretion. Am J Physiol. 1991;260(6 Pt 1):C1233–44.
51. Nakamura T, et al. M(3) muscarinic acetylcholine receptor plays a critical role in parasympathetic control of salivation in mice. J Physiol. 2004;558(Pt 2):561–75.
52. Gautam D, et al. Cholinergic stimulation of salivary secretion studied with M1 and M3 muscarinic receptor single- and double-knockout mice. Mol Pharmacol. 2004;66(2):260–7.
53. Glavind K, Chancellor M. Antimuscarinics for the treatment of overactive bladder: understanding the role of muscarinic subtype selectivity. Int Urogynecol J. 2011;22(8):907–17.
54. Dmochowski RR, Gomelsky A. Update on the treatment of overactive bladder. Curr Opin Urol. 2011;21(4):286–90.
55. Kaplan SA, Schneider T, Foote JE, et al. Superior efficacy of fesoterodine over tolterodine extended release with rapid onset: a prospective, head-to-head, placebo-controlled trial. BJU Int. 2011;107(9):1432–40.
56. Chung SD, Chang HC, Chiu B, et al. The efficacy of additive tolterodine extended release for 1-year in older men with storage symptoms and clinical benign proastatic hyperplasia. NeurourolUrodyn. 2011;30(4):568–71.
57. Oki T, Takeuchi C, Yamada S. Comparative evaluation of exocrine muscarinic receptor binding characteristics and inhibition of salivation of solifenacin in mice. Biol Pharm Bull. 2006;29(7):1397–400.
58. Versi E, et al. Dry mouth with conventional and controlled-release oxybutynin in urinary incontinence. The Ditropan XL Study Group. Obstet Gynecol. 2000;95(5):718–21.
59. Casaburi R, et al. The spirometric efficacy of once-daily dosing with tiotropium in stable COPD: a 13-week multicenter trial. The US Tiotropium Study Group. Chest. 2000; 118(5):1294–302.
60. Tashkin D, Kesten S. Long-term treatment benefits with tiotropium in COPD patients with and without short-term bronchodilator responses. Chest. 2003;123(5):1441–9.
61. Vogelmeier C, Banerji D. NVA237, a long-acting muscarinic antagonist, as an emerging therapy for chronic obstructive pulmonary disease. Ther Adv Respir Dis. 2011;5(3):163–73. Epub 2011 Apr 20.
62. Leonard B, Richelson H. Synaptic effects of antidepressants: relationship to their therapeutic and adverse effects. In: Buckley P, Waddington JL, editors. Schizophrenia and mood disorders: the new drug therapies in clinical practice. Oxford: Butterworth- Heinemann; 2000.
63. Trindade E, et al. Use of granulocyte macrophage colony stimulating factor in children after orthotopic liver transplantation. J Hepatol. 1998;28(6):1054–7.
64. Bertram U, et al. Saliva secretion following long-term antidepressant treatment with nortriptyline controlled by plasma levels. Scand J Dent Res. 1979;87(1):58–64.

65. von Knorring L, Mornstad H. Qualitative changes in saliva composition after short-term administration of imipramine and zimelidine in healthy volunteers. Scand J Dent Res. 1981;89(4):313–20.
66. Hunter KD, Wilson WS. The effects of antidepressant drugs on salivary flow and content of sodium and potassium ions in human parotid saliva. Arch Oral Biol. 1995;40(11):983–9.
67. Bradley RM, Fukami H, Suwabe T. Neurobiology of the gustatory-salivary reflex. Chem Senses. 2005;30:I70–1.
68. Ishizuka KI, et al. Multi-source inputs converge on the superior salivatory nucleus neurons in anaesthetized rats. Auton Neurosci. 2010;156(1–2):104–10.
69. Ueda H, et al. Muscarinic receptor immunoreactivity in the superior salivatory nucleus neurons innervating the salivary glands of the rat. Neurosci Lett. 2011;499(1):42–6.
70. Renzi A, De Luca Jr LA, Menani JV. Lesions of the lateral hypothalamus impair pilocarpine-induced salivation in rats. Brain Res Bull. 2002;58(5):455–9.
71. Takakura AC, et al. Effects of AV3V lesion on pilocarpine-induced pressor response and salivary gland vasodilation. Brain Res. 2005;1055(1–2):111–21.
72. Takakura AC, et al. Activation of alpha(2)-adrenoceptors in the lateral hypothalamus reduces pilocarpine-induced salivation in rats. Neurosci Lett. 2009;450(3):225–8.
73. Moreira TS, et al. Central moxonidine on salivary gland blood flow and cardiovascular responses to pilocarpine. Brain Res. 2003;987(2):155–63.
74. Phillips MA, Szabadi E, Bradshaw CM. Comparison of the effects of clonidine and yohimbine on pupillary diameter at different illumination levels. Br J Clin Pharmacol. 2000;50(1):65–8.
75. Moreira Tdos S, et al. Inhibition of pilocarpine-induced salivation in rats by central noradrenaline. Arch Oral Biol. 2002;47(6):429–34.
76. Gotrick B, Giglio D, Tobin G. Effects of amphetamine on salivary secretion. Eur J Oral Sci. 2009;117(3):218–23.
77. Abdelmawla AH, et al. Comparison of the effects of venlafaxine, desipramine, and paroxetine on noradrenaline- and methoxamine-evoked constriction of the dorsal hand vein. Br J Clin Pharmacol. 1999;48(3):345–54.
78. Hassan SM, Wainscott G, Turner P. A comparison of the effect of paroxetine and amitriptyline on the tyramine pressor response test. Br J Clin Pharmacol. 1985;19(5):705–6.
79. Michna E, et al. Systematic literature review and meta-analysis of the efficacy and safety of prescription opioids, including abuse-deterrent formulations, in non-cancer pain management. Pain Med. 2014;15(1):79–92.
80. Gotrick B, Tobin G. The xerogenic potency and mechanism of action of tramadol inhibition of salivary secretion in rats. Arch Oral Biol. 2004;49(12):969–73.
81. Fox PC, et al. Pilocarpine treatment of salivary gland hypofunction and dry mouth (xerostomia). Arch Intern Med. 1991;151(6):1149–52.
82. Greenspan D, Daniels TE. Effectiveness of pilocarpine in postradiation xerostomia. Cancer. 1987;59(6):1123–5.
83. Gotrick B, et al. Oral pilocarpine for treatment of opioid-induced oral dryness in healthy adults. J Dent Res. 2004;83(5):393–7.
84. Thomson WM, et al. Shortening the xerostomia inventory. Oral Surg Oral Med Oral Pathol Oral Radiol Endod. 2011;112(3):322–7.
85. Wolff A, Zuk-Paz L, Kaplan I. Major salivary gland output differs between users and non-users of specific medication categories. Gerodontology. 2008;25(4):210–6.
86. Furness S, et al. Interventions for the management of dry mouth: topical therapies. Cochrane Database Syst Rev. 2011;12:CD008934.
87. Bots CP, et al. The management of xerostomia in patients on haemodialysis: comparison of artificial saliva and chewing gum. Palliat Med. 2005;19(3):202–7.
88. Davies AN. A comparison of artificial saliva and chewing gum in the management of xerostomia in patients with advanced cancer. Palliat Med. 2000;14(3):197–203.
89. Gomez-Moreno G, Aguilar-Salvatierra A, Guardia J, et al. The efficacy of a topical sialogogue spray containing 1 % malic acid in patients with antidepressant-induced dry mouth: a double-blind, randomized clinical trial. Depress Anxiety. 2013;30(2):137–42.

# Cancer-/Cancer Treatment-Related Salivary Gland Dysfunction

# 4

Andrew N. Davies

**Abstract**

Salivary gland dysfunction (xerostomia, salivary gland hypofunction) is common in patients with cancer and is associated with significant morbidity/impairment of quality of life in this group of patients. This chapter will review the medical literature on the epidemiology, aetiology, clinical features and management of salivary gland dysfunction in patients with cancer.

## Definitions

Xerostomia is defined as "the subjective sensation of dryness of the mouth" [1], whilst salivary gland hypofunction is defined as "any objectively demonstrable reduction in either whole and/or individual gland flow rates" [2]. Salivary gland dysfunction (SGD) has been defined as "any alteration in the qualitative or quantitative output of saliva caused by an increase (hyperfunction) or decrease (hypofunction) in salivary output [3]. However, SGD is more often used as an umbrella term to describe patients with xerostomia and/or salivary gland hypofunction [4].

## Epidemiology

### General Oncology Population

The prevalence of xerostomia is 22–26 % in the general population [5, 6], whereas the prevalence of xerostomia is 54–55 % in mixed oncology populations

A.N. Davies, FRCP
Supportive & Palliative Care Team,
Royal Surrey County Hospital,
Egerton Road, Guildford, Surrey GU2 7XX, UK
e-mail: adavies12@nhs.net



G. Carpenter (ed.), *Dry Mouth: A Clinical Guide on Causes, Effects and Treatments*, DOI 10.1007/978-3-642-55154-3_4

**Table 4.1** Prevalence of xerostomia by type of radiotherapy and time since radiotherapy

| Type of study | During radiotherapy (%) | 1–3 months post radiotherapy (%) | 3–6 months post radiotherapy (%) | 6–12 months post radiotherapy (%) | 1–2 years post radiotherapy (%) | >2 years post radiotherapy (%) |
|---|---|---|---|---|---|---|
| All studies | 93.0 | 73.6 | 79.0 | 82.9 | 77.6 | 85.3 |
| Conventional radiotherapy | 81.4 | 70.9 | 83.2 | 71.5 | 83.8 | 90.9 |
| 3-D conformal radiotherapy | None reported | 46.7 | 74.5 | 90.3 | 75.4 | 69.4 |
| Intensity-modulated radiation therapy | 100 | 89.4 | 72.7 | 90.1 | 66.0 | 68.1 |

Adapted from reference [15]

[7, 8] and 78–82 % in advanced oncology populations [9, 10]. Thus, xerostomia is one of the most common symptoms experienced by all groups of oncology patients [7–10].

Investigators have found a disparity between the recorded prevalence of xerostomia and the true prevalence of xerostomia [11]. It is unclear why there is such a disparity, but this probably reflects both healthcare professional-related factors (e.g. perception that the symptom is unimportant) and patient-related factors (e.g. perception that other symptoms are more important) [12]. It should be noted that the aforementioned figures are based on studies where patients were specifically asked about the presence of xerostomia, rather than studies where patients were expected to spontaneously report the presence of xerostomia.

The prevalence of salivary gland hypofunction has been reported to be 82–83 % in advanced oncology populations [13, 14]. In the study by Davies et al., 82 % of the patients had a low unstimulated whole salivary flow rate (UWSFR), whilst 42 % of the patients had a low stimulated whole salivary flow rate (SWSFR) [14]. There are no analogous studies involving less advanced oncology populations.

## Radiotherapy to the Head and Neck Region

Xerostomia is extremely common in patients that have received radiotherapy to the head and neck region; Table 4.1 shows the weighted prevalence of xerostomia following different types of radiotherapy [15].

## Radioactive Iodine

The prevalence of xerostomia 1–2 years post radioactive iodine has been estimated to be 33.6 % [15].

## Chemotherapy

The prevalence of xerostomia during chemotherapy has been estimated to be 49.9 % [15]. It appears (from the limited literature) that xerostomia is usually an acute complication of chemotherapy, i.e. the xerostomia improves following cessation of the chemotherapy.

## Aetiology

There are numerous causes of SGD in the general population [16], with the most common cause being drug treatment [17]. SGD is a side effect of many drugs [18], including many of the drugs used in day-to-day clinical practice [19]. Similarly, there are numerous causes of SGD in the oncology population (Box 4.1) [9, 20–28],

**Box 4.1 Causes of Salivary Gland Dysfunction in Patients with Cancer**

Related to Cancer

- Tumour infiltration[1]
- Paraneoplastic syndrome[1] [20]

Related to Cancer Treatment

- Surgery[1] [21]
- Radiotherapy
- Radionuclide therapy (e.g. $I^{131}$ therapy) [22]
- Chemotherapy
- Biological therapy (e.g. interleukin-2) [23]
- Graft versus host disease [24]

Additional Causes

- Drug treatment[2] [9]
- Dehydration [25]
- Malnutrition
- Decreased oral intake (e.g. PEG feeding)
- Decreased mastication (e.g. liquid diet) [26]
- Anxiety [27]
- Depression [28]
- Sjögren's syndrome
- Other disorders of salivary glands
- Neurological disorders

[1]Uncommon causes.

[2]Most common cause.

with the most common cause again being drug treatment [9]. SGD is a side effect of many of the drugs used in supportive care/palliative care (e.g. analgesics, anti-emetics) [9]. Drug-induced SGD is discussed in detail in Chap. 3.

### Radiotherapy to the Head and Neck Region

The development of salivary gland dysfunction is related to the cumulative dose of radiotherapy and the volume of salivary gland tissue included in the treatment field [15]. Salivary flow rates decrease during the radiotherapy (with a reduction occurring in the first week of treatment) and then further decrease in the 1–3 months post radiotherapy [15]. Over time, there is some limited improvement in salivary flow rates, and SWSFRs are generally higher than UWSFRs.

Parotid-sparing intensity-modulated radiotherapy (IMRT) can reduce the prevalence/severity of salivary gland dysfunction, but does not prevent the development of xerostomia due to damage to the minor salivary glands and the submandibular glands (which are the major sources of salivary mucin, i.e. intraoral lubrication). IMRT is discussed in detail in Chap. 9. Currently, it is unclear whether concomitant chemotherapy has any effect on the development of salivary gland dysfunction [15].

## Pathophysiology

Xerostomia is usually the result of a decrease in the volume of saliva secreted (i.e. salivary gland hypofunction). Indeed, normal subjects usually complain of a dry mouth when their UWSFR falls by 50 % [29]. However, xerostomia may also result from a change in the composition of the saliva secreted [30]. Indeed, Davies et al. reported that 15 % of advanced cancer patients with xerostomia had a "normal" UWSFR (i.e. $\geq$ 0.1 ml/min) and that 53 % of advanced cancer patients with xerostomia had a "normal" SWSFR (i.e. $\geq$ 0.5 ml/min) [9].

## Clinical Features

The clinical features of SGD are very variable (Table 4.2) [31] and reflect the differing functions of saliva [16]. SGD is associated with a number of oral problems but is also associated with more generalised problems. Indeed, SGD is associated with a significant negative impact on quality of life (Box 4.2) [15, 32].

The clinical features of SGD vary from individual to individual and may vary within an individual over time. Patients with xerostomia may have some or none of the aforementioned clinical features. In addition, the xerostomia may be of varying frequency and varying severity and lead to varying levels of distress (Table 4.3) [9]. Similarly, patients with salivary gland hypofunction may have some or none of the aforementioned clinical features (including xerostomia).

**Table 4.2** Complications of salivary gland dysfunction [31]

| | |
|---|---|
| General problems | Oral discomfort |
| | Lip discomfort |
| | Cracking of lips |
| Eating-related problems | Anorexia |
| | Taste disturbance |
| | Difficulty chewing |
| | Difficulty swallowing |
| | Decreased intake of nutrition |
| Speech-related problems | Difficulty speaking |
| Oral hygiene | Poor oral hygiene |
| | Halitosis |
| Oral infections | Oral candidosis |
| | Dental caries |
| | Periodontal disease |
| | Salivary gland infections |
| Systemic infections | Secondary to oral infection (e.g. pneumonia, septicaemia) |
| Dental/denture problems | Dental erosion (leading to dental sensitivity/trauma to oral mucosa) |
| | Poorly fitting dentures (leading to trauma to oral mucosa) |
| Psychosocial problems | Embarrassment |
| | Anxiety |
| | Depression |
| | Social isolation |
| Miscellaneous problems | Sleep disturbance |
| | Difficulty using oral transmucosal medication (i.e. sublingual/ buccal medication) |
| | Oesophagitis |
| | Urinary frequency (secondary to increased intake of fluid) |

**Box 4.2 Quotations from Cancer Patients with Xerostomia [32]**

"It's so dry and sticky, my mouth glues, sometimes I have difficulties even opening my mouth".

"Eating takes a long time, I stayed there at the table for 30–45 min after everybody else. I had to sip before each swallowing, totally about 1 l of water".

"My voice disappears totally as a consequence of dryness of the mouth, and it is very tiresome to talk".

"We were to celebrate my birthday and I had helped to prepare salmon and looked forward to have dinner with the family. The taste alteration was incredible, the food tasted of absolutely nothing or possibly of wheat flour; I was disappointed and depressed and felt sorry for myself, I couldn't feel or share happiness with my family during that occasion".

"…the problems are there constantly, my illness is there constantly, I am never free".

**Table 4.3** Clinical features of xerostomia in patients with advanced cancer [9]

| Characteristic | Descriptor | Percentage |
|---|---|---|
| Frequency | "Rarely" | 4 |
| | "Occasionally" | 20 |
| | "Frequently | 40 |
| | "Almost constantly" | 36 |
| Severity | "Slight" | 14 |
| | "Moderate" | 37 |
| | "Severe" | 33 |
| | "Very severe" | 16 |
| Distress | "Not at all" | 16 |
| | "A little bit" | 21 |
| | "Somewhat" | 23 |
| | "Quite a bit" | 26 |
| | "Very much" | 14 |

It is important to emphasise that there may be a discrepancy between the symptoms experienced by patients and the signs identified by healthcare professionals. The "classic" signs of salivary gland hypofunction include dryness of the oral mucosa, dryness of the lips, absence of a "pool" of saliva in the floor of the mouth, fissuring of the oral mucosa (especially of the tongue) and cracking of the lips [2]. However, patients with xerostomia, and some patients with salivary gland hypofunction, may have no obvious abnormalities on examination. Hence, a normal oral examination does not preclude a diagnosis of SGD (see below).

## Assessment

A wide range of investigations may be employed in the management of SGD in the general population. Some of these investigations are used to diagnose SGD (e.g. measurement of salivary flow rates), whilst other investigations are used to determine the cause of the SGD (e.g. detection of autoantibodies). However, most of these investigations are not indicated in the assessment of SGD in the cancer population. Indeed, a diagnosis of SGD can invariably be made on the basis of routine clinical skills, i.e. taking a history and performing an examination [2].

Table 4.4 shows the relevant National Cancer Institute Common Terminology Criteria for Adverse Events (CTCAE) relating to cancer treatment [33]. These criteria are widely used in clinical practice/clinical trials and are recommended by organisations such as the Food and Drug Administration (United States of America). However, research suggests that similar observer-completed assessment tools may have poor interobserver reliability, may not correlate with objective measures of SGD and (particularly) may not correlate with subjective measures of SGD [34].

**Table 4.4** National Cancer Institute Common Toxicity Criteria for Adverse Events (CTCAE) version 3

| Adverse event (AE) | Grade 1 – "mild" AE | Grade 2 – "moderate" AE | Grade 3 – "severe" AE | Grade 4 – life-threatening/ life-disabling AE | Grade 5 – death due to AE |
|---|---|---|---|---|---|
| Dry mouth/ salivary gland (xerostomia)<br><br>Short name – dry mouth | Symptomatic (dry or thick saliva) without significant dietary alteration; unstimulated salivary flow >0.2 ml/min | Symptomatic and significant oral intake alteration (e.g. copious water, other lubricants, diet limited to purees and/or soft, moist foods); unstimulated saliva 0.1–0.2 ml/min | Symptoms leading to inability to adequately aliment orally, IV fluids, tube feedings or TPN indicated; unstimulated saliva <0.1 ml/min | – | – |
| Salivary gland changes/saliva<br><br>Short name – salivary gland changes | Slightly thickened saliva; slightly altered taste (e.g. metallic) | Thick ropy, sticky saliva; markedly altered taste; alteration in diet indicated; secretion-induced symptoms not interfering with ADL | Acute salivary gland necrosis; severe secretion-induced symptoms interfering with ADL | Disabling | – |

Adapted from reference [33]

## Management

SGD is a heterogeneous condition and so requires individualised management. The management of SGD depends on a variety of different factors, including the aetiology/pathophysiology of the SGD, the clinical features of the SGD, the general condition of the patient, the dental status of the patient, the treatment preferences of the patient, the availability of specific interventions and the affordability of specific interventions [31]. The management of SGD involves a number of different strategies, including: (a) the prevention of SGD, (b) the treatment of the cause of SGD, (c) the symptomatic treatment of SGD, (d) the prevention of the complications of SGD and (e) the treatment of the complications of SGD [31].

## Prevention of SGD

As discussed above, SGD is extremely common in patients that have received conventional radiotherapy to the head and neck region. A number of strategies have been used to try to prevent radiotherapy-related SGD, including surgical transfer of salivary glands (i.e. submandibular glands) [35], use of novel radiotherapy techniques (e.g. IMRT) and use of radioprotectors (e.g. amifostine) [36]. Recently, the Oral Care Study Group of Multinational Association of Supportive Care in Cancer (MASCC) reviewed the data on these strategies and recommended the use of IMRT but was unable to make recommendations about the surgical transfer of salivary glands or the use of amifostine [37].

## Treatment of the Cause of SGD

Box **4.1** shows the main causes of cancer-related SGD. Some of these causes may be amenable to a specific intervention, although most are not amenable to any intervention. Drug treatment is the most common cause of cancer-related SGD [9]. In theory, it is possible to discontinue or substitute the relevant drugs. However, it is often difficult to discontinue these drugs, since they are needed to manage the underlying cancer or another serious condition. Similarly, it is usually futile to substitute these drugs, since the SGD is a side effect of the class of drug, rather than a side effect of the individual drug [18].

It should be noted that researchers are starting to investigate novel techniques to repair damaged salivary glands, including the utilisation of gene therapy and tissue engineering [38].

## Symptomatic Treatment of SGD

The symptomatic treatment of SGD involves the use of saliva stimulants (agents that promote saliva secretion) and saliva substitutes (agents that replace missing saliva). There are good reasons for prescribing saliva stimulants rather than saliva substitutes [4]. Thus, saliva stimulants increase the secretion of "normal" saliva and so will ameliorate xerostomia and the other clinical features of SGD. In contrast, saliva substitutes, which are very different from normal saliva (i.e. physically, chemically), will usually only ameliorate xerostomia. Moreover, in studies that have compared saliva stimulants with saliva substitutes, patients have generally expressed a preference for the saliva stimulants [39, 40]. Nevertheless, some patients do not respond to treatment with saliva stimulants and so will require treatment with saliva substitutes (e.g. some patients with radiation-induced SGD).

## Saliva Stimulants

- Chewing gum

  Chewing gum increases salivary flow by two mechanisms: ~85 % of the increase is related to stimulation of chemoreceptors within the oral cavity (i.e. taste effect), whilst ~15 % of the increase is related to stimulation of mechanoreceptors in/around the oral cavity (i.e. chewing effect) [41]. Patients with SGD should use "sugar-free" chewing gum, and patients with dental prostheses should use "low-tack" (less sticky) chewing gum.

  Chewing gum has been reported to be effective in the management of xerostomia in various groups of patients, including patients with radiation-induced SGD [40] and advanced cancer patients with drug-induced SGD [42]. Moreover, chewing gum has been reported to be more effective than organic acids and artificial saliva in studies involving mixed groups of patients with SGD [39, 40]. It should be noted that studies involving patients with radiation-induced SGD have produced variable results, with some reporting good results [40] and others less good results [39].

  Chewing gum is generally well tolerated. However, side effects can occur and may be related to: (a) chewing, e.g. jaw discomfort and headache; (b) inappropriate ingestion, e.g. respiratory tract obstruction and gastrointestinal obstruction; (c) non-allergic reactions to additives, e.g. oral discomfort and flatulence; and (d) allergic reactions to additives, e.g. stomatitis and perioral dermatitis. Chewing gum is an acceptable form of treatment for most patients, including most elderly patients [42, 43].
- Organic acids

  Various organic acids have been used as saliva stimulants, including ascorbic acid (vitamin C), citric acid (the acid in citrus fruits) and malic acid (the acid in apples and pears). Organic acids increase salivary flow through stimulation of chemoreceptors within the oral cavity.

  The use of organic acids is associated with the development of oral discomfort [39, 40]. Thus, organic acids should not be used in patients with dry mucosae, cracked mucosae, stomatitis and/or mucositis. Moreover, the use of organic acids may be associated with the exacerbation of certain pH-related complications of SGD (i.e. demineralisation of the teeth, dental caries, oral candidosis) [4, 44]. Thus, organic acids should not be used in patients with teeth and should be used with caution in edentulous patients.

- Parasympathomimetic drugs

  Parasympathomimetic drugs stimulate the part of the autonomic nervous system responsible for the secretion of saliva from the salivary glands. The parasympathomimetic drugs include choline esters (e.g. pilocarpine, cevimeline) that have a direct effect and cholinesterase inhibitors (e.g. distigmine, pyridostigmine) that that have an indirect effect by inhibiting the metabolism of endogenous acetylcholine.

  Pilocarpine has been reported to be effective in the management of SGD due to salivary gland disease (e.g. Sjögren's syndrome), drug treatment (in cancer patients) [45], radiotherapy [46, 47] and graft versus host disease [48, 49]. Indeed, it has been reported to be more effective than artificial saliva in the management of SGD secondary to drug treatment [45] and radiotherapy [50].

  A recent Cochrane systematic review investigated the role of parasympathomimetic drugs in the management of radiation-induced SGD [51]. The reviewers concluded that "there is limited evidence to support the use of pilocarpine hydrochloride in the treatment of radiation-induced salivary gland dysfunction" and that "currently, there is little evidence to support the use of other parasympathomimetic drugs in the treatment of this condition".

  The systematic review found that 49–52 % patients respond to pilocarpine [46, 47]. However, the response rate in the included studies may not reflect the response rates in the general population. Thus, one of the inclusion criteria for the two main included studies was "some evidence of residual salivary function" [46, 47], which is clearly not a universal finding in patients with radiation-induced SGD. It is reasonable to suppose that patients with evidence of salivary gland functioning would be more likely to respond to pilocarpine, since such findings confirm that the salivary glands are still functioning to an extent and so still capable of responding to a stimulant.

  Overall, the response rates were similar for patients taking the standard (5 mg tds) and the higher dose (10 mg tds) in the main fixed-dose study [46]. Nevertheless, some patients only appeared to respond to the higher doses (10 mg tds) in the main dose-titration study [47]. There are two possible explanations for the latter finding: (a) some patients improved because of the increase in dose; or (b) some patients improved because of the increase in time on the drug, i.e. some patients had a delayed response to the drug. It is difficult to determine the importance of these two factors, although it is clear from the data that some patients do have a delayed response to the drug, i.e. up to 12 weeks [46].

  The systematic review also found that many patients develop side effects. The side effects are usually related to generalised parasympathetic stimulation and include sweating, headache, urinary frequency and vasodilatation. The incidence of side effects is dose related, i.e. the higher the dose of pilocarpine, the higher the incidence of side effects. However, the systematic review found that few (6 %) patients discontinue pilocarpine due to side effects at the standard dose of 5 mg tds [46].

  The other choline esters that have been used in clinical practice include bethanechol, carbacholine and cevimeline. Bethanechol has been reported to be effective in the management of drug-induced SGD [52] and of radiotherapy-induced SGD [53, 54]. Similarly, cevimeline has been reported to be effective in the management of Sjögren's syndrome, radiotherapy-induced SGD [55, 56] and graft versus host disease [57].

- Acupuncture

  Acupuncture has been reported to be useful in the management of SGD secondary to benign salivary gland disease, drug treatment (in cancer patients) [58] and radiotherapy [59, 60]. In addition, a recent study has reported that acupuncture given during radiotherapy may ameliorate the development of radiation-induced SGD [61].

  Investigators have reported the use of diverse acupuncture points (number/type of points) and diverse treatment schedules (number/duration of treatments). The effect of acupuncture often increases during a course of treatment [58] and often continues for some time after the end of the course of treatment [59]. Moreover, the effect of acupuncture may be maintained by single treatments given on an as-required basis (e.g. 1–2 monthly) [62]. The mechanism of action of acupuncture has yet to be elucidated, although increases in relevant neuropeptide secretion and intraoral blood flow have been reported [58].

  Acupuncture is generally well tolerated, although it can cause local haemorrhage and also local/systemic infection. Hence, acupuncture should be used with caution in patients with bleeding diatheses and in patients that are immunocompromised. Some patients report feeling tired after treatment [59], whilst other patients report coincidental health-related benefits from the treatment [59].

## Saliva Substitutes

- Water

  Patients often use water to treat dryness of the mouth. However, in studies, patients have reported that water is less effective than "artificial saliva" [63, 64]. Moreover, in one study, patients reported that the mean duration of improvement of dryness of the mouth was only 12 min (range 4–29 min) [65].

  In spite of the above, many patients choose to use water rather than other saliva substitutes [66]. The reasons for this phenomenon include familiarity, efficacy (moderate), tolerability, availability and affordability [66]. The use of water is not associated with side effects per se, although polydipsia is inevitably associated with polyuria (and nocturia) [4].

- "Artificial saliva"

  It is common practice for healthcare professionals to prescribe "artificial saliva" for the treatment of SGD. A number of commercial products have been developed, which differ in formulation (e.g. spray, gel, lozenge), lubricant (e.g. carboxymethylcellulose, hydroxyethylcellulose, mucin) and additives (e.g. flavourings, fluoride, antimicrobial factors). It should be noted that most of these commercial products have not been formally tested in cancer patients with SGD or indeed in any group of patients with SGD.

The "ideal" artificial saliva should be easy to use, pleasant to use, effective and well tolerated [66]. Moreover, it should have a neutral pH (to prevent demineralisation of the teeth) and contain fluoride (to enhance remineralisation of the teeth). Unfortunately, some commercial products have an acidic pH, and these should definitely not be prescribed in dentate patients and should probably not be prescribed in any patient with SGD.

A commercial mucin-based spray (Saliva Orthana®) has been reported to be relatively effective/well tolerated in patients with radiation-induced SGD [67, 68] and in cancer patients with drug-induced SGD [42, 45]. Indeed, Saliva Orthana® was reported to be more effective/better tolerated than a carboxymethylcellulose-based artificial saliva in patients with radiation-induced SGD [67, 68]. However, the duration of effect of the Saliva Orthana® was only ~30 min, which necessitated repeated use of the product during the day and night [67]. (The duration of effect of the carboxymethylcellulose-based artificial saliva was ~10 min [67].)

Similarly, two commercial hydroxyethylcellulose-based gels containing lactoperoxidase, lysozyme and lactoferrin (Oral Balance®, bioXtra®) have been reported to be relatively effective/well tolerated in patients with radiation-induced SGD [69, 70]. Indeed, the Oral Balance® gel and associated toothpaste were reported to be more effective/better tolerated than a carboxymethylcellulose-based artificial saliva and conventional toothpaste in patients with radiation-induced SGD [69]. It should be noted that there is little evidence that the presence of antimicrobial factors in these products actually prevents/ameliorates the infectious complications of SGD (Table 4.2) [71]. Other products that have shown promise in patients with radiation-induced SGD include one based on linseed extract (Salinum®) [72] and another one based on hydroxyethylcellulose with citric acid (Optimoist®) [73].

Artificial saliva is generally well tolerated, although some patients report local problems (e.g. oral irritation, taste disturbance), whilst some patients even report systemic problems (e.g. nausea, diarrhoea) [45, 66]. The duration of effect of artificial saliva is invariably short, which necessitates the repeated use of these products during the day and night. Indeed, the short duration of effect is one of the main reasons why patients do not continue to use artificial saliva.

## Prevention of the Complications of SGD

The main complications of SGD are shown in Table 4.2. Adequate management of SGD may prevent the development of these complications. Nevertheless, the following preventative strategies should be considered in all patients with SGD:

1. Maintenance of oral hygiene – dentate patients need to clean their teeth at least twice a day, and edentulous patients need to clean their dentures at least once a day and to remove their dentures at night-time [74].

2. Use of fluoridated toothpaste – all dentate patients should use a toothpaste with at least 1,000 ppm fluoride, whilst dentate patients with radiation-induced SGD should use a specialist toothpaste with 5,000 ppm fluoride.
3. Avoidance of acidic drinks/foods/medication – acidic products will contribute to complications such as dental erosion, dental caries and oral candidosis.
4. Avoidance of sugar-sweetened drinks/foods/medication – sugar-sweetened products will contribute to complications such as dental caries and oral candidosis.
5. Avoidance of xerostomic medication – it should be noted that some oral care products contain alcohol, which may further aggravate the situation.
6. Regular dental review – patients should have regular dental reviews (with a dentist/dental hygienist).

## References


1. Edgar WM, O'Mullane DM, editors. Saliva and oral health. 2nd ed. London: British Dental Association; 1996.
2. Navazesh M, Christensen C, Brightman V. Clinical criteria for the diagnosis of salivary gland hypofunction. J Dent Res. 1992;71:1363–9.
3. Millard HD, Mason DK, editors. Perspectives on the 3rd world workshop on oral medicine. Ann Arbor: University of Michigan; 2000.
4. Davies A. Salivary gland dysfunction. In: Davies A, Finlay I, editors. Oral care in advanced disease. Oxford: Oxford University Press; 2005. p. 97–113.
5. Billings RJ, Proskin HM, Moss ME. Xerostomia and associated factors in a community-dwelling adult population. Community Dent Oral Epidemiol. 1996;24:312–6.
6. Nederfors T, Isaksson R, Mornstad H, Dahlof C. Prevalence of perceived symptoms of dry mouth in an adult Swedish population – relation to age, sex and pharmacotherapy. Community Dent Oral Epidemiol. 1997;25:211–6.
7. Portenoy RK, Thaler HT, Kornblith AB, McCarthy Lepore JM, Friedlander-Klar H, et al. Symptom prevalence, characteristics and distress in a cancer population. Qual Life Res. 1994;3:183–9.
8. Chang VT, Hwang SS, Feuerman M, Kasimis BS, Thaler HT. The Memorial Symptom Assessment Scale Short Form (MSAS-SF). Cancer. 2000;89:1162–71.
9. Davies AN, Broadley K, Beighton D. Xerostomia in patients with advanced cancer. J Pain Symptom Manag. 2001;22:820–5.
10. Tranmer JE, Heyland D, Dudgeon D, Groll D, Squires-Graham M, Coulson K. Measuring the symptom experience of seriously ill cancer and noncancer hospitalized patients near the end of life with the Memorial Symptom Assessment Scale. J Pain Symptom Manag. 2003;25:420–9.
11. Shah S, Davies AN. Medical records vs. patient self-rating. J Pain Symptom Manag. 2001;22:805–6.
12. Shorthose K, Davies A. Symptom prevalence in palliative care. Palliat Med. 2003;17:723–4.
13. Chaushu G, Bercovici M, Dori S, Waller A, Taicher S, Kronenberg J, et al. Salivary flow and its relation with oral symptoms in terminally ill patients. Cancer. 2000;88:984–7.
14. Davies AN, Broadley K, Beighton D. Salivary gland hypofunction in patients with advanced cancer. Oral Oncol. 2002;38:680–5.
15. Jensen SB, Pedersen AM, Vissink A, Andersen E, Brown CG, Davies AN, et al. A systematic review of salivary gland hypofunction and xerostomia induced by cancer therapies: prevalence, severity and impact on quality of life. Support Care Cancer. 2010;18:1039–60.

16. Anonymous. Saliva: its role in health and disease. FDI Working Group 10 of the Commission on Oral Health, Research and Epidemiology (CORE). Int Dent J. 1992;42(4 Suppl 2): 291–304.
17. Sreebny LM, Valdini A, Yu A. Xerostomia. part II: relationship to nonoral symptoms, drugs, and diseases. Oral Surg Oral Med Oral Pathol. 1989;68:419–27.
18. Sreebny LM, Schwartz SS. A reference guide to drugs and dry mouth – 2nd edition. Gerodontology. 1997;14:33–47.
19. Smith RG, Burtner AP. Oral side-effects of the most frequently prescribed drugs. Spec Care Dentist. 1994;14:96–102.
20. Folli F, Ponzoni M, Vicari AM. Paraneoplastic autoimmune xerostomia. Ann Intern Med. 1997;127:167–8.
21. Schubert MM, Izutsu KT. Iatrogenic causes of salivary gland dysfunction. J Dent Res. 1987;66(Spec Iss):680–8.
22. Solans R, Bosch JA, Galofre P, Porta F, Rosello J, Seva-O'Callagan A, et al. Salivary and lacrimal gland dysfunction (sicca syndrome) after radioiodine therapy. J Nucl Med. 2001; 42:738–43.
23. Nagler RM, Gez E, Rubinov R, Laufer D, Ben-Aryeh H, Gaitini D, et al. The effect of low-dose interleukin-2-based immunotherapy on salivary function and composition in patients with metastatic renal cell carcinoma. Arch Oral Biol. 2001;46:487–93.
24. Nagler R, Marmary Y, Krausz Y, Chisin R, Markitziu A, Nagler A. Major salivary gland dysfunction in human acute and chronic graft-versus-host disease (GVHD). Bone Marrow Transplant. 1996;17:219–24.
25. Gregersen MI, Bullock LT. Observations on thirst in man in relation to changes in salivary flow and plasma volume. Am J Physiol. 1933;105:39–40.
26. Johansson I, Ericson T. Effects of a 900-kcal liquid or solid diet on saliva flow rate and composition in female subjects. Caries Res. 1989;23:184–9.
27. Bergdahl M, Bergdahl J. Low unstimulated salivary flow and subjective oral dryness: association with medication, anxiety, depression, and stress. J Dent Res. 2000;79:1652–8.
28. Antilla SS, Knuuttila ML, Sakki TK. Depressive symptoms as an underlying factor of the sensation of dry mouth. Psychosom Med. 1998;60:215–8.
29. Dawes C. Physiological factors affecting salivary flow rate, oral sugar clearance, and the sensation of dry mouth in man. J Dent Res. 1987;66(Spec):648–53.
30. Pankhurst CL, Smith EC, Rogers JO, Dunne SM, Jackson SHD, Proctor G. Diagnosis and management of the dry mouth: part 1. Dent Update. 1996;23:56–62.
31. Davies A. Salivary gland dysfunction. In: Davies AN, Epstein JB, editors. Oral complications of cancer and its management. Oxford: Oxford University Press; 2010. p. 203–23.
32. Rydholm M, Strang P. Physical and psychosocial impact of xerostomia in palliative cancer care: a qualitative interview study. Int J Palliat Nurs. 2002;8:318–23.
33. National Cancer Institute Common Terminology Criteria for Adverse Events (CTCAE). Available from National Cancer Institute (US National Institutes of Health) website: http://www.cancer.gov/.
34. Meirovitz A, Murdoch-Kinch CA, Schipper M, Pan C, Eisbruch A. Grading xerostomia by physicians or by patients after intensity-modulated radiotherapy of head-and-neck cancer. Int J Radiat Oncol Biol Phys. 2006;66:445–53.
35. Jha N, Seikaly H, Harris J, Williams D, Liu R, McGaw T, et al. Prevention of radiation induced xerostomia by surgical transfer of submandibular salivary gland into the submental space. Radiother Oncol. 2003;66:283–9.
36. Sasse AD, Clark LG, Sasse EC, Clark OA. Amifostine reduces side effects and improves complete response rate during radiotherapy: results of a meta-analysis. Int J Radiat Oncol Biol Phys. 2006;64:784–91.
37. Jensen SB, Pedersen AM, Vissink A, Andersen E, Brown CG, Davies AN, et al. A systematic review of salivary gland hypofunction and xerostomia induced by cancer therapies: management strategies and economic impact. Support Care Cancer. 2010;18:1061–79.

38. Atkinson JC, Baum BJ. Salivary enhancement: current status and future therapies. J Dent Educ. 2001;65:1096–101.
39. Bjornstrom M, Axell T, Birkhed D. Comparison between saliva stimulants and saliva substitutes in patients with symptoms related to dry mouth. A multi-centre study. Swed Dent J. 1990;14:153–61.
40. Stewart CM, Jones AC, Bates RE, Sandow P, Pink F, Stillwell J. Comparison between saliva stimulants and a saliva substitute in patients with xerostomia and hyposalivation. Spec Care Dentist. 1998;18:142–8.
41. Abelson DC, Barton J, Mandel ID. Effect of sorbitol sweetened breath mints on salivary flow and plaque pH in xerostomic subjects. J Clin Dent. 1989;1:102–5.
42. Davies AN. A comparison of artificial saliva and chewing gum in the management of xerostomia in patients with advanced cancer. Palliat Med. 2000;14:197–203.
43. Aagaard A, Godiksen S, Teglers PT, Schiodt M, Glenert U. Comparison between new saliva stimulants in patients with dry mouth: a placebo-controlled double-blind crossover study. J Oral Pathol Med. 1992;21:376–80.
44. Newbrun E. Xerostomia. Oral Surg Oral Med Oral Pathol. 1981;52:262.
45. Davies AN, Daniels C, Pugh R, Sharma K. A comparison of artificial saliva and pilocarpine in the management of xerostomia in patients with advanced cancer. Palliat Med. 1998; 12:105–11.
46. Johnson JT, Ferretti GA, Nethery WJ, Valdez IH, Fox PC, Ng D, et al. Oral pilocarpine for post-irradiation xerostomia in patients with head and neck cancer. N Engl J Med. 1993;329:390–5.
47. LeVeque FG, Montgomery M, Potter D, Zimmer MB, Rieke JW, Steiger BW, et al. A multicentre, randomized, double-blind, placebo-controlled, dose-titration study of oral pilocarpine for treatment of radiation-induced xerostomia in head and neck cancer patients. J Clin Oncol. 1993;11:1124–31.
48. Singhal S, Mehta J, Rattenbury H, Treleaven J, Powles R. Oral pilocarpine hydrochloride for the treatment of refractory xerostomia associated with chronic graft-versus-host disease. Blood. 1995;85:1147–8.
49. Nagler RM, Nagler A. Pilocarpine hydrochloride relieves xerostomia in chronic graft-versus-host disease: a sialometrical study. Bone Marrow Transplant. 1999;23:1007–11.
50. Davies AN, Singer J. A comparison of artificial saliva and pilocarpine in radiation-induced xerostomia. J Laryngol Otol. 1994;108:663–5.
51. Davies AN, Shorthose K. Parasympathomimetic drugs for the treatment of salivary gland dysfunction due to radiotherapy. Cochrane Database Syst Rev. 2007;(3):CD003782.
52. Everett HC. The use of bethanechol chloride with tricyclic antidepressants. Am J Psychiatry. 1975;132:1202–4.
53. Epstein JB, Burchell JL, Emerton S, Le ND, Silverman Jr S. A clinical trial of bethanechol in patients with xerostomia after radiation therapy. A pilot study. Oral Surg Oral Med Oral Pathol. 1994;77:610–4.
54. Gorsky M, Epstein JB, Parry J, Epstein MS, Le ND, Silverman Jr S. The efficacy of pilocarpine and bethanechol upon saliva production in cancer patients with hyposalivation following radiation therapy. Oral Surg Oral Med Oral Pathol Oral Radiol Endod. 2004;97:190–5.
55. Chambers MS, Posner M, Jones CU, Biel MA, Hodge KM, Vitti R, et al. Cevimeline for the treatment of postirradiation xerostomia in patients with head and neck cancer. Int J Radiat Oncol Biol Phys. 2007;68:1102–9.
56. Witsell DL, Stinnett S, Chambers MS. Effectiveness of cevimeline to improve oral health in patients with postradiation xerostomia. Head Neck. 2012;34:1136–42.
57. Carpenter PA, Schubert MM, Flowers ME. Cevimeline reduced mouth dryness and increased salivary flow in patients with xerostomia complicating chronic graft-versus-host disease. Biol Blood Marrow Transplant. 2006;12:792–4.
58. Rydholm M, Strang P. Acupuncture for patients in hospital-based home care suffering from xerostomia. J Palliat Care. 1999;15:20–3.

59. Blom M, Dawidson I, Fernberg JO, Johnson G, Angmar-Mansson B. Acupuncture treatment of patients with radiation-induced xerostomia. Eur J Cancer B Oral Oncol. 1996;32B: 182–90.
60. Simcock R, Fallowfield L, Monson K, Solis-Trapala I, Parlour L, Langridge C, et al. ARIX: a randomised trial of acupuncture v oral care sessions in patients with chronic xerostomia following treatment of head and neck cancer. Ann Oncol. 2013;24:776–83.
61. Meng Z, Garcia MK, Hu C, Chiang J, Chambers M, Rosenthal DI, et al. Randomized controlled trial of acupuncture for prevention of radiation-induced xerostomia among patients with nasopharyngeal carcinoma. Cancer. 2012;118:3337–44.
62. Johnstone PA, Niemtzow RC, Riffenburgh RH. Acupuncture for xerostomia: clinical update. Cancer. 2002;94:1151–6.
63. Duxbury AJ, Thakker NS, Wastell DG. A double-blind cross-over trial of a mucin-containing artificial saliva. Br Dent J. 1989;166:115–20.
64. Wiesenfeld D, Stewart AM, Mason DK. A critical assessment of oral lubricants in patients with xerostomia. Br Dent J. 1983;155:155–7.
65. Olsson H, Axell T. Objective and subjective efficacy of saliva substitutes containing mucin and carboxymethylcellulose. Scand J Dent Res. 1991;99:316–9.
66. Epstein JB, Stevenson-Moore P. A clinical comparative trial of saliva substitutes in radiation-induced salivary gland hypofunction. Spec Care Dentist. 1992;12:21–3.
67. Vissink A, 's-Gravenmade EJ, Panders AK, Vermey A, Petersen JK, Visch LL, et al. A clinical comparison between commercially available mucin- and CMC-containing saliva substitutes. Int J Oral Surg. 1983;12:232–8.
68. Visch LL, 's-Gravenmade EJ, Schaub RM, Van Putten WL, Vissink A. A double-blind crossover trial of CMC- and mucin-containing saliva substitutes. Int J Oral Maxillofac Surg. 1986;15:395–400.
69. Epstein JB, Emerton S, Le ND, Stevenson-Moore P. A double-blind crossover trial of Oral Balance gel and Biotene toothpaste versus placebo in patients with xerostomia following radiation therapy. Oral Oncol. 1999;35:132–7.
70. Shahdad SA, Taylor C, Barclay SC, Steen IN, Preshaw PM. A double-blind, crossover study of Biotene Oralbalance and BioXtra systems as salivary substitutes in patients with post-radiotherapy xerostomia. Eur J Cancer Care. 2005;14:319–26.
71. Tenovuo J. Clinical applications of antimicrobial host proteins lactoperoxidase, lysozyme and lactoferrin in xerostomia: efficacy and safety. Oral Dis. 2002;8:23–9.
72. Andersson G, Johansson G, Attstrom R, Edwardsson S, Glantz PO, Larsson K. Comparison of the effect of the linseed extract Salinum and a methyl cellulose preparation on the symptoms of dry mouth. Gerodontology. 1995;12:12–7.
73. Rhodus NL, Bereuter J. Clinical evaluation of a commercially available oral moisturizer in relieving signs and symptoms of xerostomia in postirradiation head and neck cancer patients and patients with Sjogren's syndrome. J Otolaryngol. 2000;29:28–34.
74. Sweeney P. Oral hygiene. In: Davies A, Finlay I, editors. Oral care in advanced disease. Oxford: Oxford University Press; 2005. p. 21–35.

# Part III

# Effects

# Oral Dryness, Dietary Intake, and Alterations in Taste

# 5

Anja Weirsøe Dynesen

**Abstract**

Xerostomia and decreased salivary secretion may give rise to a number of oral complications. These include dry, atrophic and tender oral mucosa; impaired mastication, food bolus formation, and swallowing; altered sensation of taste; as well as increased risk of developing dental caries and erosion that could be followed by tooth loss. These are all complications that theoretically may have a negative impact on dietary intake. Although the literature does not present a direct association between decreased salivary secretion and malnutrition, it is concluded that salivary gland dysfunction may add to the conditions that make it difficult to maintain an adequate dietary intake in some individuals. Also, the opposite can occur. Thus, persons with an inadequate dietary intake may present with xerostomia and decreased salivary secretion. Therefore, clinical recommendations for counseling of dry mouth patients should draw attention to the impact of an unbalanced diet on salivary secretion and emphasize that oral dryness may have a negative impact on food consumption.

Impaired salivary secretion is most often associated with the subjective feeling of dry mouth (xerostomia). The etiology of decreased salivary secretion is diverse. Some of the most common causes are intake of xerogenic medications or polypharmacy, a number of diseases (e.g. Sjögren's syndrome, mental depression, diabetes mellitus (not regulated), and hyper- and hypothyroidism), chemotherapy, and radiotherapy to the head and neck region. Accordingly, the prevalence of oral dryness increases with age. Thus, it is estimated that 30 % of the population aged 65 years and above is suffering from oral

A.W. Dynesen, DDS, MSc. Human Nutrition, PhD
Department of Odontology, Faculty of Health and Medical Sciences,
University of Copenhagen, Nørre Allé 20, Copenhagen, DK-2200 N, Denmark
e-mail: awd@sund.ku.dk



G. Carpenter (ed.), *Dry Mouth: A Clinical Guide on Causes, Effects and Treatments*, DOI 10.1007/978-3-642-55154-3_5

dryness of some degree, while on an overall population base, it is assumed that at least 10 % of all adults live with the sensation of dry mouth [1].

Saliva secretion plays a major role in maintaining a healthy oral cavity and in oral functioning. Thus, decreased salivary secretion increases the risk of dental caries and erosion and oral mucosal infections. Also, functions such as perception of taste, chewing, food bolus making, swallowing, and initial digestion are highly dependent on a sufficient salivary secretion. Since both the health condition of the oral cavity and oral functioning are essential for the intake of food, the condition of decreased salivary secretion and its oral consequences may potentially have an influence on what people are able to eat and enjoy eating. The following chapter will focus on the complex relationship between salivary gland dysfunction/oral dryness and dietary intake.

## The Relation between Salivary Secretion and Dietary Intake and Nutritional Status

The functions of saliva that play a role toward the intake of food are several but can be divided into three superior categories. The first category is related to *oral pain and discomfort*: Thus, oral health and comfort is essential for the pleasure of eating; therefore, in cases where persons present with dry, atrophic, and tender oral mucosa due to a decreased salivary secretion, oral discomfort, and pain may have a negative influence on dietary intake. The second category is related to a *challenged chewing and swallowing process*: Thus, saliva is important in the chewing process, since saliva binds food fragments together and a food bolus is formed, which is eventually swallowed. Lack or decreased amount of saliva would very likely challenge this procedure and therefore possibly influence the dietary intake. The third category concerns *altered taste*: Thus, saliva serves as a transport media for taste substances and holds a number of digestive and other enzymes that are involved in taste perception. Therefore, decreased salivary secretion may lead to altered or impaired perception of taste, which could also have an impact on food intake. The possible consequences of oral dryness and interrelations between the different parameters are illustrated in Fig. 5.1.

Although, theoretically several conditions related to oral dryness potentially could impair dietary intake, the literature evaluating the relationship between xerostomia or decreased salivary secretion and dietary intake/nutritional status is sparse and, in addition, mostly concerns elderly populations.

The overall association between salivary flow rate and xerostomia and various nutritional parameters has been studied by the use of malnutrition screening tools like the Mini-Nutritional Assessment Index [2] and the subjective global assessment (SGA) [3] or other anthropometric measurements like body mass index (BMI), triceps skinfold thickness, and mid-arm circumference [4]. These tools are used to identify the state of nutrition and categorize subjects as being well nourished, at risk of malnutrition, or actually malnourished. Thus, studies have shown that xerostomia is significantly more prevalent in subjects at risk of malnutrition and malnourished subjects [5–8]. However, when measuring the actual salivary flow rate, results contradict. Thus, a study measuring both stimulated and unstimulated whole saliva flow rates in a group of Finnish community-dwelling elderly found no

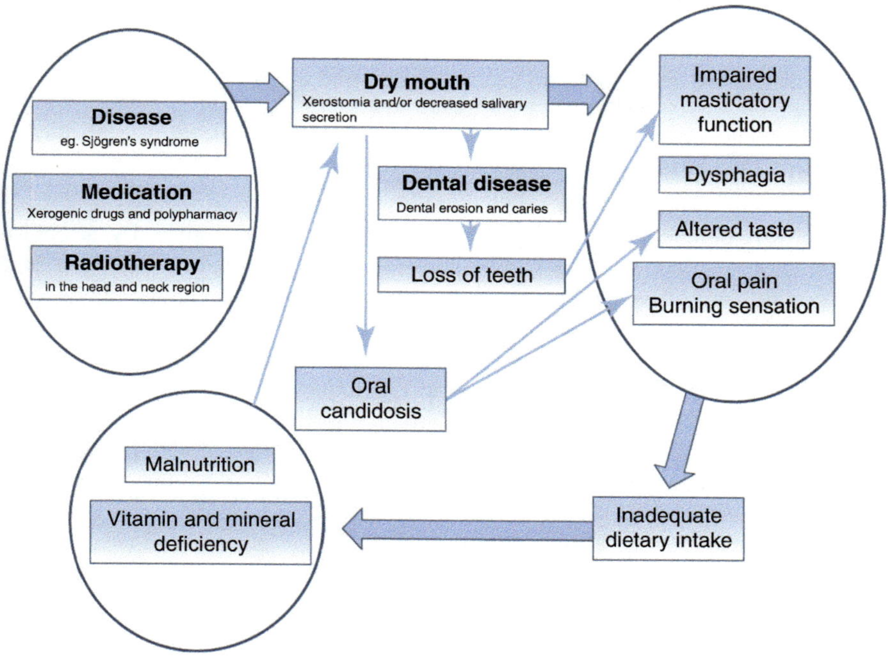


**Fig. 5.1** Dry mouth and dietary intake. The figure illustrates by arrows possible interactions between dry mouth and dietary intake

association between low unstimulated and stimulated whole saliva flow rates and risk of malnutrition [9], while others report that low stimulated whole saliva flow rates (<0.7 ml/min) are associated with nutritional deficit in older noninstitutionalized people [10] and that persons with hyposalivation (defined as unstimulated whole saliva flow rates <0.1 ml/min and stimulated whole saliva flow rates <0.5 ml/min) present with lower nutritional scores than person with a normal salivary secretion [11]. Concerning the actual dietary intake, the impact of oral dryness has also been studied. Thus, xerostomia in older adults has been associated with inadequate intakes of fiber, potassium, vitamin B6, iron, calcium, and zinc [12], and in patients with Sjögren's syndrome, the intake of protein, dietary fibers, potassium vitamin A, vitamin C, thiamin, riboflavin, vitamin B6, calcium, iron, and zinc was significantly lower compared with a healthy control group [13]. However, when investigating elderly without xerostomia, comparable deficiencies may be present indicating that elderly generally may be at risk of malnutrition due to other causes than xerostomia and decreased salivary secretion [12]. A study measuring the dietary intake by the healthy eating index (HEI-2005) [14, 15] showed that those with xerostomia were significantly more likely to meet recommendations for total fruit intake (which includes fruit juices) and significantly less likely to meet recommendations for whole-grain products. Additionally, modification of foods has been shown to be more prevalent in the persons with the most severe xerostomia [16]. In a British study including food data based on a list of 16 food items varying from considered easy to difficult to eat, the dietary intake of dentate participants with perceived oral dryness did not seem to be affected, while the edentate participants reported more difficulty to eat the food items that required more chewing [17]. Thus, in general the picture relating dietary intake and salivary secretion is blurred.

## Oral Pain and Discomfort

If the salivary deficiency is pronounced, the oral mucosa can appear dry, atrophic, and sometimes inflamed. Major complaints from patients with xerostomia and decreased salivary secretion are a burning sensation, pain and dryness of the mouth, cracking of lips and commissures, and fissuring of the tongue. Additionally, the xerostomic condition is often accompanied by opportunistic microbial infections such as oral candidiasis [18]. Not surprisingly, pain in the mouth due to xerostomia has been associated with malnutrition in a group of institutionalized elderly [8], and in a group of head and neck cancer patients who had been treated with radiotherapy, mucosal sensitivity has been associated with reduced oral energy and protein intake [19].

## Challenged Chewing and Swallowing Process

Oral health and comfort is necessary for good masticatory function. Thus, saliva is important in the chewing process, since saliva lubricates food and binds food fragments together in a food bolus which is eventually swallowed. When suffering from decreased salivary secretion, chewing comfort will be diminished, and food will tend to stick to the oral mucosa rather than forming a bolus. Additionally, the swallowing process will be challenged when the lubricating effect of saliva is missing. Accordingly, it has been reported that elderly individuals with xerostomia had difficulty in chewing and swallowing and were significantly more likely to avoid crunchy foods such as carrots and sticky foods such as peanut butter as compared with individuals without xerostomia [20]. These findings are supported in a study investigating mastication, which showed that persons with decreased stimulated parotid saliva flow required twice as many chewing cycles before initial swallowing of two almonds of standardized size as compared with controls with normal salivary flow rate. These dry mouth patients also indicated that their food preferences changed after developing xerostomia. Thus, they reported to cut food into smaller portions and to avoid certain foods such as certain dry breads and foods difficult to chew like carrots [21]. Also, perception of low salivary flow has been associated with poor self-assessed chewing ability [22].

While decreased salivary secretion apparently has some direct impact on chewing ability and dietary intake, one could argue that there is an indirect relation as well. That is because decreased salivary secretion increases the risk of caries [23], which could be followed by loss of teeth, as seen in irradiated head and neck cancer patients [24]. Accordingly, mastication could be impaired, and decreased salivary secretion may therefore indirectly affect dietary intake [25].

To conclude on the association between salivary secretion and dietary intake, it is generally difficult to make unquestionable statements about the impact of salivary gland dysfunction on dietary intake on the basis of the present literature. Depending on the subjects included, which vary between elderly community-dwelling, hospitalized, healthy, and diseased individuals and the methods used for estimating the state of malnutrition or dietary intake, results describe different conditions and situations. However, although the picture is unclear, it is likely that decreased salivary secretion and xerostomia, which could lead to challenged chewing and swallowing, burning, as well as tender oral mucosa, may have a negative impact on dietary intake and nutritional status in some individuals.

## Dry Mouth and Sensation of Taste

Saliva contributes to the perception of taste in various ways. Firstly, on the short term, saliva dilutes, digests, or chemically reacts with food stuffs and further transports taste substances to the taste buds and receptors. Secondly, saliva takes part in the long-term maintenance and protection of the taste receptors [26]. Accordingly, decreased salivary secretion and dry mouth may in different ways have an impact on the perception of taste.

The oral taste buds that hold the taste receptor cells are distributed mainly in the oral mucosa although taste buds are also scattered throughout the larynx, pharynx, and epiglottis. In the oral cavity taste buds are primarily situated on the tongue in the foliate and circumvallate papillae but also in the fungiform papillae (Fig. 5.2) and the mucosa of the soft palate. When food is entering the oral cavity, saliva either

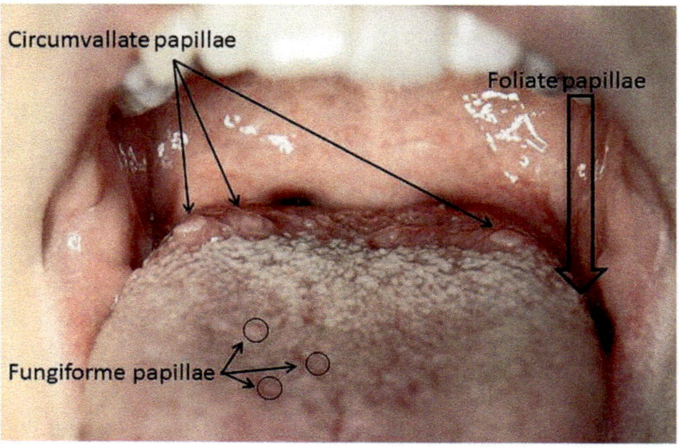


**Fig 5.2** A tongue. The papillae that hold taste buds are marked. Around 10–12 circumvallate papillae are located distally on the dorsum of tongue. The fungiform papillae are scattered on the anterior part of the tongue dorsum, while the foliate papillae cannot be seen directly on this picture, since these papillae are situated on the lateral border of the posterior part of tongue. The *wide arrow* marks the approximate location

dilutes, digests, or chemically reacts with food substances and further helps to transport molecules perceived as taste to the taste receptors. Taste sensation is classified into five modalities: sour, sweet, bitter, salt, and umami [27]. Sour taste is primarily caused by acids [28], while a typical sweet stimulus is that of sucrose although other sugars and proteins can also bring about the taste of sweet [29]. The taste of salt classically involves NaCl [30], while bitter taste that is the most sensitive of all taste qualities is caused by both naturally and synthetic compounds, e.g., caffeine, quinine, and strychnine [29].

## Effects of Saliva on Taste Substances

The strongest salivary stimulus is induced by the sour taste modality. It is well known that increased salivary flow rate is associated with a higher bicarbonate concentration and accordingly a higher salivary pH. Bicarbonate is the major buffering ion in stimulated saliva. Since the perception of sour taste is dependent on the presence of H+, an increase in the salivary pH caused by the bicarbonate buffering effect will have a diminishing effect on sour taste perception. Thus, when salivary flow rates were artificially reduced by administration of atropine, the registration threshold of sour taste was lowered [31, 32]. Additionally, higher sour taste threshold has been measured in individuals with higher whole saliva flow rates compared with individuals with lower flow rates [31]. Accordingly, it could be argued that sour taste sensitivity is influenced by salivary flow rate, although the clinical value of this relation needs further investigation.

In addition to salivary bicarbonate, some organic substances in saliva can interact with taste substances. Thus, carbonic anhydrase VI (also named gustin) plays an essential role in taste perception, and a deficiency in this protein has been associated with an overall decreased taste perception [33]. Since carbonic anhydrase VI has been associated with taste bud growth and development, it is suggested that inhibition of synthesis of carbonic anhydrase VI is related to development of taste bud abnormalities followed by loss of taste function [34]. Also, the cyclic nucleotides cAMP and cGMP in parotid saliva have been recognized as playing important roles in maintaining taste function [35], while basic proline-rich proteins and histidine-rich proteins through their binding to polyphenols are involved in the sensation of astringency, which is suggested to be a result of both taste and tactile mechanisms working together [36].

Little is known about the digestive functions of saliva in relation to taste perception. However, the presence of lipase and lipolysis in the oral cavity may play a role in fat perception and liking [37]. The digestion of polysaccharides by amylase starts in the oral cavity [38], and salivary amylase activity may be involved in specific flavor and texture sensations through the enzymatic breakdown of starch [39]. Additionally, the composition of saliva has been associated with the bitter taste sensation [40, 41].

## Altered Taste in Dry Mouth Patients

In studies describing clinical characteristics of patients with dry mouth complaints of altered taste are often mentioned [42–44]. Thus, it has been described by several studies that patients with Sjögren's syndrome present with reduced taste perception [45–47] like irradiated head and neck cancer patients often present with taste alterations [19, 48, 49], although some investigators have observed complete recovery of taste function after 6–12 months after radiation therapy [50]. Concerning the latter group of patients, it has been suggested that loss or alteration of taste may rather be related to the proportion of the tongue contained within the radiation treatment field than the decreased salivary secretion [51]. According to this, there has been described a significant correlation between atrophic tongue mucosa and both salivary flow deficiency and taste function in a group of Sjögren's syndrome patients [52], which propose that damage to the taste buds or taste receptor sites due to irradiation or decreased salivary secretion additionally may play a role in alterations of taste described in relation to dry mouth.

However, not all patients with xerostomia experience an impaired perception of taste [53]. Likewise, the severity of taste disorder does not necessarily correlate with the degree of parotid and submandibular gland dysfunction [54]. This supports that it is unlikely that the decrease in taste sensitivity can be explained simply by a reduced diffusion of taste substances to the receptor site [55]. While the mixed saliva of the oral cavity is associated with the taste receptors of the fungiform papillae and taste receptors located in the soft palate, the foliate and circumvallate papillae are influenced by flow of von Ebner's glands [26]. Thus, dysfunction of major salivary glands does not exclude that minor or von Ebner's salivary glands are still functioning, which could explain that not all patients with xerostomia present with altered taste perception [29].

Regardless of the cause, altered and decreased taste perception is important toward the joy and the actual intake of food. Especially in frail elderly or hospitalized persons with dry mouth, attention should be paid to meal patterns and food intake to prevent inadequate dietary intake. While administration of artificial saliva based on carboxymethylcellulose may have little or no effect on gustatory function [56], it has been shown that flavor enhancement of cooked meals is an effective way to improve dietary intake and body weight in elderly nursing home residents [57].

When evaluating the overall impact of oral dryness and decreased salivary secretion on dietary intake, a prominent example that summarizes the palette of complications is irradiated head and neck cancer patients. These patients experience xerostomia and decreased salivary secretion, oral pain, challenged mastication and swallowing, and altered taste [58], which in many cases lead to a reduced and inadequate dietary intake resulting in an unintended body weight loss [19]. Furthermore, it has previously been described that salivary gland dysfunction may add to the conditions that make it difficult to maintain an adequate dietary intake in elderly populations. Thus, despite the multifactorial etiology of malnutrition in elderly or other individuals suffering from xerostomia and/or decreased salivary secretion, the impact of dry mouth and the concomitant consequences on dietary intake must not be neglected. Therefore, clinical recommendations for counseling individuals suffering from oral dryness should emphasize that this condition may have a negative impact on food consumption behaviors. Hence, questions about altered food choices and amounts as well as recent unintended weight loss may provide relevant anamnestic information in these patients.

## The Impact of Nutritional Status on Salivary Secretion

Just as decreased salivary secretion can lead to malnutrition, the opposite can also occur. Thus, persons who live on an unbalanced or inadequate diet may present with xerostomia and/or decreased salivary secretion. Dietary conditions that may prove to have an impact on salivary secretion are dehydration, general malnutrition, and micronutrient deficiencies.

### Dehydration

Dehydration is a simple cause to decreased salivary secretion especially observed in frail elderly, where dehydration is frequently associated with insufficient water intake or excessive water loss through damaged kidneys [59], but also healthy younger adults may experience decreased parotid salivary secretion as a result of dehydration [60]. The effect of dehydration on parotid salivary secretion seems to be most pronounced in the unstimulated state [61]. Xerostomia and decreased salivary secretion in persons with eating disorders like anorexia nervosa and bulimia nervosa may also in some cases be explained by dehydration caused by self-induced vomiting several times daily or the practice of excessive amounts of exercise [62].

Thus, the daily water lost by kidneys, intestines, lungs, and skin must be closely balanced by a daily intake of liquid. In general, healthy adult individuals are recommended to have a daily liquid intake of 1½–2 l. It has been suggested that patients showing oral signs of dehydration could benefit from increasing their intake of soup. Water bound to organic molecules particularly vegetable fibers is thought to pass through the gastrointestinal system more slowly than free water and thus leave a longer transit time to increase reabsorption of water [63].

### Malnutrition and Micronutrients Deficiency

Little is known about the direct effect of malnutrition and nutrient deficiencies on salivary secretion. Subjects, who were experimentally fasting, meaning a daily liquid intake of at least 3 l of commercially available herb tea, broth, and juices of fruits and vegetables (in total 300 kcal), experienced during the 8 days of fasting a feeling of dryness and foulness of the mouth [64]. More severe cases of malnutrition have been studied in children in third world countries who suffered from protein-energy malnutrition (PEM). Thus, in a group of Indian children, the stimulated salivary secretion rate was significantly lower in children with severe to moderate PEM based on height-to-age ratios, while there were no differences in unstimulated salivary secretion between the groups [65]. However, a retrospective study of the effect of early childhood PEM and adolescent nutritional status revealed that early childhood PEM and continuing chronic nutritional stress resulting in delayed growth (stunting) had a negative impact on both unstimulated and stimulated salivary secretion. Thus, it is suggested that exocrine saliva glandular systems in humans may be compromised for extended periods following early childhood PEM [66].

The impact of micronutrient deficiencies on salivary secretion in humans is sparsely investigated and with no apparent associations. Xerostomia has been linked to ascorbate status [67] and vitamin A [63] and zinc deficiency [54], however, without substantial evidence. Also, iron supplementation in iron-deficit persons has been tested toward increasing salivary flow without effect [68]. However, persons who suffer from deficiency of vitamins (riboflavin, pyridoxine, folate, cobalamin) and minerals (iron) may present with oral complications such as dry atrophic mucosa, burning sensation, and glossitis [63, 69], which are similar symptoms to those presented in persons with decreased salivary secretion.

**Conclusions**

The relationship between oral health and nutrition is multifaceted. Alterations of the structure and function of the oral cavity may have an influence on dietary intake and contribute to development of nutrient deficiency. Likewise, nutrition and dietary intake may have an impact on oral health. Salivary secretion is just a small player in this complex synergy, which also includes manifestations of systemic diseases in the oral cavity [70]. Attention to the increasing knowledge of oral and nutrition health is highly relevant for a number of health-care professionals including medical doctors, dentists, dental hygienists, dieticians, caregivers, and others who through dietary counseling, nutrition therapy, and oral health care may improve nutritional status, prevent weight loss and unnecessary oral symptoms and overall ensure a comprehensive multidisciplinary health care [71].

## References


1. Bardow A, Pedersen AM, Nauntofte B. Saliva. In: Miles T, Nauntofte B, Svensson P, editors. Clinical oral physiology. Copenhagen: Quintessence Publishing Co. Ltd.; 2004. p. 17–51.
2. Vellas B, Villars H, Abellan G, Soto ME, Rolland Y, Guigoz Y, et al. Overview of the MNA – its history and challenges. J Nutr Health Aging. 2006;10(6):456–63.
3. Detsky AS, Baker JP, Mendelson RA, Wolman SL, Wesson DE, Jeejeebhoy KN. Evaluating the accuracy of nutritional assessment techniques applied to hospitalized patients: methodology and comparisons. JPEN J Parenter Enteral Nutr. 1984;8(2):153–9.
4. Dormenval V, Budtz-Jørgensen E, Mojon P, Bruyere A, Rapin CH. Associations between malnutrition, poor general health and oral dryness in hospitalized elderly patients. Age Ageing. 1998;27(2):123–8.
5. El Osta N, Hennequin M, Tubert-Jeannin S, Abboud Naaman NB, El OL, Geahchan N. The pertinence of oral health indicators in nutritional studies in the elderly. Clin Nutr. 2014;33(2):316–21.
6. Soini H, Routasalo P, Lauri S, Ainamo A. Oral and nutritional status in frail elderly. Spec Care Dent. 2003;23(6):209–15.

7. Holm B, Söderhamn O. Factors associated with nutritional status in a group of people in an early stage of dementia. Clin Nutr. 2003;22(4):385–9.
8. Soini H, Muurinen S, Routasalo P, Sandelin E, Savikko N, Suominen M, et al. Oral and nutritional status – is the MNA a useful tool for dental clinics. J Nutr Health Aging. 2006;10(6):495–9.
9. Syrjäla AM, Pussinen PI, Komulainen K, Nykanen I, Knuuttila M, Ruoppi P, et al. Salivary flow rate and risk of malnutrition – a study among dentate, community-dwelling older people. Gerodontology. 2013;30(4):270–5.
10. Mesas AE, Andrade SM, Cabrera MA, Bueno VL. Oral health status and nutritional deficit in noninstitutionalized older adults in Londrina, Brazil. Rev Bras Epidemiol. 2010;13(3):434–45.
11. Samnieng P, Ueno M, Shinada K, Zaitsu T, Wright FAC, Kawaguchi Y. Association of hyposalivation with oral function, nutrition and oral health in community-dwelling elderly Thai. Community Dent Health 2012;29(1):117–23.
12. Rhodus NL, Brown J. The association of xerostomia and inadequate intake in older adults. J Am Diet Assoc. 1990;90(12):1688–92.
13. Rhodus NL. Qualitative nutritional intake analysis of older adults with Sjogren's syndrome. Gerodontology. 1988;7(2):61–9.
14. Guenther PM, Reedy J, Krebs-Smith SM, Reeve BB. Evaluation of the healthy eating index-2005. J Am Diet Assoc. 2008;108(11):1854–64.
15. Guenther PM, Reedy J, Krebs-Smith SM. Development of the healthy eating index-2005. J Am Diet Assoc. 2008;108(11):1896–901.
16. Quandt SA, Savoca MR, Leng X, Chen H, Bell RA, Gilbert GH, et al. Dry mouth and dietary quality in older adults in North Carolina. J Am Geriatr Soc. 2011;59(3):439–45.
17. Sheiham A, Steele JG, Marcenes W, Finch S, Walls AW. The impact of oral health on stated ability to eat certain foods; findings from the national diet and nutrition survey of older people in Great Britain. Gerodontology. 1999;16(1):11–20.
18. Vissink A, Sreebny LM. Symptoms and semiotics. In: Sreebny LM, Vissink A, editors. Dry mouth. The malevolent symptom: a clinical guide. 1st ed. Iowa: Blackwell Publishing; 2010. p. 52–63.
19. Ganzer H, Touger-Decker R, Parrott JS, Murphy BA, Epstein JB, Huhmann MB. Symptom burden in head and neck cancer: impact upon oral energy and protein intake. Support Care Cancer. 2013;21(2):495–503.
20. Loesche WJ, Bromberg J, Terpenning MS, Bretz WA, Dominguez BL, Grossman NS, et al. Xerostomia, xerogenic medications and food avoidances in selected geriatric groups. J Am Geriatr Soc. 1995;43(4):401–7.
21. Dusek M, Simmons J, Buschang PH, Al-Hashimi I. Masticatory function in patients with xerostomia. Gerodontology. 1996;13(1):3–8.
22. Ikebe K, Sajima H, Kobayashi S, Hata K, Morii K, Nokubi T, et al. Association of salivary flow rate with oral function in a sample of community-dwelling older adults in Japan. Oral Surg Oral Med Oral Pathol Oral Radiol Endod. 2002;94(2):184–90.
23. Dawes C. Salivary flow patterns and the health of hard and soft oral tissues. J Am Dent Assoc. 2008;139(Suppl):18S–24.
24. Dreizen S, Daly TE, Drane JB, Brown LR. Oral complications of cancer radiotherapy. Postgrad Med. 1977;61(2):85–92.
25. Sheiham A, Steele J. Does the condition of the mouth and teeth affect the ability to eat certain foods, nutrient and dietary intake and nutritional status amongst older people? Public Health Nutr. 2001;4(3):797–803.
26. Mese H, Matsuo R. Salivary secretion, taste and hyposalivation. J Oral Rehabil. 2007;34(10):711–23.
27. Spielman AI, Ship JA. Taste and smell. In: Miles TS, Nauntofte B, Svensson P, editors. Clinical oral physiology. 1st ed. Copenhagen: Quintessence Publishing Co. Ltd.; 2004. p. 53–70.
28. Beatty RM, Gragg LH. The sourness of acids. J Am Chem Soc. 1935;57:2347–51.
29. Spielman AI. Interaction of saliva and taste. J Dent Res. 1990;69(3):838–43.
30. Murphy C, Cardello AV, Brand J. Tastes of fifteen halide salts following water and NaCl: anion and cation effects. Physiol Behav. 1981;26(6):1083–95.

31. Norris MB, Noble AC, Pangborn RM. Human saliva and taste responses to acids varying in anions, titratable acidity, and pH. Physiol Behav. 1984;32(2):237–44.
32. Christensen CM, Navazesh M, Brightman VJ. Effects of pharmacologic reductions in salivary flow on taste thresholds in man. Arch Oral Biol. 1984;29(1):17–23.
33. Shatzman AR, Henkin RI. Gustin concentration changes relative to salivary zinc and taste in humans. Proc Natl Acad Sci U S A. 1981;78(6):3867–71.
34. Henkin RI, Martin BM, Agarwal RP. Decreased parotid saliva gustin/carbonic anhydrase VI secretion: an enzyme disorder manifested by gustatory and olfactory dysfunction. Am J Med Sci. 1999;318(6):380–91.
35. Henkin RI, Velicu I, Papathanassiu A. cAMP and cGMP in human parotid saliva: relationships to taste and smell dysfunction, gender, and age. Am J Med Sci. 2007;334(6):431–40.
36. Bajec MR, Pickering GJ. Astringency: mechanisms and perception. Crit Rev Food Sci Nutr. 2008;48(9):858–75.
37. Neyraud E, Palicki O, Schwartz C, Nicklaus S, Feron G. Variability of human saliva composition: possible relationships with fat perception and liking. Arch Oral Biol. 2012;57(5): 556–66.
38. Hoebler C, Karinthi A, Devaux MF, Guillon F, Gallant DJ, Bouchet B, et al. Physical and chemical transformations of cereal food during oral digestion in human subjects. Br J Nutr. 1998;80(5):429–36.
39. de Wijk RA, Prinz JF, Engelen L, Weenen H. The role of alpha-amylase in the perception of oral texture and flavour in custards. Physiol Behav. 2004;83(1):81–91.
40. Dsamou M, Palicki O, Septier C, Chabanet C, Lucchi G, Ducoroy P, et al. Salivary protein profiles and sensitivity to the bitter taste of caffeine. Chem Senses 2012;37:87–95.
41. Morzel M. Chabanet C, Schwartz C, Lucchi G, Ducoroy P, Nicklaus S. Salivary protein profiles are linked to bitter taste acceptance in infants. Eur J Pediatr 2014;173:575–82.
42. Cho MA, Ko JY, Kim YK, Kho HS. Salivary flow rate and clinical characteristics of patients with xerostomia according to its aetiology. J Oral Rehabil. 2010;37(3):185–93.
43. Bergdahl M. Salivary flow and oral complaints in adult dental patients. Community Dent Oral Epidemiol. 2000;28(1):59–66.
44. Toida M, Nanya Y, Takeda-Kawaguchi T, Baba S, Iida K, Kato K, et al. Oral complaints and stimulated salivary flow rate in 1188 adults. J Oral Pathol Med. 2010;39(5):407–19.
45. Kamel UF, Maddison P, Whitaker R. Impact of primary Sjogren's syndrome on smell and taste: effect on quality of life. Rheumatology (Oxford). 2009;48(12):1512–4.
46. Henkin RI, Talal N, Larson AL, Mattern CF. Abnormalities of taste and smell in Sjogren's syndrome. Ann Intern Med. 1972;76(3):375–83.
47. Weiffenbach JM, Schwartz LK, Atkinson JC, Fox PC. Taste performance in Sjogren's syndrome. Physiol Behav. 1995;57(1):89–96.
48. Mossman K, Shatzman A, Chencharick J. Long-term effects of radiotherapy on taste and salivary function in man. Int J Radiat Oncol Biol Phys. 1982;8(6):991–7.
49. Mossman KL, Henkin RI. Radiation-induced changes in taste acuity in cancer patients. Int J Radiat Oncol Biol Phys. 1978;4(7–8):663–70.
50. Ruo Redda MG, Allis S. Radiotherapy-induced taste impairment. Cancer Treat Rev. 2006;32(7):541–7.
51. Fernando IN, Patel T, Billingham L, Hammond C, Hallmark S, Glaholm J, et al. The effect of head and neck irradiation on taste dysfunction: a prospective study. Clin Oncol (R Coll Radiol). 1995;7(3):173–8.
52. Negoro A, Umemoto M, Fujii M, Kakibuchi M, Terada T, Hashimoto N, et al. Taste function in Sjogren's syndrome patients with special reference to clinical tests. Auris Nasus Larynx. 2004;31(2):141–7.
53. Weiffenbach JM, Fox PC, Baum BJ. Taste and salivary function. Proc Natl Acad Sci U S A. 1986;83(16):6103–6.
54. Tanaka M. Secretory function of the salivary gland in patients with taste disorders or xerostomia: correlation with zinc deficiency. Acta Otolaryngol Suppl. 2002;546:134–41.

55. Matsuo R. Role of saliva in the maintenance of taste sensitivity. Crit Rev Oral Biol Med. 2000;11(2):216–29.
56. Temmel AF, Quint C, Schickinger-Fischer B, Hummel T. Taste function in xerostomia before and after treatment with a saliva substitute containing carboxymethylcellulose. J Otolaryngol. 2005;34(2):116–20.
57. Mathey MF, Siebelink E, de GC, Van Staveren WA. Flavor enhancement of food improves dietary intake and nutritional status of elderly nursing home residents. J Gerontol A Biol Sci Med Sci. 2001;56(4):M200–5.
58. Jensen SB, Pedersen AM, Reibel J, Nauntofte B. Xerostomia and hypofunction of the salivary glands in cancer therapy. Support Care Cancer. 2003;11(4):207–25.
59. Massler M. Geriatric nutrition II: dehydration in the elderly. J Prosthet Dent. 1979;42(5):489–91.
60. Fischer D, Ship JA. The effect of dehydration on parotid salivary gland function. Spec Care Dent. 1997;17(2):58–64.
61. Ship JA, Fischer DJ. The relationship between dehydration and parotid salivary gland function in young and older healthy adults. J Gerontol A Biol Sci Med Sci. 1997;52(5):M310–9.
62. Dynesen AW, Bardow A, Pedersen AML, Nauntofte B. Oral findings in Anorexia nervosa and Bulimia nervosa with special reference to salivary changes. Oral Biosci Med. 2004;1:151–69.
63. Niessen LC, Jones JA. Oral health changes in the elderly. Their relationship to nutrition. Postgrad Med. 1984;75(5):231–7.
64. Johansson I, Ericson T, Steen L. Studies of the effect of diet on saliva secretion and caries development: the effect of fasting on saliva composition of female subjects. J Nutr. 1984;114(11):2010–20.
65. Johansson I, Saellstrom AK, Rajan BP, Parameswaran A. Salivary flow and dental caries in Indian children suffering from chronic malnutrition. Caries Res. 1992;26(1):38–43.
66. Psoter WJ, Spielman AL, Gebrian B, St JR, Katz RV. Effect of childhood malnutrition on salivary flow and pH. Arch Oral Biol. 2008;53(3):231–7.
67. Enwonwu CO. Ascorbate status and xerostomia. Med Hypotheses. 1992;39(1):53–7.
68. Flink H, Tegelberg A, Thorn M, Lagerlof F. Effect of oral iron supplementation on unstimulated salivary flow rate: a randomized, double-blind, placebo-controlled trial. J Oral Pathol Med. 2006;35(9):540–7.
69. Moynihan P. Nutritional impact in oral health promotion. Oral Health Prev Dent. 2003;1 Suppl 1:385–401.
70. Islam NM, Bhattacharyya I, Cohen DM. Common oral manifestations of systemic disease. Otolaryngol Clin North Am. 2011;44(1):161–82, vi.
71. Touger-Decker R, Mobley C. Position of the Academy of Nutrition and Dietetics: oral health and nutrition. J Acad Nutr Diet. 2013;113(5):693–701.

# Xerostomia and the Oral Microflora

6

Antoon J.M. Ligtenberg and Annica Almståhl

**Abstract**

Xerostomia is the feeling of a dry mouth usually caused by hyposalivation. It may occur after radiation therapy of the head and neck, in systemic diseases such as Sjögren's syndrome, or as a side effect of medication. Hyposalivation changes the oral microbiome with the most dramatic changes after radiation therapy. The number of lactobacilli and *Candida albicans* increases. Also the number of mutans streptococci increases in hyposalivated subjects, but sugar consumption is a stronger determinant for the level of mutans streptococci. Hyposalivated subjects are more susceptible to oral infections such as caries and mucosal infections. This is both caused by changes in the oral microflora and weakening of salivary protection mechanisms such as cleansing by the salivary flow and buffering capacity.

In the case of ventilated patients at intensive care units, hyposalivation leads to accumulation of dental plaque and a shift in microflora, which may cause lung infections. Oral hygiene in combination with oral antiseptics reduces the risk for lung infections in these patients.

Therapies for xerostomia consist of artificial saliva, gels, or spray. These products may contain polymers that form a microbial substrate. Application of salivary antimicrobial substances like lysozyme, lactoferrin, or lactoperoxidase in these products did not lead to lower microbial counts in vivo.

In conclusion, hyposalivation leads to changes in the oral microflora. In combination with a lower defense, this leads to a higher susceptibility to oral

A.J.M. Ligtenberg, PhD (✉)
Department of Oral Biochemistry, Academic Centre for Dentistry Amsterdam, Gustav Mahlerlaan 3004, Amsterdam 1081 LA, The Netherlands
e-mail: a.ligtenberg@acta.nl

A. Almståhl, PhD, Dental hygienist
Department of Oral Microbiology and Immunology, Sahlgrenska Academy, University of Gothenburg, Gothenburg, Sweden



G. Carpenter (ed.), *Dry Mouth: A Clinical Guide on Causes, Effects and Treatments*, DOI 10.1007/978-3-642-55154-3_6

infections such as caries and mucosal infections. There is a need for products normalizing the oral microflora and thereby decreasing the risk of oral diseases in subjects with hyposalivation.

## Introduction

Xerostomia is the medical term for the feeling of dryness of the mouth. Although this feeling of dryness is subjective, it is usually caused by hyposalivation, a reduced ability to produce saliva. This feeling may be encompassed with a decreased quality of life, because all kinds of activities, like speaking, eating, and swallowing, can be affected negatively. In addition, saliva is important for protection against dehydration of the oral cavity and microbial attacks. A reduced amount of saliva therefore also leads to oral health problems, most commonly an increased incidence of caries, oral mucosal infections, halitosis, and gingival inflammation. In general, three main causes of xerostomia are recognized [1]:

1. The first group are patients that are treated for a tumor in the head and neck region. There are 390,000 new cases of oral cancer per year in the world (WHO). Most oral cancers are treated with radiation therapy, in many cases combined with cytostatic drugs. Radiation therapy including the salivary glands leads to damage to the secretory cells and a reduced saliva production. Cytostatic drugs may also have negative effects on salivary secretion.
2. The second group are patients with systemic disease. Sjögren's syndrome, an autoimmune disease affecting glandular tissues, is the best known cause, but also other diseases, like HIV/AIDS, diabetes mellitus, and Crohn's disease, may result in reduced salivary flow.
3. The third and by far the most heterogeneous group are people who experience xerostomia as a side effect of the use of medication or drugs. Over 400 medications have been reported to cause xerostomia [2]. Since the use of medication increases with age, especially elderly people are at risk.

## Saliva and the Healthy Microbiome

To recognize the effect of hyposalivation on the oral microflora, we first need to know the composition of the healthy microflora and what the effect of saliva is on the composition and maintenance of the healthy microflora. With classical techniques as culturing and microscopy, already over 400 different species have been identified in saliva. Species belonging to the normal oral microflora are, for example, alpha-hemolytic streptococci, *Actinomyces*, *Haemophilus*, and *Neisseria*. With the availability of molecular techniques like the sequencing of 16 S ribosomal RNA, a core microbiome of over 600 species has been identified [3, 4]. Inside the mouth different habitats are recognized, each with a different microbiome. The gingival and buccal mucosae and palate have a comparable microbiome. Saliva, tongue, and supra- and subgingival plaques have their own unique microbiome [3]. The microbiome is quite stable during life and undergoes limited changes. Compared with the microbiome in the gut or on the skin, the oral microbiome shows less variation both within and between persons [5]. With a settled oral microbiome, new species, acquired by eating or social contacts, have a small chance to colonize. There are no significant differences in the oral microbiome among people of different locations worldwide showing that differences in diet among different populations have limited influence. Several selective aspects determine the survival of the oral microbiome (Fig. 6.1). For maintenance in the oral cavity, microorganisms have to (1) grow and reproduce, (2) bind to a surface to prevent from being swallowed, and (3) resist the antimicrobial activity of saliva.

1. The first selective factor in the mouth is the availability of nutrients. The most important nutrient for oral bacteria is saliva. In contrast to what is generally thought, our nutrition has little influence on our microbiome. The only exception

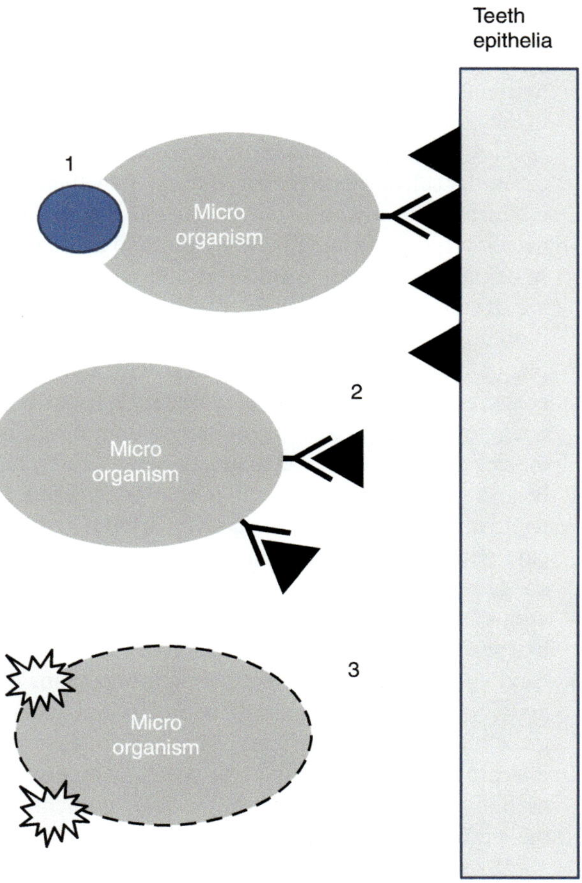


**Fig. 6.1** Effect of saliva on the colonization of microorganisms. (*1*) Salivary substances, like MUC5B, are the most important nutrients for microorganisms in the oral cavity (*blue circle*). (*2*) Saliva forms receptors for microbial attachment. Similar proteins in solution prevent their binding to the tooth surface (*black triangles*). (*3*) Saliva proteins, like histatins, lactoperoxidase, and lysozyme, have antimicrobial activity (*star symbol*)

is the frequent consumption of sucrose, glucose, and other easily fermentable carbohydrates [6]. By fermentation of sugar, acids are produced which leads to a lowering of the pH in dental plaque. This favors the growth of acidophilic and cariogenic microorganisms like *Streptococcus mutans*. In saliva especially the high-molecular-weight mucin, MUC5B, is an important nutrient source. MUC5B consists for up to 90 % of long branched carbohydrate chains. Complete degradation of these carbohydrate chains requires a large set of enzymes requiring many microbial species. The genome of a single microorganism is too limited to encode for all the enzymes. Therefore, a consortium of microbial species live in a symbiotic relationship [7–9]. In addition, some microorganisms use the waste products of other bacteria as nutrients. Also serum components, which enter the oral cavity as crevicular fluid, can be used as a substrate [9, 10]. During experimental gingivitis, the amount of plasma protein and bacterial counts on the tooth surfaces have been shown to increase [11].

2. The second selective factor is that microorganisms have to attach to a surface in the oral cavity in order to resist the saliva flow and swallowing. The continuous salivary flow constantly clears the mouth from non-attached microorganisms. The fact that the microbial composition of dental plaque is different from the microflora on soft dental surfaces or the tongue despite the availability of similar nutrients shows that microbial attachment is an important selective determinant in the oral cavity [12]. Bacteria have specific adhesins that they use for binding to salivary proteins that cover the dental surface. These bacteria recognize the same or similar salivary proteins in solution, by which adhesion to the dental surface is inhibited. The mucin MUC 7 and salivary agglutinin bind and aggregate oral bacteria thus preventing their adhesion to similar receptors on the dental surface. In dental plaque, only a small proportion of the microorganisms directly bind to the dental surface [13]. Most of the microorganisms in dental plaque grow in a biofilm, a microbial layer of hundreds of microorganisms. The bacteria in dental plaque bind to each other, a process which can be mimicked in the test tube by coaggregation [7, 14] When planktonic suspensions of two bacterial species that coaggregate are mixed, they rapidly clump which is visually observable. During the development of dental plaque, a shift in microbial composition occurs from a benign microflora of primarily Gram-positive microorganisms to a more pathogenic microflora of Gram-negative bacteria. Primary colonizers tend to coaggregate with other primary colonizers, and secondary colonizers also only tend to coaggregate other secondary colonizers. *Fusobacterium nucleatum* coaggregates with both primary and secondary colonizers thus playing a key role in the microbial shift to a more pathogenic microflora [7, 15].
3. Next to adhesion and growth, microorganisms must resist the antimicrobial activity in saliva. Saliva shows antimicrobial activity by killing and inhibition of growth but also by prevention of adhesion. There are also numerous antimicrobial proteins in saliva, like lysozyme, lactoperoxidase, lactoferrin, and antimicrobial peptides. Considering the high numbers of microorganisms in saliva, their effect is limited, but saliva is able to kill non-oral microorganisms like *Escherichia coli* [16].

## Changes in the Microbiome of Dry Mouth Patients

Since saliva is important for the microbial balance in the mouth, hyposalivation may lead to disturbances of the microbial ecology. Under normal conditions about 0.2–0.4 ml/min of unstimulated saliva is produced. A secretion rate ≤0.1 ml/min is considered to be hyposalivation. Corresponding figures for stimulated whole saliva are 1–3 ml/min and ≤0.7 ml/min. Below are results from studies of the oral microflora both in rinsing samples and in samples collected from specific sites in subjects with hyposalivation of different origins presented.

## Oral Microflora in Subjects with Radiation-Induced Hyposalivation

The oral microflora in subjects undergoing radiation therapy was investigated already in the 1970s [17, 18]. Brown et al. [17] showed a marked increase in numbers of lactobacilli, *Candida*, and staphylococci and a decrease in *Streptococcus sanguinis* and *Fusobacterium*, after completed radiation therapy (RT). These alterations remained 30 months later. Also Llory et al. [18] reported persisting high numbers and proportions of acidogenic microorganisms 1–4 years after completed radiation therapy. In these earlier studies, very low salivary secretion rates, a mean of 0.08 ml/min, were reported in subjects who had undergone radiation therapy in the head and neck region [17]. Since then, cancer treatment has improved markedly with more accurate focusing techniques, the use of three-dimensional planning of the radiation field, brachytherapy (iridium implant in the tumor), intensity modulated radiotherapy and sparing of the parotid glands on the contralateral side. These factors have decreased the negative effects on the salivary glands, and higher salivary secretion rates can be regained compared with those 40–50 years ago. Consequently, radiation therapy may have less pronounced effects on the oral microflora than it used to have.

The oral microflora in subjects with radiation-induced hyposalivation has been investigated also in the latest decades [19–23]. In the study by Almståhl et al. [19], the oral microflora in rinsing samples in groups with hyposalivation of different origins was compared. Compared with subjects with primary Sjögren's syndrome and subjects with hyposalivation due to medication or of unknown origin, the group with hyposalivation due to radiation therapy (6 months after completed treatment) had the highest numbers and proportions of lactobacilli and *Candida albicans*. About one third of the patients had very high levels of mutans streptococci, while in one third of the patients, this bacterium was not detected. An increase in salivary numbers of bacteria associated with caries and *Candida* has also been reported by others [20, 21]. Hu et al. [23] followed the changes in the oral microbiome of patients undergoing radiation therapy. Pooled supragingival plaque from the maxillary first molar was collected before and during radiation therapy and analyzed by pyrosequencing of the 16S rRNA. The variation in species was reduced by radiation therapy. Higher doses of radiation lead to a stronger species reduction. Also a change in bacterial species was observed. Before radiation therapy the most abundant phyla were, in order of prevalence, Proteobacteria, Firmicutes, Bacteroidetes, and Actinobacteria. During radiation therapy the order was changed to Firmicutes, Actinobacteria, Proteobacteria, and Bacteroidetes [23]. Six genera were found in all subjects at the start of the study: *Streptococcus*, *Actinomyces*, *Capnocytophaga*, *Neisseria*, *Granulicatella*, and *Gemella*. Of these, only *Streptococcus* and *Actinomyces* were always found in all subjects across the different time points of the therapy.

In a few studies the oral microflora in different ecosystems has been analyzed using cultivation techniques [21, 22]. Al-Nawas and Grötz [21] found no significant changes in the frequencies of bacteria associated with periodontal diseases in the gingival crevice region during the 12 months' follow-up period after radiation therapy.

In a study by Almståhl et al. [22], the oral microflora in five ecosystems (the dorsum of the tongue, buccal mucosa, vestibulum in the molar region, supragingival plaque, and gingival crevice region) was analyzed. Samples were taken from subjects 6 months after completed radiation therapy (RT group) and compared with the microflora in controls matched according to age, sex, and number of teeth and with normal salivary secretion rate. The cancer patients had received radiation doses ranging between 64.6 and 76.6 Gy, and the major salivary glands were included in the radiation field. Twelve of the 13 subjects in the study were also treated with brachytherapy (between 6 and 30 Gy). The subjects showed severe hyposalivation—the mean unstimulated salivary secretion rate was $0.005 \pm 0.02$ ml/min (median 0 ml/min) and the mean stimulated secretion rate $0.32 \pm 0.32$ ml/min (median 0.23 ml/min).

## Dorsum of the Tongue

The mean total count and the numbers of streptococci, *Streptococcus salivarius*, and *Fusobacterium nucleatum* were significantly lower in the RT group than in the control group, while the numbers of *C. albicans* and enterococci were significantly higher.

## Buccal Mucosa

The RT group tended to have lower numbers of *Streptococcus sanguinis/oralis*, associated with good oral health. Also the proportion of *S. sanguinis/oralis* of the total number of streptococci was lower. *C. albicans* and *Staphylococcus aureus* on the buccal mucosa were only detected in the RT group and not in the healthy group.

## Vestibulum in the Molar Region

The mean proportion of streptococci tended to be lower in the RT group than in the controls. The mucosal pathogens *C. albicans*, *S. aureus*, Gram-negative enteric rods, and enterococci were more frequently detected in the RT group. The numbers of *C. albicans* and enterococci were significantly higher in the RT group.

## Supragingival Plaque

In the supragingival plaque, the most marked difference was in the number and proportion of lactobacilli (Tables 6.1 and 6.2). Of the controls only one had detectable levels of lactobacilli, whereas in the radiation therapy group, 92 % showed growth of lactobacilli. The proportions of mutans streptococci and *C. albicans* tended to be higher in the RT group than in the control group.

## Gingival Crevice Region

The total number of anaerobically growing bacteria was significantly higher, but the number of *Prevotella intermedia/nigrescens*, associated with gingivitis, was significantly lower in the RT group than in the controls. *Porphyromonas gingivalis* and *Aggregatibacter actinomycetemcomitans*, both associated with periodontitis, were not detected in any of the RT subjects.

It can be concluded that the most dramatic changes in the oral microflora after radiation therapy in the head and neck region are a marked increase in aciduric and acidogenic lactobacilli, *C. albicans*, and enterococci [21]. It should be noted that the subjects included were taking good care of their oral health: they had a good oral hygiene and went to the dental clinic at least once a year, and many of them used fluoride rinse several times per week.

**Table 6.1** Numbers (log10) of microorganisms in supragingival plaque in groups with hyposalivation of different origins

| | RT (6 months) (*n*=13) | RT (3 years) (*n*=11) | pSS (*n*=20) | Unknown (*n*=20) | Controls (*n*=29) |
|---|---|---|---|---|---|
| Total count | 6.68±0.59 (6.64) | 6.29±0.65 (6.40) | 6.45±0.49 (6.47) | 6.65±0.65 (6.59) | 6.10±0.87 (6.40) |
| Streptococci | 5.88±0.59 (5.94) | 5.73±0.88 (5.68) | 5.90±0.52 (5.91) | 6.00±0.59 (6.02) | 5.54±0.78 (5.63) |
| *S. sanguinis/oralis* | 4.13±2.12 (4.78) | 4.14±1.54 (4.60) | 4.97±1.40 (5.34) | 5.32±0.86 (5.34) | 4.68±1.42 (4.87) |
| Mutans streptococci | 3.38±2.25 (4.15) | 4.13±1.75 (4.64) | 4.44±1.44 (4.44) | 4.24±1.14 (4.09) | 2.32±1.76 (2.81) |
| Lactobacilli | 4.70±1.70 (4.98) | 4.10±2.40 (4.95) | 2.62±2.15 (2.87) | 1.87±2.08 (1.70) | 0.18±0.71 (0.00) |
| *Actinomyces* | 4.17±2.25 (4.41) | 4.47±2.13 (4.98) | 3.67±1.89 (3.90) | 4.63±1.42 (4.69) | 3.96±1.50 (4.39) |
| *C. albicans* | 1.69±2.10 (0.00 | 2.59±1.55 (2.98) | 1.60±1.47 (1.70) | 1.31±1.31 (1.70) | 0.46±1.06 (0.00) |

Data for the RT group 6 months post RT are from Almståhl et al. [22], RT 3 years from Almståhl et al 2014, submitted for publication for the pSS group from Almståhl et al. [27], for the unknown group from Almståhl and Wikström [30], and for the controls from all three studies.
Mean ± SD and median values (parenthesis) are given
*RT* radiation therapy, *pSS* primary Sjögren's syndrome, *Unknown* hyposalivation due to medicines or of unknown origin

**Table 6.2** Proportion of microorganisms in the supragingival plaque in groups with hyposalivation of different origins

| | RT (6 months) (*n*=13) | RT (3 years) (*n*=11) | pSS (*n*=20) | Unknown (*n*=20) | Controls (*n*=29) |
|---|---|---|---|---|---|
| *Proportion of the total count* | | | | | |
| Streptococci | 27±28 (22) | 33±33 (32) | 35±28 (30) | 38±37 (17) | 40±32 (28) |
| Lactobacilli | 10±19 (1.4) | 12±13 (2.5) | 7.6±24 (0.02) | 0.7±1.8 (0.0) | 0.02±0.09 0.0) |
| *Actinomyces* | 6.4±12 (1.4) | 16±32 (4.0) | 3.3±5.0 (0.4) | 11±26 (1.8) | 6.5±19 (1.1) |
| *C. albicans* | 0.9±2.9 (0.0) | 0.22±0.33 (0.1) | 0.04±0.07 (0.003) | 0.009±0.01 (0.0) | 0.004±0.01 (0.0) |
| *Proportion of total number of streptococci* | | | | | |
| *S. sanguinis* | 19±28 (5.2) | 17±29 (4.5) | 33±29 (25) | 33±26 (28) | 33±27 (28) |
| Mutans streptococci | 6.2±5.9 (6.1) | 22±35 (5.1) | 26±39 (5.9) | 12±24 (3.4) | 4.7±16 (0.1) |

Data for the RT group 6 months post RT are from Almståhl et al. [22]. RT 3 years from Almståhl et al 2014, submitted for publication for the pSS group from Almståhl et al. [27], for the Unknown group from Almståhl and Wikström [30], and for the controls from Almståhl all three studies. Mean ± SD and median values (in parenthesis) are given

*RT* radiation therapy, *pSS* primary Sjögren's syndrome, *Unknown* hyposalivation due to medicines or of unknown origin

Preliminary results from our longitudinal study on the oral microflora in subjects with radiation-induced hyposalivation indicate that the high numbers and proportions of lactobacilli and mutans streptococci detected in the supragingival plaque 6 months post RT persist up to 3 years post RT (Tables 6.1 and 6.2), while the frequency of mucosal pathogens decreases over time (Almståhl et al. submitted for publication).

## Oral Microflora in Primary Sjögren's Syndrome

Primary Sjögren's syndrome (pSS) is as previously mentioned an autoimmune disease directed against glandular tissues. One of the diagnostic criteria is the presence of inflammatory cells in the salivary glands. All secretory glands including the salivary glands are affected. Nine out of ten patients with pSS are women. The oral microflora in subjects with pSS has been analyzed in several studies [19, 24–28]. High levels of mutans streptococci and lactobacilli were reported by both Lundström and Lindström [24] and Kolavic et al. [25]. Also Leung et al. [29] found increased levels of lactobacilli in saliva of patients with Sjögren's syndrome. *Lactobacillus* species frequently found were *L. acidophilus*, *L. fermentum*, and *L. minutus*. *Candida* were detected on the tongue in 59 % of pSS subjects [24]. In the study by Leung et al. [29], also the microflora in supragingival plaque was examined. They found a significantly higher proportion of *Lactobacillus* species, especially *L. acidophilus*, compared to controls with normal salivary secretion rate. No significant differences in prevalence, number, or proportion of *S. mutans* or anaerobic Gram-negative rods were detected. In the study by Almståhl et al. [19], the microflora in rinsing samples from different groups with hyposalivation was examined. The pSS group included showed the second highest level of lactobacilli. Mutans streptococci were detected in 95 % of the subjects in pSS group and mostly in high numbers.

In another study, the microflora in five ecosystems (the dorsum of the tongue, buccal mucosa, vestibulum in the molar region, supragingival plaque, and gingival crevice region) was analyzed in 20 subjects with pSS (≥16 teeth and no removable dentures) and compared with the microflora in matched controls with normal salivary secretion rate [27]. Their unstimulated salivary secretion rate was 0.02±0.02 ml/min (median 0.01 ml/min) and the stimulated salivary secretion rate 0.47±0.38 ml/min median (0.40 ml/min).

On the dorsum of the tongue, the pSS group had a higher proportion of streptococci of the total microbial count and a higher proportion of *S. salivarius* of the total number of streptococci than the controls, while the proportion of *F. nucleatum* of the total count was lower. On the buccal mucosa, the pSS group had a higher total microbial count and a higher number of streptococci. In the vestibulum in the molar region, there were no statistically significant differences in the numbers or proportions. In the supragingival plaque, the pSS group showed a significantly higher number and proportion of mutans streptococci compared with the controls. Also the numbers of lactobacilli and *C. albicans* were significantly higher, and the proportion of lactobacilli tended to be higher. In the gingival crevice region, there were no statistically significant differences in the numbers or proportions of the microorganisms. The periodontal pathogens *P. gingivalis* and *A. actinomycetemcomitans* were not detected in any of the pSS subjects. As for the RT group, the most marked change in oral microflora in the pSS group was an increase in acidogenic and aciduric microorganisms, especially in the supragingival plaque.

## Oral Microflora in Subjects with Hyposalivation due to Medication

The knowledge on the oral microflora in subjects with hyposalivation due to medicines is scarce. This might be due to the fact that it is a very heterogenous group. In three studies subjects with hyposalivation due to medicines or of unknown origin were examined [19, 30, 31]. The subjects included in this group had undergone biopsy of the labial minor gland for investigation of a possible Sjögren's syndrome but had not shown any signs of inflammation. Therefore, they did not get the diagnosis of Sjögren's syndrome. For some of the patients, medication might explain their hyposalivation. Other possible reasons for their hyposalivation might have been hormonal changes or depression.

In rinsing samples, this group showed increased numbers of lactobacilli compared with subjects with normal salivary secretion rate [19]. However, their levels of lactobacilli were considerably lower than for the subjects with pSS and radiation-induced hyposalivation. This is most likely due to the fact that this group had a much higher stimulated salivary secretion rate, 0.93±0.54 ml/min, compared with the other groups, 0.47±0.38 ml/min in the pSS group and 0.35±0.38 ml/min in the RT group.

As for subjects with radiation-induced hyposalivation and pSS, the microflora in five ecosystems in subjects with hyposalivation of unknown origin was studied [30]. To be included the subjects had ≥16 teeth and no removable dentures and an unstimulated secretion rate of ≤0.1 ml/min. The mean unstimulated secretion rate was 0.04±0.04 ml/min (median 0.04 ml/min) and the stimulated secretion rate 0.98±0.51 ml/min (median 0.97 ml/min).

On the dorsum of the tongue, the hyposalivated group had a lower number of *F. nucleatum*. On the buccal mucosa, there were no significant differences in the numbers or proportions of microorganisms. In the vestibulum in the molar region, the number of enterococci tended to be higher in the hyposalivated group. In the supragingival plaque, the hyposalivated group had significantly higher numbers of mutans streptococci and lactobacilli and tended to have an increased number of *C. albicans*, but no significant differences in proportions of microorganisms were detected. In the gingival crevice, no significant differences in the numbers of proportions of microorganisms were detected.

To summarize the findings of the oral microflora in subjects with hyposalivation of different origins, a common feature was an increase in lactobacilli [19, 22, 27, 30]. The most dramatic increase was seen for the RT subjects followed by the pSS subjects. In the RT group the aggressive cancer treatment, rapid decrease in salivary secretion rate, and changed dietary habits during cancer treatment might have influence on the marked increase in lactobacilli. In the pSS subjects a contributing factor to the high levels of lactobacilli might be their high number of filled surfaces and crown joints, which can serve as retention sites for the lactobacilli. For mutans streptococci the differences between the hyposalivated subjects and the controls were not so clear. Mutans streptococci were however more frequently detected in the hyposalivated subjects, and many had high levels. Another interesting finding was that the frequency and number of *C. albicans* were higher in the interproximal supragingival plaque than on the tongue and mucosal membranes. This stresses the importance of interdental cleaning for subjects with hyposalivation. The group with hyposalivation due to medication or of unknown origin also had increased levels of lactobacilli, but the changes in microflora were not so marked as in the irradiated patients or the patients with Sjögren's syndrome. It is however possible that subjects with hyposalivation due to medicines or of unknown origin are pre-Sjögren's syndrome patients and that their salivary secretion rates will gradually decrease and thereby their risk of a disturbed microflora increases.

The subjects included in studies examining the oral microflora in subjects with hyposalivation have been middle aged [19, 22, 27, 28, 31, 32]. A growing group with hyposalivation, mostly due to polypharmacy, are elderly people. The proportion of elderly having natural teeth is increasing. The oral microflora was analyzed in a group of dependent elderly (79–98 years old with ≥10 teeth and no removable prosthesis [33]. Their unstimulated and stimulated salivary secretion rates were not possible to measure, but it can be suspected that it was lower than normal due to the high intake of medicines, mean 6±3 medicines (median 6). The majority of the subjects showed low labial minor gland flow rates. In the supragingival plaque, the dependent elderly showed high numbers and proportions of lactobacilli, mutans streptococci, and *Candida*, and enterococci were frequently found. This group is a challenge considering that many are not able to maintain a good oral hygiene due to decreased fine motor skills or dementia.

## Xerostomia and Ventilation

An example of what can happen with the oral microbiome when one is not able to take care of the oral hygiene is patients who are mechanically ventilated in intensive care units. Ten to thirty percent of the mechanically ventilated patients develop pneumonia, and 50 % of the antibiotics prescribed in intensive care units are related to (suspected) ventilator-associated pneumonia [34]. Ventilator-associated pneumonia is the leading cause of death from nosocomial infections in the United States [35]. One of the risk factors for the development of pneumonia is the reduced salivary flow and associated accumulation of dental plaque. The absence of oral stimulation and the use of xerogenic drugs combined with limited or hampered oral care result in the development of a microflora that is potentially pathogenic when entering the lungs. Causative agents of ventilator-associated pneumonia are Gram-negative enteric bacteria such as *E. coli* and *Klebsiella pneumoniae* and other species such as *Pseudomonas aeruginosa* and *S. aureus*. These species are usually not found in dental plaque. Comparison of dental plaque of patients in intensive care units with that of healthy controls revealed that patients had higher levels of dental plaque and this plaque included respiratory pathogens. In contrast, dental plaque of controls was rarely colonized by respiratory pathogens [36]. Somewhat unexpected is the finding that plaque of patients that recently received antibiotic treatment had a greater chance of being colonized by respiratory pathogens than plaque of those without treatment [37]. Possibly, these patients receive antibiotic treatment because they have a higher risk for developing infections. It is also possible that suppression of the commensal flora by antibiotics gives pathogens an opportunity to multiply. Treatment of these patients consists of oral care by tooth brushing combined with chlorhexidine or povidone-iodine flushing [38, 39].

## Caries

As mentioned already, many hyposalivated subjects have an increase in mutans streptococci and lactobacilli, which are associated with caries development. The occurrence of caries is the result of "an ecological disaster" as it was called by Philip Marsh [40]. Sucrose is in dental plaque fermented to primarily lactic acid that causes a decrease in pH in dental plaque. A low pH favors the growth of acidophilic bacteria like *S. mutans* and *Lactobacillus* spp. which are acidogenic at a pH lower than 4.7. This leads to demineralization of the dental enamel. The decrease in pH is more important than the availability of carbohydrates [41]. Although frequent sucrose consumption is considered the major cause of dental caries, people with hyposalivation are at high risk of developing caries [42]. In caries prediction models, for example, cariogram, saliva secretion is one of the predictive factors for caries experience [43]. Also salivary buffering capacity, which is usually lower in subjects with low saliva secretion, is one of the predictive factors in this model.

Saliva is relatively effective in protection against dental caries. Caries usually develops at sites that are not easily accessible for saliva and not on smooth surfaces. Saliva protects against caries in four ways:

1. Salivary proteins form a protective layer on the dental surface. Especially MUC5B, as a component of the mature dental pellicle, forms a coating on the dental surface that is protective against acidic attack [44]. The thickness of mucosal fluid layers of dry mouth patients was lower on the buccal mucosa, anterior tongue, and lower labial mucosa compared to age-matched controls [45]. Whether the thickness of the mucosal fluid layer on the dental surface is also lower remains to be investigated.
2. Buffering systems in saliva neutralize the acids that are formed. Saliva contains bicarbonate and phosphate buffering systems. The concentration of bicarbonate and correspondingly the pH and buffering capacity increase with a higher secretion rate of saliva [46]. At low salivary secretion both the pH and buffering capacity in saliva are lower than in controls in all groups with hyposalivation (radiation therapy, primary Sjögren's syndrome, unknown origin) [47]. The lower secretion rate of saliva combined with the lower buffering capacity leads to prolonged periods of low pH in dental plaque after the consumption of sweet beverages [48, 49] which favors the outgrowth of acidophilic microorganisms. After a sucrose rinse RT patients displayed significant lower plaque pH.
3. Saliva dilutes acids. Acidic taste stimulates saliva secretion. In healthy persons saliva secretion under the influence of citric acid can go as high as 7 ml/min [50]. With a higher saliva secretion, the acid in the mouth is diluted. High volumes of saliva lead to higher swallowing frequency and a shorter time of acids in the mouth [51]. In hyposalivated patients, dilution and neutralization of acids are much slower than in healthy persons. This favors the survival of an acidogenic microflora in dental plaque [22, 27, 31, 48]. In these patients caries also appear at smooth surfaces, which are normally not prone to caries.
4. Saliva promotes remineralization [52]. Salivary proteins like statherin and proline-rich proteins bind calcium ions thus keeping saliva supersaturated with calcium phosphate. These proteins bind to the dental surface enhancing remineralization of the tooth enamel.

## Mutans Streptococci and Dental Caries

Mutans streptococci are considered the major causative agent in dental caries. They have many virulence factors such as the ability to metabolize carbohydrates at low pH and the ability to adhere to the hard dental surfaces. For the adherence to dental surfaces, they synthesize extracellular dextrans out of sucrose. The number of mutans streptococci in saliva and supragingival dental plaque is highly depending on the frequency of sugar intake [53]. In subjects with hyposalivation induced by radiation therapy, the number of mutans streptococci was also found in higher proportions, but in about a quarter of the patients, no *S. mutans* was found [22]. Since it is well known that radiotherapy patients show a decline in saliva secretion with the corresponding dental risks, these patients follow a preventive dental care program with supplementary fluoride. They are also recommended frequent visits to the dental clinic. The patients are routinely given the advice of reducing their ingestion of easily fermentable carbohydrates, which might explain the relatively low number of mutans streptococci in this group [54]. However, preliminary longitudinal data for subjects with hyposalivation due to radiation therapy show a gradual increase in the proportion of mutans streptococci in the supragingival plaque over time. It is possible that with the persisting low saliva flow and buffering capacity, even a low intake of easily fermentable carbohydrates leads to prolonged periods of low pH favoring the growth of cariogenic microorganisms.

Other groups with hyposalivation are usually less aware of their increased risk of oral diseases. For the primary Sjögren's syndrome patients, for example, the symptoms of oral dryness precede the diagnosis for several years [24]. People with dry mouth complaints tend to stimulate their salivary flow by frequent sugar consumption or the consumption of soft drinks, as had been described for patients with Sjögren's syndrome and patients using neuroleptics [55–57] or methylenedioxymethamphetamine (XTC) [58]. Under these conditions the growth of mutans streptococci is favored.

## *Lactobacillus* Species

Just like *S. mutans*, *Lactobacillus* species are able to metabolize carbohydrates at low pH. In fact, *Lactobacillus* cultures in glucose can reach a lower pH than cultures of mutans streptococcil (3.6–4.0 vs. 4.0–4.4) [59]. Historically, lactobacilli were the first microorganisms implicated in the development of dental caries, and a strong correlation has been established between the *Lactobacillus* counts and dental caries [60–63]. Nonetheless, lactobacilli are not a causative agent in dental caries because they lack the virulence factors of mutans streptococci, namely, their ability to adhere to the dental surface and their capacity to produce insoluble glycans from glucose. Also their biofilm-forming capacity is low compared with that of oral streptococci.

High proportions of lactobacilli are frequently found in the saliva and supragingival plaque of subjects with hyposalivation, either due to medicines, Sjögren's syndrome, or radiation therapy [22, 27, 31, 64]. The lactobacilli in the supragingival plaque of these subjects were identified using restriction fragment length polymorphism [65]. The most prevalent *Lactobacillus* species detected were *Lactobacillus fermentum* (7 subjects), *L. casei* (7 subjects), and *L. rhamnosus* (6 subjects). *L. fermentum* and *L. casei* were the most prevalent species in anterior sites and *L. rhamnosus* and *L. fermentum* in posterior sites. In anterior sites, hyposalivated subjects with high *Lactobacillus* counts had an increased plaque acidogenicity compared to those with low counts. In posterior sites, subjects with high *Lactobacillus* counts had a lower final pH compared with those with low counts. No specific species could be related to plaque acidogenicity. Further studies including more subjects need to be performed to increase our knowledge on *Lactobacillus* species in subjects with hyposalivation.

Lactobacilli have been studied extensively for improvement of the intestinal flora, and now they are also applied as a probiotic for improvement of oral health [66, 67]. Probiotics are viable microorganisms that when administered in adequate amounts are beneficial to the health of the host [68]. Daily intake of milk supplemented with *L. rhamnosus* stimulated the reversal of root caries [69], and daily doses of a *L. reuteri* formulation reduced plaque scores and gingivitis in a group with moderate to severe gingivitis [70]. Also endogenous lactobacilli might have such beneficial effects on gingivitis, although in this case it is important to consider the cariogenic potential of the strains [71]. To use lactobacilli as probiotics in subjects with hyposalivation and already high proportions of lactobacilli might not be the best alternative. In an in vitro study, the ability of 50 *Lactobacillus* strains isolated from the supragingival plaque to ferment sugars and sugar alcohols was tested [72]. Twenty-five strains had been isolated from subjects who had undergone radiation therapy 3–5 years earlier, 16 strains came from subjects with primary Sjögren's syndrome, and nine had been isolated from subjects with normal salivary secretion rate. As can be seen in Table 6.3, about 50 % of the strains were able to lower the pH ≤5.5 using mannitol and sorbitol and 36 % using xylitol. In subjects with hyposalivation and very high counts of lactobacilli, it is possible that frequent intake of products containing sugar alcohols will enhance the growth of lactobacilli.

## Oral Mucosal Infections

Hyposalivation patients show an increased number of oral mucosal infections. Microorganisms associated with oral mucosal infections are *Candida* spp., *S. aureus*, Gram-negative anaerobic rods, and enterococci. The frequency and number of *C. albicans* is increased in most types of hyposalivation [19, 22, 27, 29, 30]. *C. albicans* is a dimorphic fungus, which is present in the globular yeast form and rodlike hyphal form. In general, the yeast form is less virulent but disseminates easier than the hyphal form. The hyphal form is more adhesive and able to penetrate the tissues.

A high number of individuals carry *C. albicans* without any complaints [73–75]. When the oral defense is disturbed, *C. albicans* can outgrow and cause infections. This may be the case in denture wearers, people undergoing antibiotic treatment, immunocompromised people or people under immunosuppressive therapy, and subjects with hyposalivation. There are several forms of oral candidosis, but it is usually characterized by the presence of white pseudomembranous plaques on an erythematous surface or erythematous lesions [74]. Oral immunity against candidosis is largely cell mediated. In people receiving immunosuppressive therapy, candidosis is one of the side effects, and candidosis is one of the first manifestations of HIV infection. Saliva, on the other hand, is also important in protection against candidosis. Antimicrobial peptides in saliva kill *C. albicans*, and salivary statherin keeps *C. albicans* in the non-virulent yeast form [76, 77]. *C. albicans* colonization is increased in subjects with hyposalivation, both the number of colonized individuals, as well as the microbial counts, and also the occurrence of oral candidosis is increased [19, 78]. After radiation therapy of the head and neck region, a temporal shift to non-albicans *Candida* species occurs, such as *C. glabrata*, *C. tropicalis*, *C. dubliniensis*, and *C. krusei* [79, 80]. *Candida* counts were higher in subjects with less than 6 months hyposalivation than in subjects with longer than 6 months hyposalivation [78]. Probably, in the long term, some immune defense is triggered thus reducing the numbers of *Candida*. However, preliminary results show an increased prevalence of *C. albicans* in the supragingival plaque in subjects with radiation-induced hyposalivation over time.

As mentioned earlier, also bacteria can be involved in or cause oral mucosal infections. *S. aureus* is a Gram-positive coccoid bacteria which belongs to the normal flora on the skin, intestinal tract, and nasopharynx. *S. aureus* is associated with, for example, wound infections and food poisoning. Gram-negative anaerobic rods include *Escherichia* and *Klebsiella*, which belong to the intestinal flora. Enterococci are Gram-positive coccoid bacteria, which are resistant to many antibiotics and antiseptics and therefore difficult to get rid of. Enterococci were frequently found especially in subjects with radiation-induced hyposalivation [22]. Microbial diagnosis is therefore important so that the right treatment can be given.

**Table 6.3** pH after 24 h of fermentation of mannitol, sorbitol, and xylitol for different *Lactobacillus* species

| Species | Mannitol | Sorbitol | Xylitol |
|---|---|---|---|
| *L. fermentum* ($n=12$) | 6.4±0.6[a] (5.1–6.9) (15) | 6.5±0.5[a](5.5–7.0) (8) | 6.5±0.4 (5.7–7.0) (8) |
| *L. casei* ($n=10$) | 5.2±0.7 (4.7–6.8) (80) | 5.6±0.7 (5.0–7.1) (80) | 5.7±0.6 (5.2–7.0) (70) |
| *L. rhamnosus* ($n=8$) | 5.1±0.4 (4.8–6.0) (88) | 5.3±0.3 (5.0–6.1) (88) | 5.6±0.3 (5.2–6.1) (38) |
| *L. paracasei* ($n=7$) | 5.2±0.8 (4.6–6.9) (86) | 5.3±0.7[b](4.7–6.8) (86) | 5.6±0.6 (4.9–6.9) (57) |
| *L. salivarius* ($n=2$) | 5.5 (4.9–6.0) (50) | 5.4 (5.0–5.8) (50) | 5.7 (5.3–6.1) (50) |
| *L. acidophilus* ($n=1$) | 6.2 | 5.9 | 6.3 |
| *L. gasseri* ($n=1$) | 6.1 | 6.1 | 6.2 |
| Unidentified ($n=9$) | 5.9±0.8 (4.8–6.9) (33) | 6.1±0.7 (5.2–7.0) (22) | 6.2±0.6 (5.4–6.9) (33) |
| All 50 strains | 5.7±0.8 (4.7–6.9) (52) | 5.8±0.7 (4.8–7.1) (50) | 6.0±0.6 (5.1–7.0) (36) |

Data from Almståhl et al. [72]

Mean ± SD, and range are presented as well as proportions of strains giving a pH ≤5.5 (in parenthesis)

[a]Higher compared with *L. rhamnosus* and *L. casei* ($p<0.01$ for both)

[b]Lower compared with *L. paracasei* ($p<0.01$)

## Gingivitis and Periodontitis

Decreased salivary secretion is thought to promote plaque accumulation and thus gingival inflammation. However, both the degree of gingivitis and the numbers of microorganisms associated with gingivitis were comparable with healthy controls [22, 28, 30, 31]. The periodontal pathogens *P. gingivalis* and *A. actinomycetemcomitans* were rarely detected in hyposalivated subjects [22, 27, 30]. Probably the increase in acid-producing bacteria in many subjects with hyposalivation suppresses bacteria associated with gingivitis and periodontitis. A contributing factor to the low level of gingivitis in these studies might have been that those willing to participate were interested in their oral health and had a good oral hygiene. They visited the dental clinic at least once a year and often more frequently. In other studies it was shown that subjects with primary Sjögren's syndrome in the long term, after 8.8 years, showed more clinical attachment loss and leakage of gingival crevicular fluid [81, 82].

## Effect of Treatment of Xerostomia on the Oral Microflora

There are several types of products for relieving the symptoms of dry mouth, such as tablets, chewing gum, spray, and gel. For subjects whose salivary glands still function, stimulation of their own saliva production is the most effective regimen. Sugar-free chewing gum is one of the safest and easiest saliva-stimulating agents. It stimulates the salivary glands both through chewing and taste, which is usually menthol-like. Some people use tablets or candies with acidic taste, but these are not recommended because of their erosive potential. Pharmaceutical saliva-stimulating agents like cevimeline and pilocarpine are effective but may have adverse systemic side effects.

Toothpastes, chewing gum, and products for relieving dry mouth may contain sugar substitutes like mannitol, sorbitol, and xylitol. In an in vitro study, these sugar alcohols were fermented by *Lactobacillus* strains isolated from the supragingival plaque from subjects with hyposalivation [72] (Table 6.3). Whether this also happens in vivo remains to be investigated.

## The Effect of Artificial Saliva on the Oral Microflora

For subjects who are unable to produce saliva or have a very low salivary secretion rate, the use of artificial saliva can be an option to relieve the symptoms of oral dryness. There are also sprays working in the same way or gels that are mostly used during the night.

These substitutes try to mimic the composition and properties of the natural saliva with the aim to relief dry mouth complaints and to protect the oral tissues against microbial infections that may result in tooth decay or candidosis [83]. Numerous saliva substitutes exist, varying in viscosity, base substance, and therapeutic additions. Base substance may consist of pig gastric mucins, bovine submaxillary mucins, carboxymethylcellulose, or xanthan gum. Especially both types of mucins may be used as substrates by dental plaque bacteria [84, 85]. It was suggested that these mucin-containing substitutes might add in restoring the normal oral microflora [86], but this was not supported by experimental data. Coating of hydroxyapatite surfaces with pig gastric mucin, bovine submaxillary mucin, or carboxymethylcellulose led to significantly lower numbers of adherent bacteria than pellicles formed from human saliva [87]. Most saliva substitutes have therapeutic additives that should suppress microbial growth or kill bacteria. Caution should be taken when applying these additives, because, just like natural saliva, artificial saliva is swallowed and comes into the digestive system. Aggressive antimicrobials might lead to a disturbed microflora in the gastrointestinal tract. Several saliva substitutes contain antimicrobial components also found in human saliva, like lysozyme, lactoferrin, and lactoperoxidase [88]. In vitro these products inhibited the growth of oral microorganisms and *C. albicans*, but there was limited effect on microbial counts in vivo [88–92].

**Conclusions**

Hyposalivation changes the oral microbiome, which corresponds to the degree of hyposalivation. Especially acidophilic lactobacilli, *S. mutans*, and *C. albicans* are increased which, combined with a decreased protection by saliva, adds to an increased risk for caries and mucosal infections. With modern techniques like pyrosequencing, the microbiome of the healthy oral cavity has been described. Application of these techniques in studies of hyposalivated subjects offers excellent opportunities to further increase our knowledge about the changes in the microflora in the dry mouth. There is a need for products normalizing the oral microflora and thereby decreasing the risk of oral diseases in subjects with hyposalivation.

## References

1. Tschoppe P, Wolgin ABM, Pischon N, Kielbassa AM. Etiologic factors of hyposalivation and consequences for oral health. Quintessence Int. 2010;41:321–33.
2. Turner RJ, Sugiya H. Understanding salivary fluid and protein secretion. Oral Dis. 2002;8:3–11.
3. Dewhirst FE, Chen T, Izard J, Paster BJ, Tanner AC, Yu WH, Lakshmanan A, Wade WG. The human oral microbiome. J Bacteriol. 2010;192:5002–17.
4. Zaura E, Keijser BJF, Huse SM, Crielaard W. Defining the healthy "core microbiome" of oral microbial communities. BMC Microbiol. 2009;9:259.
5. Costello EK, Lauber CL, Hamady M, Fierer N, Gordon JI, Knight R. Bacterial community variation in human body habitats across space and time. Science. 2009;326:1694–7.
6. Wade WG. The oral microbiome in health and disease. Pharmacol Res. 2013;69:137–43.
7. Kolenbrander PE. Multispecies communities: interspecies interactions influence growth on saliva as sole nutritional source. Int J Oral Sci. 2011;3:49–54.
8. Wickström C, Herzberg MC, Beighton D, Svensater G. Proteolytic degradation of human salivary MUC5B by dental biofilms. Microbiology. 2009;155:2866–72.
9. van der Hoeven JS, van den Kieboom CWA, Camp PJM. Utilization of mucin by oral *Streptococcus* species. Antonie Van Leeuwenhoek. 1990;57:165–72.

10. Biyikoglu B, Ricker A, Diaz PI. Strain-specific colonization patterns and serum modulation of multi-species oral biofilm development. Anaerobe. 2012;18:459–70.
11. Rudiger SG, Dahlen G, Carlen A. Pellicle and early dental plaque in periodontitis patients before and after surgical pocket elimination. Acta Odontol Scand. 2012;70:615–21.
12. Gibbons RJ. Role of adhesion in microbial colonization of host tissues: a contribution of oral microbiology. J Dent Res. 1996;75:866–70.
13. Li J, Helmerhorst EJ, Leone CW, Troxler RF, Yaskell T, Haffajee AD, Socransky SS, Oppenheim FG. Identification of early microbial colonizers in human dental biofilm. J Appl Microbiol. 2004;97:1311–8.
14. Kolenbrander PE, Palmer Jr RJ, Rickard AH, Jakubovics NS, Chalmers NI, Diaz PI. Bacterial interactions and successions during plaque development. Periodontol 2000. 2006;42:47–79.
15. Nobbs AH, Jenkinson HF, Jakubovics NS. Stick to your gums: mechanisms of oral microbial adherence. J Dent Res. 2011;90:1271–8.
16. Davison G, Allgrove J, Gleeson M. Salivary antimicrobial peptides (LL-37 and alpha-defensins HNP1-3), antimicrobial and IgA responses to prolonged exercise. Eur J Appl Physiol. 2009;106:277–84.
17. Brown LR, Dreizen S, Handler S, Johnston DA. Effect of radiation-induced xerostomia on human oral microflora. J Dent Res. 1975;54:740–50.
18. Llory H, Dammron A, Gioanni M, Frank RM. Some population changes in oral anaerobic microorganisms, *Streptococcus mutans* and yeasts following irradiation of the salivary glands. Caries Res. 1972;6:298–311.
19. Almståhl A, Wikström M, Stenberg I, Jakobsson A, Fagerberg-Mohlin B. Oral microbiota associated with hyposalivation of different origins. Oral Microbiol Immunol. 2003;18:1–8.
20. Grotz KA, Genitsariotis S, Vehling D, Al-Nawas B. Long-term oral Candida colonization, mucositis and salivary function after head and neck radiotherapy. Support Care Cancer. 2003;11:717–21.
21. Al-Nawas B, Grotz KA. Prospective study of the long term change of the oral flora after radiation therapy. Support Care Cancer. 2006;14:291–6.
22. Almståhl A, Wikström M, Fagerberg-Mohlin B. Microflora in oral ecosystems in subjects with radiation-induced hyposalivation. Oral Dis. 2008;14:541–9.
23. Hu YJ, Shao ZY, Wang Q, Jiang YT, Ma R, Tang ZS, Liu Z, Liang JP, Huang ZW. Exploring the dynamic core microbiome of plaque microbiota during head-and-neck radiotherapy using pyrosequencing. PLoS One. 2013;8:e56343.
24. Lundström IM, Lindström FD. Subjective and clinical oral symptoms in patients with primary Sjögren's syndrome. Clin Exp Rheumatol. 1995;13:725–31.
25. Kolavic SA, Gibson G, Al-Hashimi I, Guo IY. The level of cariogenic micro-organisms in patients with Sjögren's syndrome. Spec Care Dentist. 1997;17:65–9.
26. Leung WK, Jin LJ, Yam WC, Samaranayake LP. Oral colonization of aerobic and facultatively anaerobic gram-negative rods and cocci in irradiated, dentate, xerostomic individuals. Oral Microbiol Immunol. 2001;16:1–9.
27. Almståhl A, Wikström M, Kroneld U. Microflora in oral ecosystems in primary Sjögren's syndrome. J Rheumatol. 2001;28:1007–13.
28. Almståhl A, Kroneld U, Tarkowski A, Wikström M. Oral microbial flora in Sjögren's syndrome. J Rheumatol. 1999;26:110–4.
29. Leung KC, Leung WK, McMillan AS. Supra-gingival microbiota in Sjögren's syndrome. Clin Oral Investig. 2007;11:415–23.
30. Almståhl A, Wikström M. Microflora in oral ecosystems in subjects with hyposalivation due to medicines or of unknown origin. Oral Health Prev Dent. 2005;3:67–76.
31. Almståhl A, Wikström M. Oral microflora in subjects with reduced salivary secretion. J Dent Res. 1999;78:1410–6.
32. Eliasson L, Almståhl A, Lingstrom P, Wikström M, Carlen A. Minor gland saliva flow rate and proteins in subjects with hyposalivation due to Sjögren's syndrome and radiation therapy. Arch Oral Biol. 2005;50:293–9.

33. Almståhl A, Kareem KL, Carlen A, Wardh I, Lingstrom P, Wikström M. A prospective study on oral microbial flora and related variables in dentate dependent elderly residents. Gerodontology. 2012;29:e1011–8.
34. Bergmans DC, Bonten MJ, Gaillard CA, Paling JC, van der Geest S, van Tiel FH, Beysens AJ, de Leeuw PW, Stobberingh EE. Prevention of ventilator-associated pneumonia by oral decontamination: a prospective, randomized, double-blind, placebo-controlled study. Am J Respir Crit Care Med. 2001;164:382–8.
35. Scannapieco FA. Pneumonia in nonambulatory patients. The role of oral bacteria and oral hygiene. J Am Dent Assoc. 2006;137(Suppl):21S–5.
36. Scannapieco FA, Bush RB, Paju S. Associations between periodontal disease and risk for nosocomial bacterial pneumonia and chronic obstructive pulmonary disease. A systematic review. Ann Periodontol. 2003;8:54–69.
37. Scannapieco FA, Rethman MP. The relationship between periodontal diseases and respiratory diseases. Dent Today. 2003;22:79–83.
38. Labeau SO, Van de Vyver K, Brusselaers N, Vogelaers D, Blot SI. Prevention of ventilator-associated pneumonia with oral antiseptics: a systematic review and meta-analysis. Lancet Infect Dis. 2011;11:845–54.
39. Labeau SO, Blot SI. Toothbrushing for preventing ventilator-associated pneumonia. Crit Care. 2013;17:417.
40. Marsh PD. Are dental diseases examples of ecological catastrophes? Microbiology. 2003;149:279–94.
41. Marsh PD. Dental diseases–are these examples of ecological catastrophes? Int J Dent Hyg. 2006;4 Suppl 1:3–10.
42. Guggenheimer J, Moore PA. Xerostomia: etiology, recognition and treatment. J Am Dent Assoc. 2003;134:61–9.
43. Petersson GH, Twetman S, Bratthall D. Evaluation of a computer program for caries risk assessment in schoolchildren. Caries Res. 2002;36:327–40.
44. Nieuw Amerongen AV, Oderkerk CH, Driessen AA. Role of mucins from human whole saliva in the protection of tooth enamel against demineralization in vitro. Caries Res. 1987;21:297–309.
45. Pramanik R, Osailan SM, Challacombe SJ, Urquhart D, Proctor GB. Protein and mucin retention on oral mucosal surfaces in dry mouth patients. Eur J Oral Sci. 2010;118:245–53.
46. Edgar WM, Higham SM, Manning RH. Saliva stimulation and caries prevention. Adv Dent Res. 1994;8:239–45.
47. Almståhl A, Wikström M. Electrolytes in stimulated whole saliva in individuals with hyposalivation of different origins. Arch Oral Biol. 2003;48:337–44.
48. Lingstrom P, Birkhed D. Plaque pH and oral retention after consumption of starchy snack products at normal and low salivary secretion rate. Acta Odontol Scand. 1993;51:379–88.
49. Johansson AK, Lingstrom P, Birkhed D. Effect of soft drinks on proximal plaque pH at normal and low salivary secretion rates. Acta Odontol Scand. 2007;65:352–6.
50. Watanabe S, Dawes C. The effects of different foods and concentrations of citric-acid on the flow-rate of whole saliva in man. Arch Oral Biol. 1988;33:1–5.
51. Rudney JD, Ji Z, Larson CJ. The prediction of saliva swallowing frequency in humans from estimates of salivary flow rate and the volume of saliva swallowed. Arch Oral Biol. 1995;40:507–12.
52. Siqueira WL, Custodio W, McDonald EE. New insights into the composition and functions of the acquired enamel pellicle. J Dent Res. 2012;91:1110–8.
53. Ruxton CH, Gardner EJ, McNulty HM. Is sugar consumption detrimental to health? A review of the evidence 1995–2006. Crit Rev Food Sci Nutr. 2010;50:1–19.
54. Tong HC, Gao XJ, Dong XZ. Non-mutans streptococci in patients receiving radiotherapy in the head and neck area. Caries Res. 2003;37:261–6.
55. Brunstrom JM. Effects of mouth dryness on drinking behavior and beverage acceptability. Physiol Behav. 2002;76:423–9.
56. Soto-Rojas AE, Kraus A. The oral side of Sjögren syndrome. Diagnosis and treatment. A review. Arch Med Res. 2002;33:95–106.

57. Hede B, Petersen PE. Self-assessment of dental health among Danish noninstitutionalized psychiatric patients. Spec Care Dentist. 1992;12:33–6.
58. Brand HS, Dun SN, Nieuw Amerongen AV. Ecstasy (MDMA) and oral health. Br Dent J. 2008;204:77–81.
59. Takahashi N, Nyvad B. The role of bacteria in the caries process: ecological perspectives. J Dent Res. 2011;90:294–303.
60. Granath L, Cleaton-Jones P, Fatti LP, Grossman ES. Salivary lactobacilli explain dental caries better than salivary mutans streptococci in 4–5-year-old children. Scand J Dent Res. 1994;102:319–23.
61. Zickert I, Emilson CG, Krasse B. *Streptococcus mutans*, lactobacilli and dental health in 13–14-year-old Swedish children. Community Dent Oral Epidemiol. 1982;10:77–81.
62. Kohler B, Bjarnason S. Mutans streptococci, lactobacilli and caries prevalence in 11- and 12-year-old Icelandic children. Community Dent Oral Epidemiol. 1987;15:332–5.
63. Shi S, Zhao Y, Hayashi Y, Yakushiji M, Machida Y. A study of the relationship between caries activity and the status of dental caries: application of the Dentocult LB method. Chin J Dent Res. 1999;2:34–7.
64. Eliasson L, Carlen A, Almståhl A, Wikström M, Lingstrom P. Dental plaque pH and micro-organisms during hyposalivation. J Dent Res. 2006;85:334–8.
65. Almståhl A, Carlen A, Eliasson L, Lingstrom P. *Lactobacillus* species in supragingival plaque in subjects with hyposalivation. Arch Oral Biol. 2010;55:255–9.
66. Stamatova I, Meurman JH. Probiotics: health benefits in the mouth. Am J Dent. 2009;22:329–38.
67. Twetman S. Are we ready for caries prevention through bacteriotherapy? Braz Oral Res. 2012;26 Suppl 1:64–70.
68. Bernardeau M, Vernoux JP. Overview of differences between microbial feed additives and probiotics for food regarding regulation, growth promotion effects and health properties and consequences for extrapolation of farm animal results to humans. Clin Microbiol Infect. 2013;19:321–30.
69. Petersson LG, Magnusson K, Hakestam U, Baigi A, Twetman S. Reversal of primary root caries lesions after daily intake of milk supplemented with fluoride and probiotic lactobacilli in older adults. Acta Odontol Scand. 2011;69:321–7.
70. Krasse P, Carlsson B, Dahl C, Paulsson A, Nilsson A, Sinkiewicz G Decreased gum bleeding and reduced gingivitis by the probiotic Lactobacillus reuteri. Swed Dent J. 2006;30:55–60.
71. Bosch M, Nart J, Audivert S, Bonachera MA, Alemany AS, Fuentes MC, Cune J. Isolation and characterization of probiotic strains for improving oral health. Arch Oral Biol. 2012;57:539–49.
72. Almståhl A, Lingstrom P, Eliasson L, Carlen A. Fermentation of sugars and sugar alcohols by plaque *Lactobacillus* strains. Clin Oral Investig. 2013;17:1465–70.
73. Cannon RD, Chaffin WL. Oral colonization by *Candida albicans*. Crit Rev Oral Biol Med. 1999;10:359–83.
74. Williams D, Lewis M. Pathogenesis and treatment of oral candidosis. J of Oral Microbiol. 2011;3: 5771 DOI: 10.3402/jom.v3i0.5771.
75. Williams DW, Kuriyama T, Silva S, Malic S, Lewis MA. *Candida* biofilms and oral candidosis: treatment and prevention. Periodontol 2000. 2011;55:250–65.
76. den Hertog AL, van Marle J, van Veen HA, van't Hof W, Bolscher JG, Veerman EC, Nieuw Amerongen AV. Candidacidal effects of two antimicrobial peptides: histatin 5 causes small membrane defects, but LL-37 causes massive disruption of the cell membrane. Biochem J. 2005;388:689–95.
77. Leito JT, Ligtenberg AJ, Nazmi K, Veerman EC. Identification of salivary components that induce transition of hyphae to yeast in *Candida albicans*. FEMS Yeast Res. 2009;9:1102–10.
78. Guobis Z, Kareiviene V, Baseviciene N, Paipaliene P, Niedzelskiene I, Sabalys G, Kubilius R, Gervickas A. Microflora of the oral cavity in patients with xerostomia. Medicina (Kaunas). 2011;47:646–51.

79. Redding SW. The role of yeasts other than *Candida albicans* in oropharyngeal candidiasis. Curr Opin Infect Dis. 2001;14:673–7.
80. Redding SW, Dahiya MC, Kirkpatrick WR, Coco BJ, Patterson TF, Fothergill AW, Rinaldi MG, Thomas Jr CR. *Candida glabrata* is an emerging cause of oropharyngeal candidiasis in patients receiving radiation for head and neck cancer. Oral Surg Oral Med Oral Pathol Oral Radiol Endod. 2004;97:47–52.
81. Antoniazzi RP, Miranda LA, Zanatta FB, Islabao AG, Gustafsson A, Chiapinotto GA, Oppermann RV. Periodontal conditions of individuals with Sjögren's syndrome. J Periodontol. 2009;80:429–35.
82. Rhodus NL, Michalowicz BS. Periodontal status and sulcular *Candida albicans* colonization in patients with primary Sjögren's Syndrome. Quintessence Int. 2005;36:228–33.
83. Hahnel S, Behr M, Handel G, Burgers R. Saliva substitutes for the treatment of radiation-induced xerostomia–a review. Support Care Cancer. 2009;17:1331–43.
84. van der Hoeven JS, Camp PJM. Synergistic degradation of mucin by *Streptococcus oralis* and *Streptococcus sanguis* in mixed chemostat cultures. J Dent Res. 1991;70:1041–4.
85. Wong L, Sissons CH. Human dental plaque microcosm biofilms: effect of nutrient variation on calcium phosphate deposition and growth. Arch Oral Biol. 2007;52:280–9.
86. Weerkamp AH, Wagner K, Vissink A, Gravenmade EJ. Effect of the application of a mucin-based saliva substitute on the oral microflora of xerostomic patients. J Oral Pathol. 1987;16:474–8.
87. Wolinsky LE, Seto B, Cerveny R. Effect of saliva substitutes upon binding of selected oral bacteria to hydroxyapatite. Caries Res. 1985;19:507–11.
88. Sugiura Y, Soga Y, Tanimoto I, Kokeguchi S, Nishide S, Kono K, Takahashi K, Fujii N, Ishimaru F, Tanimoto M, Yamabe K, Tsutani S, Nishimura F, Takashiba S. Antimicrobial effects of the saliva substitute, Oralbalance, against microorganisms from oral mucosa in the hematopoietic cell transplantation period. Support Care Cancer. 2008;16:421–4.
89. Kirstila V, Lenander-Lumikari M, Soderling E, Tenovuo J. Effects of oral hygiene products containing lactoperoxidase, lysozyme, and lactoferrin on the composition of whole saliva and on subjective oral symptoms in patients with xerostomia. Acta odontol Scan. 1999;54:391–7.
90. Epstein JB, Stevenson-Moore P. A clinical comparative trial of saliva substitutes in radiation-induced salivary gland hypofunction. Spec Care Dentist. 1992;12:21–3.
91. Gil-Montoya JA, Guardia-Lopez I, Gonzalez-Moles MA. Evaluation of the clinical efficacy of a mouthwash and oral gel containing the antimicrobial proteins lactoperoxidase, lysozyme and lactoferrin in elderly patients with dry mouth–a pilot study. Gerodontology. 2008;25:3–9.
92. Sugiura Y, Soga Y, Yamabe K, Tsutani S, Tanimoto I, Maeda H, Kokeguchi S, Fujii N, Ishimaru F, Tanimoto M, Nishimura F, Takashiba S. Total bacterial counts on oral mucosa after using a commercial saliva substitute in patients undergoing hematopoietic cell transplantation. Support Care Cancer. 2010;18:395–8.

# Subjective Aspects of Dry Mouth

# 7

W. Murray Thomson

**Abstract**

Xerostomia is not a trivial condition: it affects the day-to-day lives of sufferers in important ways. Appropriate definition and accurate measurement are critical for better understanding, monitoring and treatment of xerostomia. This chapter describes and evaluates the various measurement approaches. These range from single-item methods to multi-item summated rating scales. All have advantages and disadvantages. The one which is chosen depends on the use to which the data will be put, the need to minimise respondent burden, the ability to make comparisons with the findings of others and the research question being investigated.

## Defining Dry Mouth: What Are We Talking About?

Much of the literature on dry mouth either fails to adequately define the condition or is predicated on the assumption that everyone who feels dry mouth has demonstrably low salivary flow and everyone with low flow suffers the symptoms of dry mouth. Dry mouth has two possible manifestations. *Xerostomia* is the subjective feeling of dry mouth and can therefore be assessed only by directly questioning individuals [10]. *Salivary gland hypofunction* (SGH) results in salivary output (flow rate) which is lower than normal; it can therefore be determined by sialometry [21]. Individuals whose salivary flow rate is below a designated clinical threshold are categorised as having SGH. Given these definitions, xerostomia is a symptom, and SGH is a sign (a sign is observed by the clinician; a symptom can be detected only by asking the patient). The empirical evidence suggests that the two are not

W.M. Thomson, BSc, BDS, MA, MComDent, PhD
Dental Epidemiology and Public Health, Oral Sciences, Faculty of Dentistry, Sir John Walsh Research Institute, The University of Otago
280 Great King St, Dunedin, Otago 9054, New Zealand
e-mail: murray.thomson@otago.ac.nz



G. Carpenter (ed.), *Dry Mouth: A Clinical Guide on Causes, Effects and Treatments*, DOI 10.1007/978-3-642-55154-3_7

necessarily concurrent. For example, an epidemiological study of older South Australians found that approximately one in five had either xerostomia or SGH but that the two coincided in only one-sixth of those with either condition [31]. Thus, it is important to be specific when describing the occurrence of dry mouth. This chapter deals with the measurement and occurrence of xerostomia, the subjective manifestation of dry mouth.

## Principles of (and Challenges in) Subjective Measurement

By definition, measuring symptoms requires asking the individual: self-report is the only method available. Eight important attributes of self-report measures have been described [28], and they apply just as much to measuring xerostomia as they do to measuring entities such as oral-health-related quality of life. Those important attributes are having a conceptual model, reliability, validity, responsiveness, interpretability, respondent and administrative burden, alternative forms and cross-cultural applicability. A *conceptual model* is essential: any measure which is used should have a sound theoretical underpinning. That is, it should be based on a thorough understanding of the entity which is being measured [43]. This makes it more likely that the measurements made will be clinically meaningful and relevant to the condition being assessed. The notion of *reliability* is concerned with both repeatability (also known as reproducibility) and precision. Repeatability encompasses both (a) the stability of measurements over time (assuming that the entity being measured has not changed during that time) and (b) intra- and inter-rater agreement. Precision encompasses the intercorrelation of the various items which make up a multi-item scale. *Validity* is defined as the degree to which the instrument measures what it purports to measure; it includes domains of relevance to its intended use, appropriate score gradients in relation to a 'gold standard' measure and the ability to relate the score range to theoretical understanding of the construct being measured (and interpret it accordingly). The other characteristics are also important but are less so for the current discussion.

The individual can be asked about his/her dry mouth symptoms in a number of ways, such as using a single-item (known as a 'global' item) method or any one of a number of multi-item methods. Each of these is considered below.

## Single-Item Approaches

A global item is a single question or statement which requires the respondent to integrate their perceptions, experiences and behaviours in respect of the entity being measured and to come up with an overall summary judgement. It has been said that such single-item measures integrate subjective perceptions and objective observations into a unified summary measure [17, 42]. Thus, a global item on dry mouth would require the individual to consider all of those aspects of the condition in order to arrive at a summary judgement of his/her dry mouth status. Examples of the global dry mouth questions which have been used are presented in Table 7.1.

**Table 7.1** Single (global) items which have been used in assessing xerostomia

| Item | Response options | Author(s) first using it | Utility? |
|---|---|---|---|
| Does your mouth feel distinctly dry? | Yes/no | Osterberg et al. [24] | Questionable |
| Do you sip liquids to aid in swallowing dry foods? | Yes/no | Fox et al. [10] | Acceptable[a] |
| Does your mouth feel dry when eating a meal? | Yes/no | Fox et al. [10] | Acceptable[a] |
| Do you have difficulties swallowing any foods? | Yes/no | Fox et al. [10] | Acceptable[a] |
| Does the amount of saliva in your mouth seem to be too little, too much, or you don't notice it? | Yes/no | Fox et al. [10] | Acceptable[a] |
| Do you feel dryness in the mouth at any time? | Not actually reported, but likely to be yes/no | Fure and Zickert [11] | Questionable |
| Do you have mouth dryness? | Yes/no | Osterberg et al. [25] | Questionable |
| Is your mouth sometimes dry? | Yes/no | Gilbert et al. [13] | Questionable |
| How often does your mouth feel dry? | Never, occasionally, frequently or always[b] | Thomson et al. [30] | Acceptable |
| During the last 4 weeks, have you had any of the following: | ….dryness of mouth? | Locker (1993) [45] | Acceptable |
| Does your mouth feel dry? | Yes/no—used as a gate to 3 others | Narhi [20] | Questionable |
| Does your mouth usually feel dry? | Not actually reported, but likely to be yes/no | Nederfors et al. [22] | Acceptable |
| Have you had a dry mouth sensation every day for the last 6 months? | Yes/no—used as a gate to 3 others | Carda et al. [3] | Questionable |

[a]With the caveat that the validity of these measures was demonstrated only with sufferers of *both* xerostomia and SGH; their utility for identifying all xerostomia sufferers remains unclear.
[b]Xerostomics are identified as those responding 'Frequently' or 'Always'.

About half of those in the table appear to be of questionable utility (although it may perhaps be that something had been lost in the translation from the original language to English). For example, that used by Osterberg et al. [24] would most likely cause the respondent to enquire along the lines of 'Do you mean now, or usually?' (as would the one reported by the same group in 1992). It could be argued that the one used by Fure and Zickert [11] could conceivably result in a prevalence estimate of 100 %, given that everyone is likely to experience transitory dry mouth at some stage. A similar problem is evident with the one reported by Gilbert et al. in 1993 [13], and the one used by Narhi in 1994 [20]. By contrast, that used by Carda et al. [3] may, in fact, be too stringent, tending to underestimate the prevalence of xerostomia.

Of the items which appear to be acceptable, those first described by Fox et al. [10] were actually validated only with people who had low salivary flow rates, and there is some evidence that those people may be only a minority of those who suffer

**Table 7.2** Overview of item content of battery-type approaches to measuring xerostomia

| Authors and year when first used | |
|---|---|
| Locker (2003)[a] | Pai et al. [26][b] |
| Have you had a dry mouth or tongue during the daytime? | The difficulty in speaking due to dryness |
| Difficulty talking | The difficulty in swallowing due to dryness |
| Difficulty swallowing | How much saliva is in your mouth |
| Difficulty chewing | The dryness of your mouth |
| Needed to drink water during the daytime | The dryness of your throat |
| Needed to drink water with meals | The dryness of your lips |
| Needed to chew gum to relieve dryness | The dryness of your tongue |
| | The level of your thirst |
| Response format 'Yes'/'No' | Response format VAS |

[a]All refer to the previous 4 weeks.
[b]All prefixed with 'Rate…'

from xerostomia [32]. There is also the concern that there are four of those questions, and each may result in a different prevalence estimate. The authors gave no guidance as to whether (or how) the four items might be used together as a battery or a scale (see below). To date, there has been no systematic examination of their properties in this respect. The items used by Thomson et al. [30] and Nederfors [22]) may be more valid because they include a temporal component. Someone who reports dry mouth 'Frequently' or 'Always'—or whose mouth usually feels dry—is likely to be a chronic sufferer of the condition. To date, no study has used both measures together.

Global items which measure xerostomia have been used extensively and can be very useful, providing that the appropriate one is used. They can be used alone or in conjunction with multi-item methods, in which case they are very useful in checking the validity of the latter (as described below).

## Multi-Item Approaches

Multi-item approaches to measuring xerostomia include both (a) batteries of items and (b) summated rating scales. Each will be described briefly.

### Batteries of Items

With these, participants respond to each item in a list, usually with a 'yes'/'no' response format. At the analysis stage, the number of positive responses is counted and used as an index score, either as a simple count or after recoding of that count into ordinal categories. Such methods have been used by a number of workers (Table 7.2). For example, [46] used a list of seven questions (sourced from the literature) and a simple 'yes'/'no' response format to assign nursing home residents to the following three groups: no xerostomia (0 positive responses), mild xerostomia (1–2) or marked xerostomia (3–7). The battery was found to have acceptable internal consistency reliability and was able to distinguish respondents with poorer OHRQoL from those with better OHRQoL, but there was no comparison with a global xerostomia item, meaning that no judgement of its validity as a xerostomia scale could be made.

Another such approach is the Challacombe scale [23], which was designed for clinical use as an objective score for oral dryness, based entirely upon the clinical observations of the examining clinician. Strictly speaking, it should not be included here because it purports to measure salivary gland hypofunction and has no subjective aspect; the individual being assessed is not asked about his/her symptoms. However, it is included here for completeness, because it is likely to turn up on any literature search for xerostomia indices. That particular scale appears to be a checklist which has arisen from experienced clinicians' observations over many years. Some clinical validity has been demonstrated, but its utility remains unclear because of the wide range of entities which comprise it. Included in the 10-item checklist are observations on instruments adhering to mucosal surfaces, saliva frothiness, whether saliva pools in the floor of the mouth, tongue appearance, gingival architecture, mucosal appearance, palatal debris and recent experience of root surface caries. The provenance of that combination was not directly specified, but it is likely to have arisen from direct clinical observations by the experienced clinicians who were involved in its development. As with the battery used by Locker, the index score is a simple count of the number of signs observed and can range from 0 to 10. Its initial validation was undertaken against measurements of salivary flow rate and oral mucosal wetness in convenience samples of Sjögren syndrome patients and a comparison group (also a convenience sample) of university staff and rest home residents. The scale showed promising validity, but it should be further examined in population-based samples and against subjective measures of dry mouth. Until that has occurred, its utility remains unclear.

Battery-type approaches can yield meaningful scores and useful data for exploring the determinants of xerostomia. However, a battery of items suffers from the problem of being really just a 'present/absent' checklist of items or issues which may or may not relate to an underlying construct (such as the experience of dry mouth).

A modification of the battery-type approach was that used by Pai et al. [26], who used a battery of eight items, with each scored using a visual analogue scale (VAS). A VAS employs a line upon which the respondent places a mark to indicate the point which represents their position between the two extremes. That particular instrument had eight xerostomia-related items, each of which had a VAS response format (ranging from 0 to 100 mm, with 100 being the worst score). Other than the use of a VAS (rather than a Likert scale, which has ordered categories) for the responses, this is essentially just a variation on the abovementioned two. It is, if anything, more restricted in its use because the individual item scores are not used together. Gerdin et al. [12] used the same VAS instrument to measure xerostomia among Swedish nursing home residents. The point of difference with this particular study was that the individual item VAS scores were then summed to give an overall score (which could range from 0 to 800 scale points). Those scores were then used to allocate respondents to one of two symptom severity categories ('no or weak dry mouth symptoms' or 'symptoms') using a cut-off value determined from responses to the item 'Does your mouth feel dry?' first used by Fox et al. [10]. The resultant scale scores showed strong correlations with other dry mouth self-reports but no association at all with salivary flow rate. Summing the responses from a VAS-type response format is uncommon but has been described as acceptable [7].

A problem with the scales described above is that their constituent items were assembled somewhat arbitrarily, from the literature, clinical experience or a combination of the two. They may have a degree of empirical validity (as evident in score gradients and associations in the hypothesised direction when they are tested clinically), but there may still be a considerable amount of error and unexplained variance which is due to the inclusion of less relevant items (or indeed the omission of others which might have been more useful). This is where summated rating scales have distinct advantages.

## Summated Rating Scales

A summated rating scale is a multi-item scale which purports to measure an underlying construct (known as a 'latent variable'). It is essentially a more refined, focused development of the item battery, with the distinction that the items have all been shown to be correlated with the latent variable and that the number of items in the scale has been demonstrated to be adequate. The idea behind using such a scale is to be able to place respondents on a continuum which represents the range of experience of the entity being measured (from the minimum to the maximum). Everyone should be able to be placed somewhere on that continuum.

Least possible ———————————————————— Most possible

The advantage of using such a scale score is that more subtle differences in health states can be explored; the data are used as a continuous variable rather than as a binary or ordinal variable.

The developmental sequence for such scales involves a fairly standard series of steps: conceptual development, in terms of the underlying theory and models; generation of an item pool, which is a comprehensive list of all issues which are relevant to the domain which it is planned to measure (from the literature, clinical experience, interviews with sufferers, and so on); item pool reduction and psychometric testing (using methods such as exploratory factor analysis to determine whether the items do actually relate to the underlying latent construct); and field testing and validation. Subsequent steps (which are generally useful) may be the development of short-form versions and validation/adaptation for use in cultures other than that in which the measure was first developed.

The Xerostomia Inventory (XI) is such a summated rating scale [31]. It is an 11-item scale (Table 7.3) which was developed during the mid-1990s as part of an investigation into the question of whether medications which cause dry mouth (xerogenic drugs) among older people are associated with great caries experience. At the time, it was realised that there was no satisfactory way of allocating participants to a continuum of symptom experience; that is, to give them a continuous

**Table 7.3** The Xerostomia Inventory—original (XI) and short-form (SXI-D) versions

| Original version[a] | Short-form version[b] |
|---|---|
| I sip liquids to aid in swallowing food | |
| My mouth feels dry when eating a meal | My mouth feels dry when eating a meal |
| I get up at night to drink | |
| My mouth feels dry | My mouth feels dry |
| I have difficulty in eating dry foods | I have difficulty in eating dry foods |
| I suck sweets or cough lollies to relieve dry mouth | |
| I have difficulties swallowing certain foods | I have difficulties swallowing certain foods |
| The skin of my face feels dry | |
| My eyes feel dry | |
| My lips feel dry | My lips feel dry |
| The inside of my nose feels dry | |

[a]Response options: 'Never' (scoring 1), 'Hardly ever' (2), 'Occasionally' (3), 'Frequently' (4) or 'Always' (5)
[b]Response options: 'Never' (scoring 1), 'Occasionally' (2) or 'Often' (3)

score which could capture more subtle interpersonal differences in dry mouth symptoms than a global item with four or five response categories. It was hoped that being able to obtain such a continuous score would then enable such a score's use in multivariate models of caries incidence and increment (the final, somewhat surprising outcome of the study was reported in [34, 35]).

The development of the XI mirrors the abovementioned sequence in most ways. Its conceptual development involved identifying the need for such a scale and fitting that into the context of contemporary knowledge of the condition at that time. It was suspected (but had not yet been confirmed) that the symptoms of dry mouth were only weakly associated with actual salivary flow rates. Item pool generation was undertaken in stages. First, a literature search revealed a number of single items which had been used previously; this informed the development of a framework for semi-structured interviews which were undertaken with four diagnosed long-term sufferers of xerostomia. Content analysis was used to identify dominant themes which were then either developed into new potential XI items—using the interviewees' own words where possible—or used to confirm and/or modify those which had been obtained from the literature. This process resulted in 19 items and ensured the following: (1) those which were used reflected many manifestations of the xerostomia experience; (2) their most appropriate wording was determined; and (3) they were grounded in the experiences of xerostomia sufferers [32].

The 19 items (with response options 'Never', 'Hardly ever', 'Occasionally', 'Frequently', or 'Always') were then field tested in the 5-year data collection phase of the South Australian Dental Longitudinal Study (SADLS), a prospective cohort study of oral health among older people [29]. The XI's development departed somewhat from the usual sequence, in that the item reduction and psychometric testing occurred at the same time as the field testing and validation. The reasons for this were purely pragmatic: there was insufficient time for the items to be tested in another sample prior to the rollout of the 5-year assessments in the SADLS study,

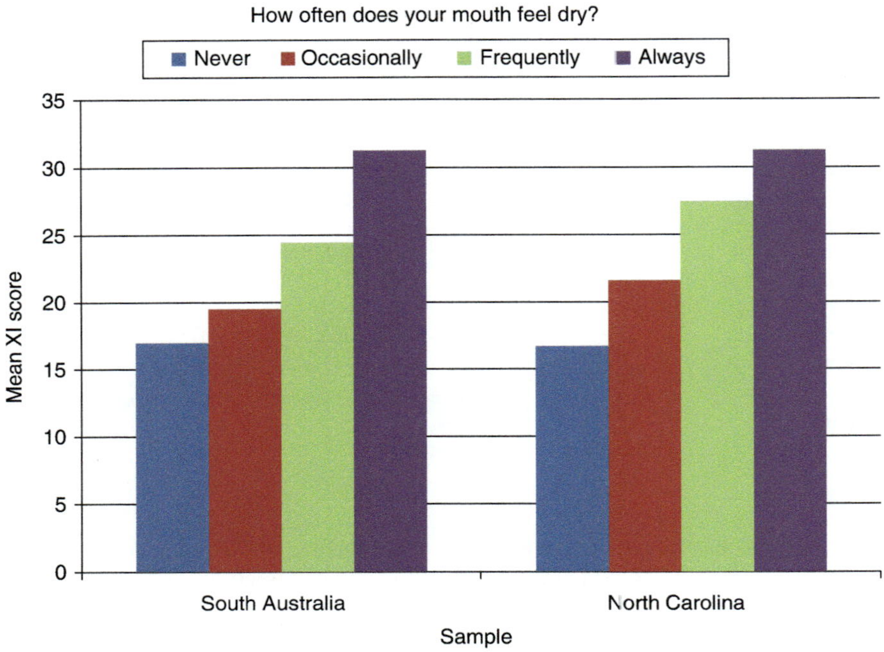


**Fig. 7.1** Validity of the 11-item Xerostomia Inventory, demonstrated in studies in South Australia [31] and North Carolina [27]

and so a not inconsiderable risk was taken. As it turned out, the gamble was justified, with the item reduction and field validation being able to be successfully completed in the same study. Exploratory factor analysis identified 11 items which appeared to represent the underlying latent construct of xerostomia; these were a mix of experiential and behavioural items, although some appeared to have more direct connection to dry mouth than others did. Among the latter were items pertaining to the eyes, the nose or the facial skin.

The concurrent validity of the XI was confirmed in the existence of a strong ascending gradient of mean scores across the response categories of the standard dry mouth question [30] which had been used at the same time. The original data are presented in Fig. 7.1, along with data from the recent study by Quandt et al. [27], which also demonstrated such a gradient. These data offer support for the scale's validity and mean that researchers and clinicians can be reasonably confident in its ability to discriminate among the various manifestations of xerostomia; that is, to place people accurately on a continuum ranging from no symptoms at all to the worst possible symptoms.

To date, the XI has been translated and used in Dutch [2], Chinese [15], Portuguese [5], Turkish [6] and Spanish [19]. Moreover, a short-form version of the Xerostomia Inventory is now available (Table 7.3). Called the SXI ('Summated Xerostomia Inventory'; [41]), it arose when Dutch researchers wished to use the XI

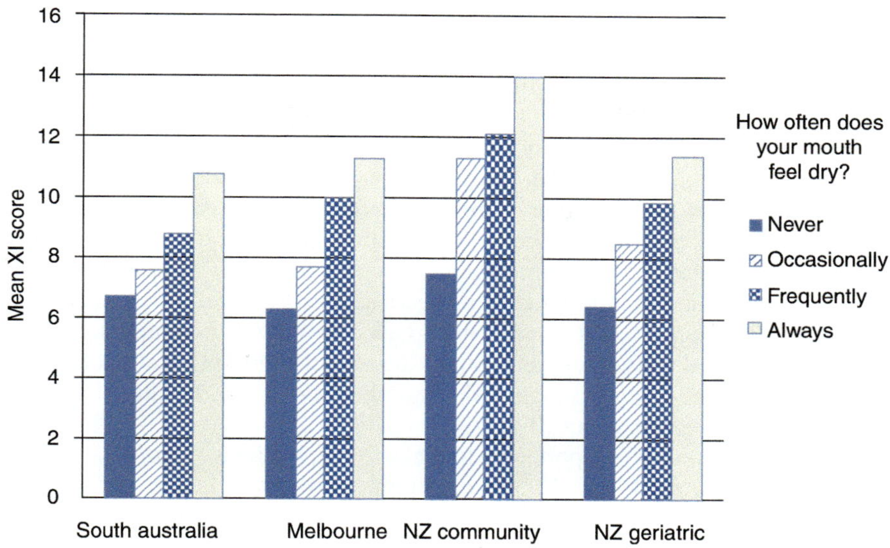


**Fig. 7.2** Validity of the 5-item SXI-D, demonstrated in studies in Australia and New Zealand (Thomson et al. [41]; reprinted with the kind permission of Elsevier Limited)

in a nursing home sample and were worried about its response format and the inclusion of some superfluous item content [44]. Accordingly, they omitted six items and reduced the number of response options from five to three ('Never', scoring 1; 'Occasionally', 2; and 'Often', 5). It was found to have acceptable validity and was easily completed by participants. Subsequently, the availability of data from a number of different countries and centres enabled an international team to investigate the validity of the SXI in Japanese, Australian and New Zealand samples, along with the original Dutch one [41]. Confirmatory factor analysis and reliability analysis confirmed the shorter scale's feasibility, and it was shown to have acceptable criterion-related validity (Fig. 7.2). Because one of the New Zealand samples was longitudinal, the responsiveness of the short-form measure was able to be demonstrated, and the minimally important difference was determined to be 4 scale points. In other words, a change in score over time by 4 or more SXI scale points can be considered to be clinically meaningful. To date, the SXI has also been validated in English, Dutch, Japanese [41] and Chinese [15].

It is important to bear in mind that none of the multi-item methods collects information on feelings of tiredness or anxiety or indeed any psychological or psychiatric traits which might be considered to be important. Researchers or clinicians wishing to explore those aspects should seek the appropriate instrument for doing so and use it concurrently with the xerostomia measure of choice. It is a simple matter to include a number of measures in a single questionnaire; after all, patients or study participants will happily complete a questionnaire without being aware of the specific instrument(s) being used.

## Is Dry Mouth Important?

On first consideration, this seems to be a fatuous question. People who have chronic dry mouth can have problems with speaking, eating and wearing dental prostheses ([4], [16]). Dry mouth is not only common; it affects sufferers' day-to-day lives, with the effects detectable at both the population level (Locker 2003; [37]) and at the individual level [9]. The latter study used a qualitative design to elicit in-depth information on people's experience of the condition and found it to be a miserable burden with devastating and debilitating impacts on well-being. Those effects arose from continual oral discomfort, eating difficulties, poor oral health (which became expensive), inadequate social support and a lack of empathy or commitment from health-care professionals. These, in turn, led to social withdrawal because of speaking difficulties and stigmatisation and restrictions in day-to-day life. Sufferers referred to being unable to enjoy living.

Such observations are supported by findings from quantitative studies. A unique investigation by Quandt et al. [27] of xerostomia and dietary intake among older North Carolina adults found that those with more severe symptoms tended to modify their intake of particular foods, avoiding those which were more difficult to eat, but that this did not affect their actual dietary quality. Locker (2003) investigated xerostomia and oral-health-related quality of life (OHRQoL) in a sample of nursing home residents, and he observed consistently poorer OHRQoL among those with xerostomia. Similar associations were noted in a sample of Swedish nursing home residents [12]. Such an association is not limited to older people either; consistently poorer QHRQoL (across all measured domains of it) was reported for a complete birth cohort of 32-year-olds by Thomson et al. [39]. A similarly strong and consistent association was observed in a nationally representative sample of adult New Zealanders (of all ages) by Benn [1].

Given that xerostomia does appear to be a burden for those who actually have the condition, the next consideration is its prevalence: how common is it? After all, a condition may have marked impacts on sufferers' lives but be relatively rare and thus of no importance at the public health level because its population burden is low. On the other hand, if it is common, a compelling case could be made for it being a public health problem. So, how common is xerostomia? Despite some variation in reported estimates from epidemiological studies of older populations, the prevalence of xerostomia tends to be about 20 %, depending upon how it was defined and measured [36]. Data from younger populations are more scarce; it was reported to be 10 % among 32-year-olds in a birth cohort and 13 % among New Zealanders aged 18 or older, in what is understood to be the only national-level estimate to date [1]. In the latter study, the highest prevalence (26 %) was among those aged 75 or more, but the next highest estimate was for those aged 25–34, at 17 %. The lowest prevalence (5 %) was among those aged 18–24. It therefore does indeed appear that, not only is xerostomia affecting sufferers' lives, but there are enough of those sufferers for the condition to be considered a public health problem as well as a personal one. This means that the condition's accurate measurement is important.

**Conclusion**

In conclusion, dry mouth is an important OHRQoL issue for sufferers, and the appropriate and accurate measurement of xerostomia is critical to better understanding, monitoring and treatment of the condition. A number of measurement instruments are available. Which one is chosen is determined by considerations such as the use to which the data will be put, the need to minimise respondent burden, the ability to make comparisons with the findings of others, and the research question being investigated.

## References

1. Benn A. Xerostomia among adult New Zealanders: a national survey. MComDent thesis. The University of Otago; 2012.
2. Bots CP, Brand HS, Veerman ECI, Korevaar JC, Valentijn-Benz M, Bezemer PD, Valentijn RM, Vos PF, Bijlsma JA, ter Wee PM, Van Amerongen BM, Nieuw Amerongen AV. Chewing gum and a saliva substitute alleviate thirst and xerostomia in patients on hemodialysis. Nephrol Dial Transplant. 2005;20:578–84.
3. Carda C, Mosquera-Lloreda N, Salom L, de Ferraris Gomez ME, Peydro A. Structural and functional salivary disorders in type 2 diabetic patients. Medicina Oral Patologia Oral Y Cirugia Bucal. 2006;11:E309–14.
4. Cassolato SF, Turnbull RS. Xerostomia: clinical aspects and treatment. Gerodontology. 2003;20:64–77.
5. da Mata A, da Silva Marques DN, Freitas F, de Almeida Rato Amaral JP, Trindade R, Barcelos F, Vaz Patto JM. Translation, validation and construct reliability of a Portuguese version of the Xerostomia Inventory. Oral Dis. 2012;18:293–8.
6. Eltas A, Tozoglu U, Keles M, Canakci V. Assessment of oral health in peritoneal dialysis patients with and without diabetes mellitus. Perit Dial Int. 2012;32:81–5.
7. Fayers PM, Machin D. Quality of life: assessment, analysis and interpretation. Chichester: Wiley; 2000.
8. Folke S, Fridlund B, Paulsson G. Views of xerostomia among health care professionals: a qualitative study. J Clin Nurs. 2009;18:791–8.
9. Folke S, Paulsson G, Fridlund B, Söderfeldt B. The subjective meaning of xerostomia—an aggravating misery. Int J Qual Stud Health Well-being. 2009;4:245–55.
10. Fox PC, Busch KA, Baum BJ. Subjective reports of xerostomia and objective measures of salivary gland performance. J Amer Dent Assoc. 1987;115:581–4.
11. Fure S, Zickert I. Salivary conditions and cariogenic microorganisms in 55, 65, and 75-year-old Swedish individuals. Scand J Dent Res. 1990;98:197–210.
12. Gerdin EW, Einarson S, Jonsson M, Aronsson K, Johansson I. Impact of dry mouth conditions on oral health-related quality of life in older people. Gerodontology. 2005;22:219–26.
13. Gilbert GH, Heft MW, Duncan RP. Mouth dryness as reported by older Floridians. Community Dent Oral Epidemiol. 1993;21:390–7.
14. Guyatt GH, Bombardier C, Tugwell PX. Measuring disease-specific quality of life in clinical trials. CMAJ. 1986;134:889–95.
15. He S, Wang J, Li M. Validation of Chinese version of the Summated Xerostomia Inventory (SXI). Qual Life Res. 2013. doi:10.1007/s11136-013-0420-y. in press.
16. Hopcraft MS, Tan C. Xerostomia: an update for clinicians. Aust Dent J. 2010;55:238–44.
17. Kaplan G, Baron-Epel O. What lies behind the subjective evaluation of health status? Soc Sci Med. 2003;56:1669–76.
18. Locker D, Wexler E, Jokovic A. What do older adults' global self-ratings of oral health measure? J Public Health Dent. 2005;65:146–52.

19. Martin-Piedra MA, Aguilar-Salvatierra A, Herrera D, Gomez-Moreno G. Effectiveness of a recent topical sialogogue in the management of drug-induced xerostomia. J Clin Exp Dent. 2011;3:268–77.
20. Närhi TO. Prevalence of subjective feelings of dry mouth in the elderly. J Dent Res. 1994;73:20–5.
21. Navazesh M. Methods for collecting saliva. Ann N Y Acad Sci. 1993;694:72–7.
22. Nederfors T, Isaksson R, Mörnstad H, Dahlöf C. Prevalence of perceived symptoms of dry mouth in an adult Swedish population - relation to age, sex and pharmacotherapy. Community Dent Oral Epidemiol. 1997;25:211–6.
23. Osailan SM, Pramanik R, Shirlaw P, Proctor GB, Challacombe SJ. Clinical assessment of oral dryness: development of a scoring system related to salivary flow and mucosal wetness. Oral Surg Oral Med Oral Pathol Oral Radiol. 2012;114:597–603.
24. Osterberg T, Landahl S, Hedegard B. Salivary flow, saliva, pH and buffering capacity in 70-year-old men and women. J Oral Rehabil. 1984;11:157–70.
25. Osterberg T, Birkhed D, Johansson C, Svanborg A. Longitudinal study of stimulated whole saliva in an elderly population. Scand J Dent Res. 1992;100:340–5.
26. Pai S, Ghezzi EM, Ship JA. Development of a visual analogue scale questionnaire for subjective assessment of salivary dysfunction. Oral Surg Oral Med Oral Pathol Oral Radiol Endod. 2001;91:311–6.
27. Quandt SA, Savoca MR, Leng X, Chen H, Bell RA, Gilbert GH, Anderson AM, Kohrman T, Arcury TA. Dry mouth and dietary quality in older adults in North Carolina. JAGS. 2011;59:439–45.
28. Scientific Advisory Committee of the Medical Outcomes Trust. Assessing health status and quality-of-life instruments: attributes and review criteria. Quality Life Res. 2002;11:193–205.
29. Slade GD, Spencer AJ. Social impact of oral conditions among older adults. Aust Dent J. 1994;39:358–64.
30. Thomson WM, Brown RH, Williams SM. Medication and perception of dry mouth in a population of institutionalised elderly people. N Z Med J. 1993;106:219–21.
31. Thomson WM, Chalmers JM, Spencer AJ, Ketabi M. The occurrence of xerostomia and salivary gland hypofunction in a population-based sample of older South Australians. Spec Care Dent. 1999;19:20–3.
32. Thomson WM, Chalmers JM, Spencer AJ, Williams SM. The Xerostomia Inventory: a multi-item approach to measuring dry mouth. Community Dent Health. 1999;16:12–7.
33. Thomson WM, Williams SM. Further testing of the xerostomia inventory. Oral Surg Oral Med Oral Pathol Oral Radiol Endod. 2000;89:46–50.
34. Thomson WM, Chalmers JM, Spencer AJ, Slade GD. Medication and dry mouth: findings from a cohort study of older people. J Public Health Dent. 2000;60:12–20.
35. Thomson WM, Spencer AJ, Slade GD, Chalmers JM. Is medication a risk factor for dental caries among older people? Evidence from a longitudinal study in South Australia. Community Dent Oral Epidemiol. 2002;30:224–32.
36. Thomson WM. Issues in the epidemiological investigation of dry mouth. Gerodontology. 2005;22:65–76.
37. Thomson WM, Poulton R, Broadbent JM, Al-Kubaisy S. Xerostomia and medications among 32-year-olds. Acta Odont Scand. 2006;64:249–54.
38. Thomson WM, Chalmers JM, Spencer AJ, Slade GD, Carter KD. A longitudinal study of medication exposure and xerostomia among older people. Gerodontology. 2006;23:205–13.
39. Thomson WM, Lawrence HP, Broadbent JM, Poulton R. The impact of xerostomia on oral-health-related quality of life among younger adults. Health Qual Life Outcomes. 2006;4:86. (7pp), http://www.hqlo.com/content/4/1/86.
40. Thomson WM. Measuring change in dry-mouth symptoms over time using the Xerostomia Inventory. Gerodontology. 2007;24:30–5.
41. Thomson WM, van der Putten G-J, de Baat C, Ikebe K, Matsuda K, Enoki K, Hopcraft M, Long G. Shortening the xerostomia inventory. Oral Surg Oral Med Oral Pathol Oral Radiol Endod. 2011;112:322–7.

42. Thomson WM, Mejia GC, Broadbent JM, Poulton R. Construct validity of Locker's global oral health item. J Dent Res. 2012;91:1038–42.
43. Tsakos G, Allen PF, Steele JG, Locker D. Interpreting oral health-related quality of life data. Community Dent Oral Epidemiol. 2012;40:193–200.
44. van der Putten G-J, Brand HS, Schools JMGA, de Baat C. The diagnostic suitability of a xerostomia questionnaire and the association between xerostomia, hyposalivation and medication use in a group of nursing home residents. Clin Oral Investig. 2010;15:185–92.
45. Locker D. Subjective reports of oral dryness in an older adult population. Comm Dent Oral Epidemiol. 1993;21:165–8.
46. Locker D. Dental status, xerostomia and the oral health-related quality of life of an elderly institutionalized population. Spec Care Dent. 2003;23:86–93.

# Part IV

# Diagnosis

# Clinical Scoring Scales for Assessment of Dry Mouth

8

Stephen J. Challacombe, Samira M. Osailan, and Gordon B. Proctor

**Abstract**

A clinical oral dryness score (CODS) for clinical *signs* has been developed and has been found to be reliable and easy to use for routine assessment of the severity of dry mouth (hyposalivation). CODS is closely related to both the unstimulated salivary flow and the thickness of the mucin layer over the epithelium (mucosal wetness) suggesting a physiological basis to the feeling of xerostomia. CODS can be incorporated into the routine clinical assessment of dry mouth patients, particularly since the clinician would normally be undertaking most aspects of the clinical assessment routinely. In general practice, a low COD score (1–3) indicates mild dryness manageable normally in practice, whereas a high CODS (7–10) is an indication for referral for further investigation. A simple index for *symptoms* of xerostomia (bother index) has also been developed and correlates well with CODS and more objective measures of hyposalivation. This strongly suggests that both types of assessment can be useful in the assessment of the dry mouth patient.

S.J. Challacombe, PhD, FRC(Path), FDSRCS, FMedSci (✉)
Department of Oral Medicine, King's College London, Guys and St Thomas' Hospital, Floor 22, Guys Tower, Guys Hospital, London SE1 9RT, UK
e-mail: stephen.challacombe@kcl.ac.uk

S.M. Osailan, BDS, PhD
Department of Oral Surgery, King Abdulaziz University, Jeddah, Saudi Arabia

G.B. Proctor, BSc, PhD
Mucosal and Salivary Biology Division, King's College London Dental Institute, Floor 17 Guy's Tower, London SE1 9RT, UK
e-mail: gordon.proctor@kcl.ac.uk





G. Carpenter (ed.), *Dry Mouth: A Clinical Guide on Causes, Effects and Treatments*, DOI 10.1007/978-3-642-55154-3_8

## Introduction

The most common cause of dry mouth is prescribed medications. However, the biological importance of saliva is perhaps best and most clearly demonstrated in those individuals with profound loss of saliva, as seen in Sjögren's syndrome (autoimmune exocrinopathy) [1] or following treatment of head and neck cancer by external beam irradiation. Under these circumstances, there is frequently general oral discomfort as well as widespread caries and candidiasis [2, 3]. Hyposalivation can be a significant health problem because it can affect nutrition and psychological well-being whilst also leading to tooth decay and other mouth infections [4]. Most 'oral' health care workers who see patients can recognise a number of signs and symptoms which suggest that the patient may have a dry mouth, but assessment of the degree of dryness is notoriously difficult. It is immediately apparent that a reproducible clinical scale of dryness might allow the clinician to determine whether the dryness is mild and could be managed with local measures and advice in the surgery (such as that secondary to xerogenic drugs) or whether it is severe and requires the patient to be referred for further investigation as to the cause and management.

The term 'xerostomia' is now generally accepted as reflecting a symptom of those patients who present with subjective complaint of oral dryness, whereas hyposalivation requires demonstration of reduced salivary flow. The assessment of xerostomia usually involves a patient history, a dry mouth questionnaire which enquires about symptoms and medications, an assessment of salivary flow and a possible use of a visual analogue scales (VAS) in order to quantify the patient's perception of the degree and severity of oral dryness and/or the adverse effects this may have on the patient's quality of life [5]. Simple functional measures can also be used such as observing if the reflective surface of the dental examination mirror adheres to the buccal mucosa or if a patient can chew and swallow a dry biscuit without water [4–6]. In order to assess glandular function, sialometry – the measurement of whole or glandular salivary flow rates – can be performed, but care must be taken to standardise the collecting conditions [7, 8]. Unstimulated whole mouth salivary flow rate is the simplest to measure and has been most frequently used but can be very variable according to the hydration of the patient or the time of day when the sample is taken [7]. Stimulated parotid salivary flow is also commonly used in the assessment of Sjögren's syndrome [9] and overall correlates well with the unstimulated flow rate.

Commonly observed signs of severe hyposalivation include depapillation or erythema of the dorsum of the tongue, fissuring of the tongue dorsum, atrophic mucosa, residual food debris and cervical caries. Mild signs of hyposalivation include frothing of saliva, mild depapillation of the sides of the tongue, thickening of the saliva and dry lips. Although these features of oral dryness are generally recognised, until recently there has been no standardised, semi-quantitative clinical method of assessment of dryness apart from assaying whole or parotid saliva flow rates (discussed elsewhere). The importance of oral disease severity scoring systems has been recognised for a variety of other oral conditions including orofacial pain, lichen planus, recurrent aphthous stomatitis (RAS) and orofacial granulomatosis (OFG) [10–12], but dry mouth scales have only recently been established [13].

These oral disease severity scoring systems generally have a semi-quantitative assessment of pain by the patient in addition to clinician, determination of the number of sites involved and the severity of disease at each site summated to give a final score out of 60. Scores above 35 might indicate that systemic therapy should be considered, whilst scores between 20 and 35 usually indicate that local therapy should be considered, and scores of below 20 may suggest that the clinician should consider whether therapy is needed at all [10–12]. They all allow assessment of the effectiveness of any therapeutic intervention to be assessed.

A semi-quantitative clinical score of dry mouth provides a means of determining disease severity and of monitoring the progress of oral dryness over time and enables comparison of the disease severity and responsiveness to therapeutic intervention. It also provides a means for correlating the clinical features of dryness with other measures such as salivary flow rates and mucosal wetness. In this chapter a clinical oral dryness score is described which can be used routinely in the assessment of patients with dry mouth symptoms. It can be shown to correlate well with salivary flow rates, mucosal wetness and patient diagnosis.

## The Clinical Oral Dryness Score (CODS)

The clinical oral dryness score (CODS) consists of a 10-point scale, each point representing a feature of dryness in the mouth. These ten features (Fig. 8.1) are:

1. Mirror sticks to buccal mucosa (Fig. 8.1a)
2. Mirror sticks to tongue (Fig. 8.1b)
3. Frothy saliva (Fig. 8.1c)
4. No saliva pooling in floor of mouth (Fig. 8.1d)
5. Tongue shows loss of papillae
6. Altered/smooth gingival architecture (Fig. 8.1e)
7. Glassy appearance to other oral mucosa especially palate (Fig. 8.1f)
8. Tongue lobulated/fissured (Fig. 8.1g)
9. Active or recently restored (last 6 months) cervical caries (more than two teeth) (Fig. 8.1h)
10. Debris on palate (excluding under dentures, Fig. 8.1i)

Although the scoring system reflects an approximate severity scale, each feature scores one point, and the total is determined. A high total score indicates increased severity of oral dryness. A specially designed form with illustrations of dry mouth features can be used for scoring oral dryness for each patient. The examiner scores the features he/she observes in the patient's mouth and thus derived a COD score of between 0 and 10 (Fig. 8.2).

*Instructions for assessment of mucosal dryness and COD score:*

1. Place the mirror head against the buccal mucosa for 2 s and gently move it away. Observe whether the mucosa pulls away with the mirror.

2. Place the mirror head against the anterior dorsum of the tongue for 2 s and gently move it away. Observe whether the tongue mucosa pulls away with the mirror.
3. Look round the mouth and observe if saliva is frothy in any areas. This can occur in the sulci as well as the floor of the mouth.
4. Saliva normally pools in the floor of the mouth. Observe if any saliva can be seen. Dryness of mucosa normally results in it being light reflective.
5. The dorsum of the tongue is very sensitive to lubrication and desquamates very consistently. Hyposalivation results initially as generalised shortening of the filiform papillae and then of patchy marginal depapillation (scores 1).

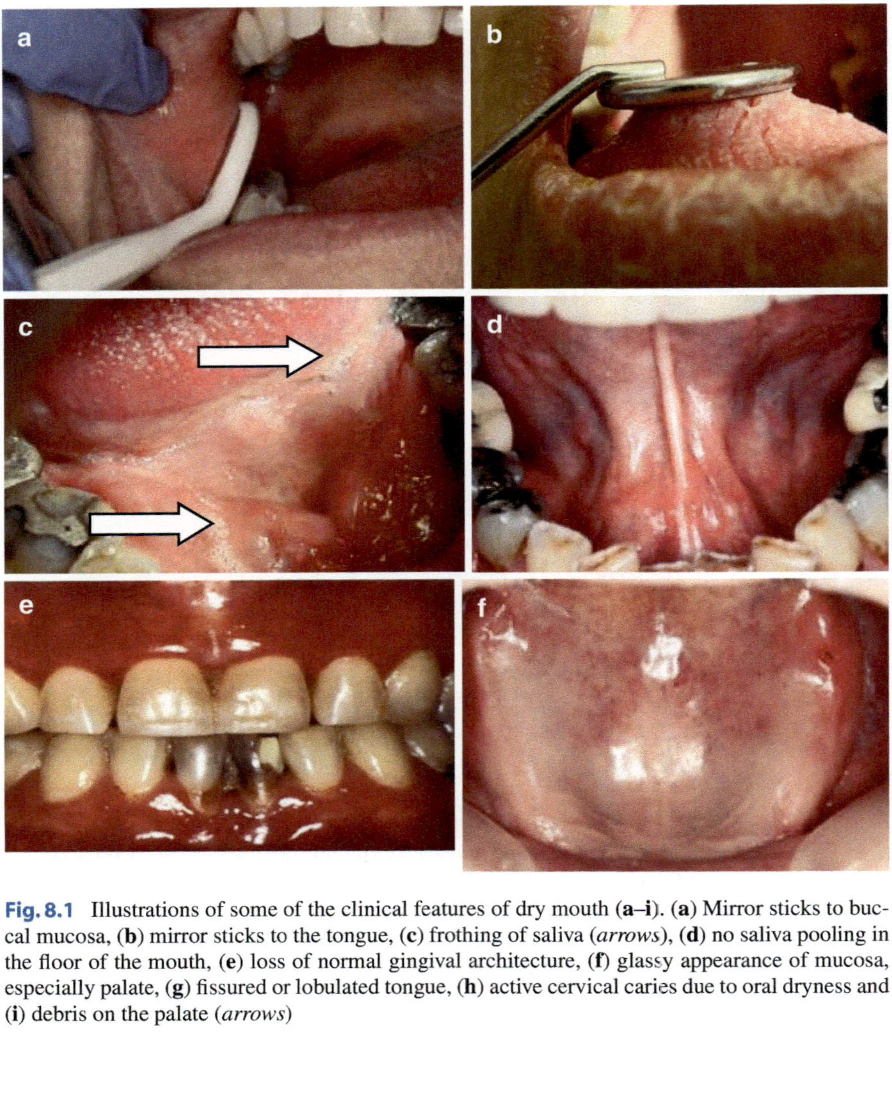


**Fig. 8.1** Illustrations of some of the clinical features of dry mouth (**a**–**i**). (**a**) Mirror sticks to buccal mucosa, (**b**) mirror sticks to the tongue, (**c**) frothing of saliva (*arrows*), (**d**) no saliva pooling in the floor of the mouth, (**e**) loss of normal gingival architecture, (**f**) glassy appearance of mucosa, especially palate, (**g**) fissured or lobulated tongue, (**h**) active cervical caries due to oral dryness and (**i**) debris on the palate (*arrows*)

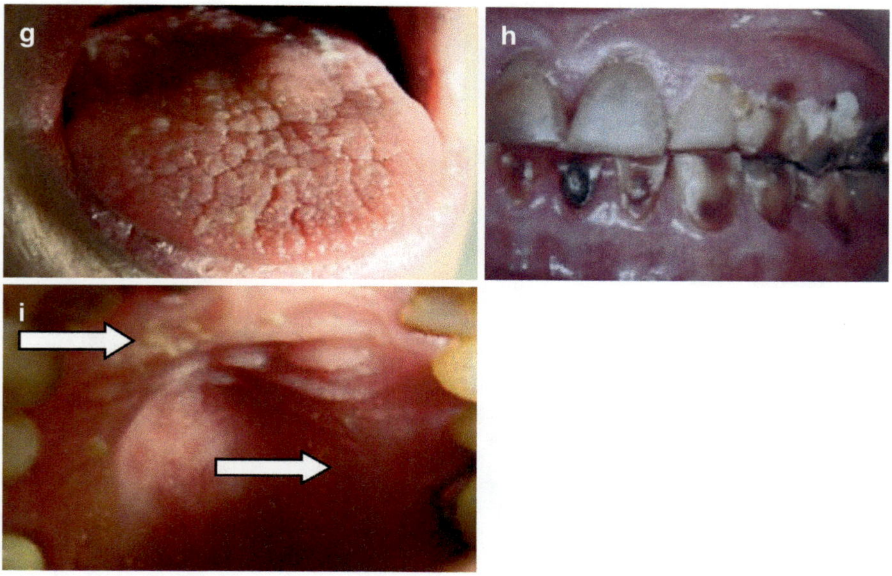


**Fig. 8.1** (continued)

6. Without adequate lubrication, gingival mucosa shows altered desquamation which is normally reflected as shiny red mucosa and loss of normal architecture such as stippling.
7. Palatal mucosa responds to lack of adequate lubrication by increased desquamation and loss of normal architecture, becoming smooth and translucent. Observe whether such changes are present.
8. In severe hyposalivation, the dorsum of the tongue becomes depapillated and then fissured and lobulated (scores a further 1).
9. Observe if there is any recent cervical caries. This scores only if two or more teeth are involved or have been filled in the last 6 months. Single cavities are not sufficiently related to hyposalivation to be discriminatory.
10. Debris such as food or desquamated epithelial cells are normally removed from the oral cavity by saliva. Presence of debris on the palate or sticking to teeth indicates loss of such function and scores 1.

## **Interpretation of the COD Score** (Fig. 8.2)

An additive score of 1–3 (Fig. 8.2) indicates *mild dryness* which may not need treatment. Sugar-free chewing gum chewed for 15–20 min twice a day may be adequate to maintain oral health and diminution of symptoms. Patients should also be advised with regard to the importance of maintaining hydration, especially the elderly.

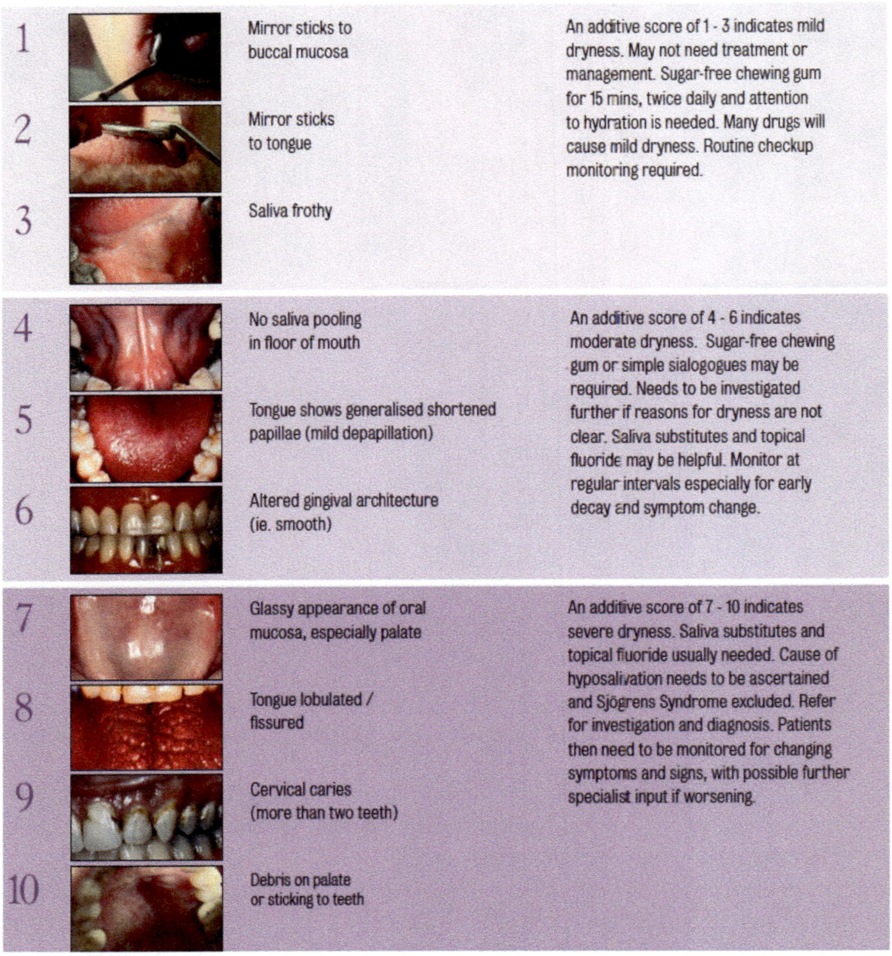


**Fig. 8.2** Clinical oral dryness scale to derive CODS assessed as mild, moderate or severe (http://www.dentalhealth.org/uploads/download/resourcefiles/download_68_1_The%20Challacombe%20Scale.pdf)

An additive score of 4–6 (Fig. 8.2) indicates *moderate dryness*. Sugar-free chewing gum or mild sialogogues may be required. Saliva substitutes and topical fluorides or fluoride toothpaste may be appropriate. If the reason for the dryness is not apparent, then these patients should be further investigated. Monitor at regular intervals to ensure that the symptoms remain unchanged and that caries development is controlled.

An additive score of 7–10 (Fig. 8.2) indicates *severe dryness*. Saliva substitutes and topical fluorides are usually needed. The cause of the hyposalivation must be determined and Sjögren's syndrome excluded [14]. This usually requires referral and investigation by a specialist in an oral medicine or rheumatology department. Patients then need to be monitored regularly to ensure maintenance of oral health, for changing symptoms and signs and further specialist advice if appropriate.

## Relationship of the CODS with Salivary Flow

In a study comparing hyposalivation subjects with controls [15], a strong correlation between the CODS score and the salivary flow was found (Fig. 8.3). Controls had a mean CODS of 1 and an unstimulated whole saliva flow rate of 0.46 ml/min, whilst xerostomia groups had mean CODS of four or greater (Fig. 8.3a) and an UWM of 0.15 ml/min or less (Fig. 8.3b). There is an inverse relationship between the COD scores and the salivary flow rates.

## Relationship Between CODS and Mucosal Wetness

Mucosal wetness is a term describing the thickness of the mucin layer protecting mucosal surfaces in the oral cavity [17, 18], and methods of assessing this are described elsewhere in this book. In essence there is a layer some 30 μm thick overlying buccal and lip mucosa, with half this thickness on the hard palate and double this thickness on the tongue (Fig. 8.4). When groups of patients are given CODS scores indicating mild, moderate or severe dryness, this correlates very well with the actual mucosal wetness [18] suggesting that the clinical assessment of dryness can be related directly to other more measureable parameters (Fig. 8.4).

The clinical oral dryness score is thus related both to salivary flow rates and to mucosal wetness. This suggests that the CODS could be used routinely in clinical oral and dental practice to assess and semi-quantify the severity of oral dryness with confidence that it is related to salivary flow and mucin thickness. In addition, although simpler than some other mucosal disease scoring systems [10–12], it should also be as suitable for monitoring longer term of disease in patients and treatment efficacy. In contrast to inflammatory diseases, long-term success with CODS would be maintenance of a low score.

The clinical features of oral dryness that are included in the CODS, for example, glassy oral mucosa, fissured or depapillated tongue and lack of saliva pooling in the floor of the mouth, are recognised as signs of hyposalivation [19]. In the CODS each feature scores 1 point, but the scale represents an approximate hierarchy of features for dry mouth, and the highest CODS tend to be associated with fissured tongue, cervical caries and the presence of food debris that is not cleared from the mouth.

### Other Clinical Scales

A set of four clinical features that, together, successfully predicted the presence or absence of salivary gland hypofunction was described by Navazesh et al. [20]. The four features were:

- Dryness of lips
- Dryness of buccal mucosa
- Absence of saliva induced by gland palpation
- Total DMFT

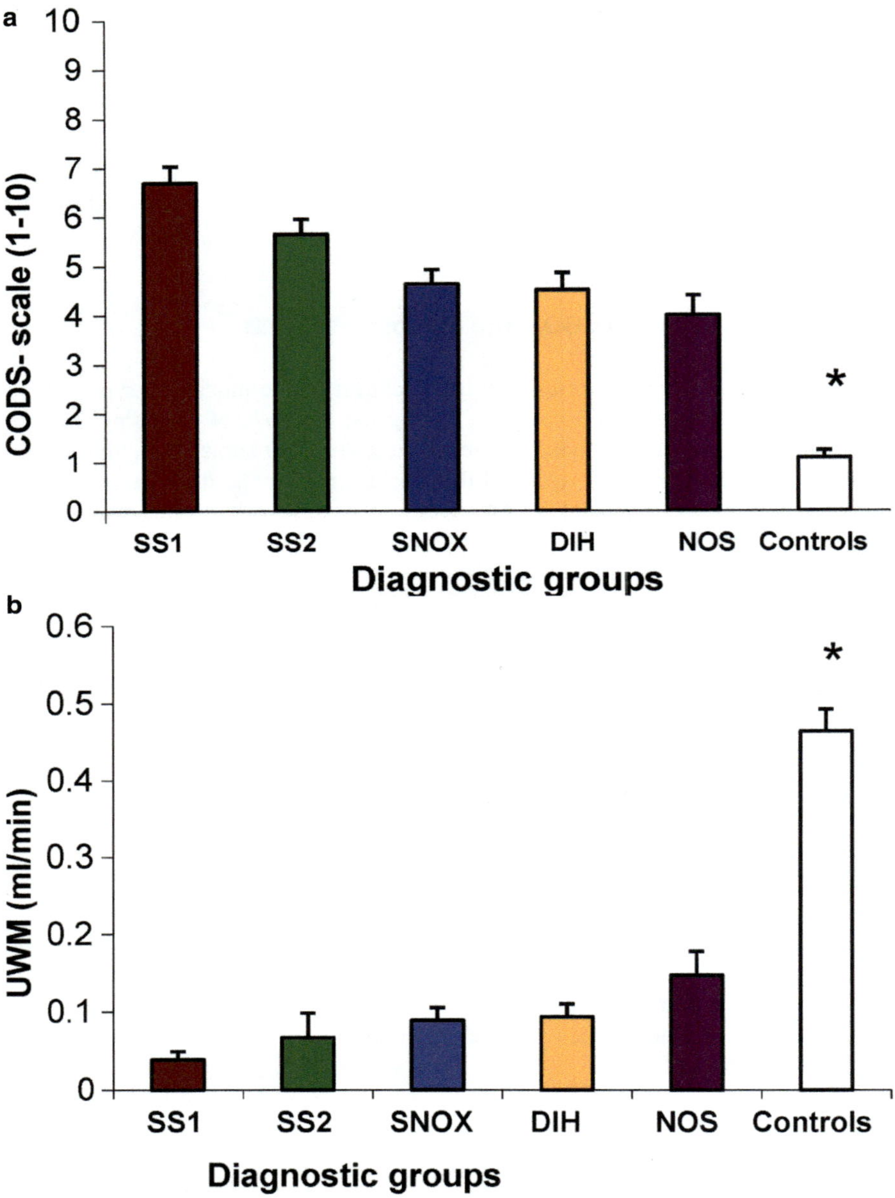


**Fig. 8.3** Comparison of clinical oral dryness score (*CODS*) and salivary flows in different patient groups and controls. (**a**) Mean CODS ± SEM. (**b**) Mean unstimulated whole salivary flow rates (ml/min). * = Mean values of were significantly higher in all patient groups compared with controls. *SS1* primary Sjögren's syndrome, *SS2* secondary Sjögren's syndrome, *SNOX* non-specific sialadenitis, generalised primary nodal osteoarthritis, xerostomia, *DIH* drug-induced hyposalivation, NOS xerostomia not otherwise specified (From Osailan et al. [7])

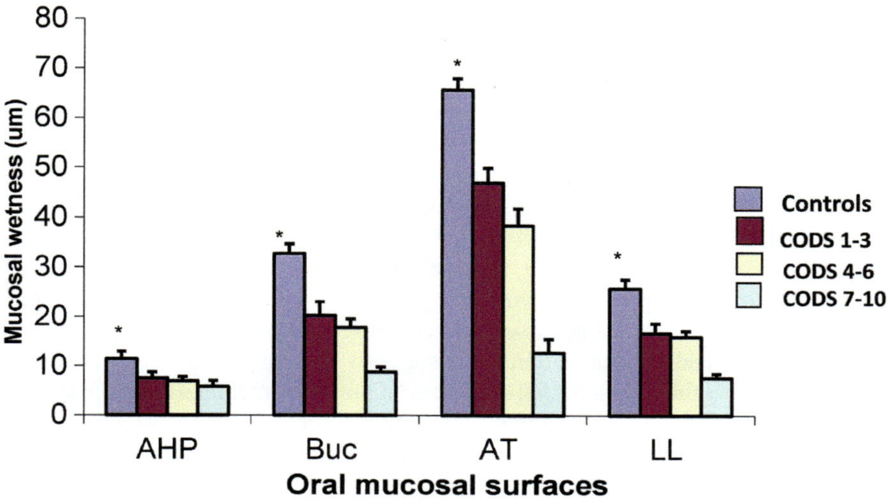


**Fig. 8.4** The relationship between CODS and wetness of oral mucosal surfaces in patients and controls. The xerostomia patients have been divided into three groups (CODS 1–3, 4–6 and 7–10). * = The mucosal wetness of the three patient groups was significantly less ($p<0.05$) than the controls for each of the four mucosal surfaces. Key: *AHP* anterior hard palate, *BUC* buccal mucosa, *AT* anterior tongue, *LL* lower lip (Figure from Osailan et al. [7])

They were not put into a scale, and all four features were necessary to predict the salivary hypofunction. Although the authors related features overall to salivary flows of less than 0.16 ml per min, the features are more consistent with severe hyposalivation. Total DMFT is very dependent on the populations being studied, especially if residing in areas served by fluoridated water. In our work on the CODS scale, dryness of lips was considered as one of the parameters, but in preliminary studies was found not to be very specific to salivary hypofunction.

Fox and colleagues [5, 19] derived a series of questions which could discriminate between those subjects with hyposalivation and a complaint of xerostomia. Questions included those designed to determine whether there was difficulty in speaking, difficulty in swallowing or altered taste. This approach has proved useful in distinguishing patients with hyposalivation from those with xerostomia alone but with salivary flows within the normal range, but was not designed to deliver a severity score. They are, however, particularly useful for surveys by telephone or questionnaire since they do not require direct clinical observation.

There have been few attempts previously to utilise clinical features to derive a semi-quantitative assessment of oral dryness in patients complaining of xerostomia with the objective of discriminating between subjects with mild, moderate or severe hyposalivation rather than detecting subjects with clear and severe reduction in salivary flow. In the CODS, additional clinical criteria have been included to give a total of ten features and scores which appear to discriminate between mild, moderate or severe hyposalivation.

## Sensitivity of CODS

The data in the study of Osailan et al. [7] suggests that the CODS can be a sensitive tool since the mean CODS correlated with the salivary flow. Since each of the diagnostic groups selected showed different mean salivary flows from the lowest in primary Sjögren's syndrome to the highest in the drug-induced group, comparison with the mean CODS allowed a direct relationship to be readily apparent. Sjögren's syndrome patients can present with some of the most severe oral dryness, and these patients had the highest CODS and the lowest salivary flow rates (UWS and SP) and least mucosal wetness. A raised COD score compared with controls was found in all patient groups who presented with xerostomia, including those with SNOX syndrome (non-specific sialadenitis and generalised nodal osteoarthritis) [13] and medication-induced hyposalivation. This suggests that most patients complaining of xerostomia do have an increased CODS, even though sometimes the salivary flow would be considered as within the normal range. Patients with xerostomia and an UWS flow rate greater than 0.2 ml/min (i.e. within normal range) nevertheless showed a significantly higher mean CODS (4–6) compared with healthy controls suggesting that symptoms are not always directly related to the salivary flow rate.

An UWS flow rate of 0.1–0.2 ml/min is frequently used as a cut-off for determining salivary hypofunction [4]. In our studies, a cut-off of 0.2 ml/min is used since this value is approximately two standard deviations below the mean of a control group consisting of 600 subjects [16]. It may also be that patients with UWS flow rates apparently within the normal flow rate range had experienced a greater than 50 % reduction in their personal baseline UWS salivary flow. It has previously been suggested that subjects need at least a 50 % reduction from their baseline resting (unstimulated) salivary flow rate in order to experience oral dryness [20, 21], although this has proved very difficult to validate.

## CODS and Mucosal Wetness

There appears to be a direct inverse relationship between CODS and mucosal wetness, suggesting that the clinical scoring reflects a measurable biological parameter. Patients with the highest CODS scores (7–10) had very low values for mucosal wetness on all mucosal surfaces. Patients grouped with CODS values between 2 and 3 and those with values between 4 and 6 also had reduced mucosal wetness, though there was a relatively small difference between them. This suggests that any of the clinical features (most commonly, mirror sticks to buccal mucosa, mirror sticks to tongue, frothy saliva, lack of saliva pooling in floor of mouth, tongue shows loss of papillae, altered gingival architecture/smooth) can be associated with moderate but significant reductions in mucosal wetness.

Thus, the CODS can provide some discrimination between patients and controls with similar salivary flow rates, patients being defined as those presenting with symptoms of xerostomia. Assessment of xerostomia by a semi-quantitative questionnaire or by a patient-reported severity scale was not always directly related to salivary flow rates, but flow rates do appear to be well correlated with CODS. This suggests that the symptoms and signs of oral dryness may not always be directly related to salivary flow rates but may be reflected in the COD score.

**Table 8.1** Oral symptoms commonly associated with xerostomia or hyposalivation

| | |
|---|---|
| Saliva | Foamy or viscous |
| Lips | Dry or cracked (cheilitis) |
| Tongue | Pain or burning (glossodynia) |
| Cheeks (buccal mucosae) | Dryness |
| Thirst | Frequent ingestion of fluids |
| Mastication | Difficulty in eating dry foods |
| Swallowing | Difficulty (dysphagia) |
| Speech | Difficulty (dysphonia) |
| Taste | Altered, usually bad (dysgeusia) |

## Semi-Quantitative Score for Symptoms of Oral Dryness: 'The Bother Index'

The CODS is a semi-quantitative assessment of oral dryness from the perspective of a clinician with the objective of determining whether it was possible to discriminate between mild, moderate and severe oral mucosal dryness. It is also possible to have an assessment from the perspective of the patient and determine whether symptoms might be related to either the CODS scores or other measureable parameters such as salivary flows. Subjective complaints of dryness do not appear to correlate well with measurable salivary gland dysfunction, but some symptoms have been found to have predictive value. In general, questions which focus on oral activities dependent on salivation, such as chewing and swallowing, seem most likely to identify patients with salivary hypofunction [6, 22]. Questionnaires such as those used by Fox et al. [5] help to define the group requiring further evaluation for disease and conditions, such as Sjögren's or SNOX syndromes. In patients identified with severe hyposalivation, the full range of tests including salivary flows, lacrimal flows and ocular evaluation (Schirmer's or lissamine green tests), labial gland biopsy and ultrasound investigations as well as serological tests need to be performed.

Common symptoms associated with xerostomia or hyposalivation are listed in Table 8.1. Whilst CODS attempts to evaluate these from the clinician's perspective, a 'bother index' can be used to quantify these from the patient's point of view. Previous investigators have used a variety of methods including: questionnaires, visual analogue scales (VAS) and simple functional measures such as difficulties in swallowing certain foods and getting up at night to drink, difficulty in eating dry food, burning or itchy sensation of tongue or gum observing if the tongue blade adheres to the buccal mucosa or if a patient can chew and swallow a dry food like biscuits without water [6, 22].

The objective of the study by Osailan et al. [23] was to design an index that assesses semi-quantitatively the degree patients are affected by their dry mouth condition and to determine whether this index ('*bother index*') correlated with different measures of dryness. Two questionnaires were designed:

(a) The bother 5 index consisted of five questions about the severity of dry mouth and any psychological effect on the patient (Table 8.2).

**Table 8.2** 'Bother 5' xerostomia index (BI5). Five questions are asked

| | |
|---|---|
| Q1 | Do you have a dry mouth problem? |
| Q2 | Does your dry mouth stop you from doing everyday activities, e.g. going out, travelling and talking on the phone? |
| Q3 | Do you avoid doing certain activities which you really like to do because of your dry mouth, e.g. wine tasting and going to the gym? |
| Q4 | Does your dry mouth stop you from eating the food you like? |
| Q5 | Do you feel embarrassed because of your dry mouth? |
| Answers are the same option to each question | Never=0, Occasionally=1, Some of the time=2, Most of the time=3, All of the time=4<br>Overall score out of 20 (4×5Qs)<br>After Osailan et al. [23] |

**Table 8.3** 'Bother 1' xerostomia index (BI1). A single question is asked

| Q. Fundamental question | On a scale of 0–10, how much is your dry mouth problem bothering you? |
|---|---|
| 0 = Does not bother me at all | 10 = Unbearable, it bothers me all the time<br>After Osailan et al. [23] |

(b) The bother 1 index consisted of a single score from 0 to 10 given by the patient after explanation (Table 8.3).

In their study, results from for 100 healthy controls were compared with 100 patients who had previously been examined and shown by sialometry to have reduced unstimulated whole mouth (UWM) salivary flow rates and increased clinical oral dryness score (CODS) and decrease mucosal wetness (MW) at four oral mucosa surfaces [22, 23].

Unsurprisingly both bother indices were markedly raised in patients compared with controls (Fig. 8.5). Interestingly, both indices were very closely correlated with no obvious increased discrimination by using bother 5 rather than bother 1. In dry mouth patients, the values of either index were significantly inversely correlated with UWM salivary flow rate and also with mucosal wetness. There was also a positive correlation with the CODS; patients with high CODS showed a positive correlation with both indices.

Thus, there appears to be a direct correlation between the semi-quantitative assessment by patients of their symptoms and the semi-quantitative clinical assessment of signs. This strongly suggests that both types of assessment can be useful in the assessment of the dry mouth patient.

**Conclusion**

A simple clinical oral dryness score (CODS) has been developed and has been found to be reliable and easy to use for routine assessment of the severity of dry mouth (hyposalivation) and possibly for the effectiveness of management methods. CODS is closely related to both the unstimulated salivary flow and the thickness of the mucin layer over the epithelium (mucosal wetness) suggesting a physiological basis to the feeling of xerostomia. CODS can be incorporated into

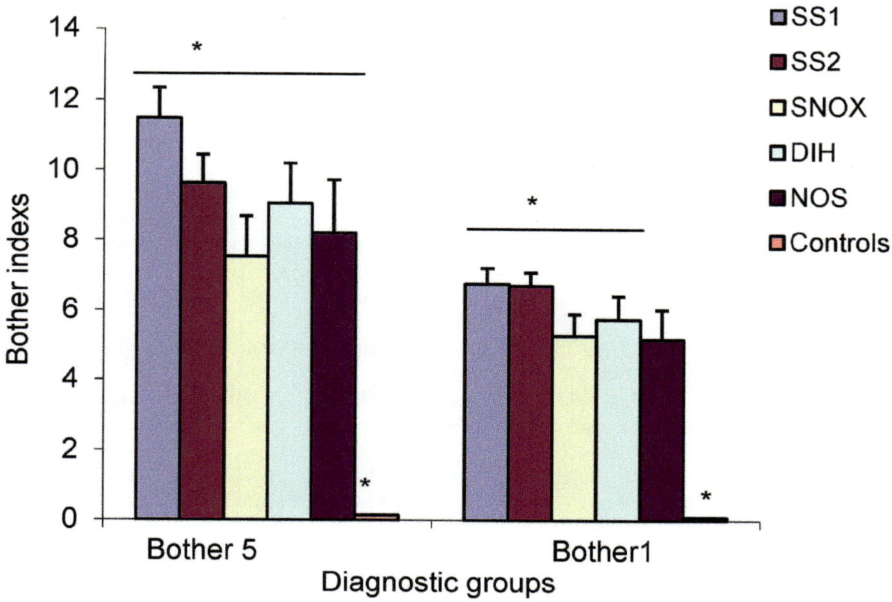


**Fig. 8.5** The relationship between bother indices and diagnostic groups. The two bother indices in all diagnostic groups were significantly ($P<0.01$) higher than controls. There were no significant differences between the diagnostic groups. *SS1* primary Sjögren's syndrome, *SS2* secondary Sjögren's syndrome, *SNOX* SNOX syndrome (primary generalised nodal osteoarthritis, xerostomia and non-specific sialadenitis), *DIH* drug-induced hyposalivation, NOS subjects complaining of xerostomia, but with no specific diagnosis) (After Osailan et al. [23])

the routine clinical assessment of dry mouth patients. Thus, the semi-quantitative CODS scoring system generally reflects both the degree of hyposalivation and the extent of reduction in mucosal wetness and should prove clinically useful both with general dentists and in specialist clinics in identifying and monitoring those patients who present with xerostomia and who will require further investigation.

A simple bother index of clinical symptoms of dryness has also been developed and appears to correlate well with more objective measures of hyposalivation as well as with the CODS. This strongly suggests that both types of assessment can be useful in the assessment of the dry mouth patient.

## References

1. Sjögren H. Zur Kenntnis der Keratoconjunctivitis sicca (Keratitis filiformis bei Hypofunktion der Tränen-drusen). Acta Ophthalmol. 1933;11:1–151.

2. Sreebny LM, Valdini A. Xerostomia part I: relationship to other oral symptoms and salivary gland hypofunction. Oral Surg Oral Med Oral Pathol. 1988;66:451–8.
3. Vissink A, Jansma J, Spijkeret FK, Burlage FR, Coppes RP. Oral sequelae of head and neck radiotherapy. Crit Rev Oral Biol Med. 2003;3:100–212.
4. Sreebny LM. Saliva in health and disease: an appraisal and update. Int Dent J. 2000;50:140–61.
5. Fox PC, Busch KA, Baum BJ. Subjective reports of xerostomia and objective measures of salivary gland performance. J Am Dent Assoc. 1987;115:581–4.
6. Fox PC. Xerostomia: recognition and management. Dent Assist. 2008;77:44–8.
7. Osailan SM, Pramanik R, Shirlaw P, Proctor GB, Challacombe SJ. Clinical assessment of oral dryness: development of a scoring system related to salivary flow and mucosal wetness. Oral Surg Oral Med Oral Pathol Oral Radiol. 2012;114:597–603.
8. Jenkins GN, Edgar WM. Effect of daily gum-chewing on salivary flow rate in man. J Dent Res. 1989;68:786–90.
9. Kassan SS, Moutsopoulos HM. Clinical manifestations and early diagnosis of Sjögren's syndrome. Arch Intern Med. 2004;164:1275–84.
10. Escudier M, Ahmed N, Shirlaw P, Setterfield J, Tappuni A, Black MM, Challacombe SJ. Scoring system for mucosal disease severity with special reference to oral Lichen Planus. Br J Dermatol. 2007;157:765–70.
11. Setterfield J, Shirlaw PJ, Bhogal BS, Tilling K, Challacombe SJ, Black MM. Cicatricial pemphigoid: serial titres of circulating IgG and IgA antibasement membrane antibodies correlate with disease activity. Br J Dermatol. 1999;140:645–50.
12. Sanderson J, Nunes C, Escudier M, Barnard K, Shirlaw P, Odell E, Chinyama C, Challacombe S. Oro-facial granulomatosis: Crohn's disease or new inflammatory bowel disease. Inflamm Bowel Dis. 2005;11:840–6.
13. Kassimos DG, Choy EHS, Challacombe SJ, Panayi GS. The prevalence of xerostomia in a population with primary generalized osteoarthritis (PGOA). Br J Rheumatol. 1995;34:132.
14. Vitali C, Bombardieri S, Jonsson R, Moutsopoulos HM, Alexander EL, Carsons SE, Daniels TE, Fox PC, Fox RI, Kassan SS, Pillemer SR, Talal N, Weisman MH. European Study Group on classification criteria for Sjogren's syndrome. Classification criteria for Sjogren's syndrome: a revised version of the European criteria proposed by the American-European Consensus Group. Ann Rheum Dis. 2002;61:554–8.
15. Whitcher JP, Shiboski CH, Shiboski SC, Heidenreich AM, Kitagawa K, Zhang S, Hamann S, Larkin G, McNamara NA, Greenspan JS, Daniels TE. Sjögren's International Collaborative Clinical Alliance Research Groups. A simplified quantitative method for assessing keratoconjunctivitis sicca from the Sjögren's syndrome international registry. Am J Ophthalmol. 2010;149:405–15.
16. Percival S, Challacombe SJ, Marsh PD. Flow rates of resting whole and stimulated parotid saliva in relation to age and gender. J Dent Res. 1994;73:1416–20.
17. Pramanik R, Osailan SM, Challacombe SJ, Urquhart D, Proctor GB. Protein and mucin retention on oral mucosal surfaces in dry mouth patients. Eur J Oral Sci. 2010;118:245–53.
18. Osailan SM, Pramanik R, Shirodaria S, Challacombe SJ, Proctor GB. Investigating the relationship between hyposalivation and mucosal wetness. Oral Dis. 2010;17:109–14.
19. Napenas JJ, Brennan MT, Fox PC. Diagnosis and treatment of xerostomia (dry mouth). Odontology. 2009;97:76–83.
20. Navazesh M, Christensen C, Brightman V. Clinical criteria for the diagnosis of salivary gland hypofunction. J Dent Res. 1992;71:1363–9.
21. Dawes C. Physiological factors affecting salivary flow rate, oral sugar clearance, and the sensation of dry mouth in man. J Dent Res. 1987;66:648–53.
22. Thomson WM, Chalmers JM, Spencer AJ, Ketabi M. The occurrence of xerostomia and salivary gland hypofunction in a population-based sample of older South Australians. Spec Care Dent. 1999;19:20–3.
23. Osailan SM, Pramanik R, Proctor GB, Challacombe SJ. Semi-quantitative score for symptoms of oral dryness: "The Bother Index" (2014 submitted).

# Imaging of Salivary Glands

**9**

Bethan Louise Thomas

**Abstract**

Imaging of the salivary glands can provide useful information on the status of the glands. Some imaging techniques provide direct evidence of the function of the glands, while others provide indirect information on gland function. This chapter aims to describe the different techniques currently available. The role each imaging modality can play in the investigation of patients with dry mouth is highlighted, along with the limitations of these imaging modalities. The current diagnostic criteria for Sjogren's syndrome include conventional sialography and scintigraphy. Other techniques that could be considered for incorporation into future diagnostic criteria, based on their proven efficacy in diagnosis of Sjogren's syndrome, are discussed.

Ultrasonography, sialography, magnetic resonance imaging (MRI) (including MRI sialography), plain radiographs, computed tomography (CT), cone beam computed tomography (CBCT), nuclear medicine (including scintigraphy), and endoscopy can all have a role to play in imaging salivary glands. Selecting the more appropriate modality based on the locally available options in a clinical setting is important to maximize their beneficial use. It should be noted that often not all of these imaging modalities are readily available in any given clinical setting, and the imaging modalities used will vary accordingly. At Guy's Hospital, London, the standard imaging protocol for patients under investigation for dry mouth and possible Sjogren's

B.L. Thomas, BDS, BSc (Hons), PhD, DDMFR RCR
Dental and Maxillofacial Radiology, Guy's Hospital, Guy's and St Thomas' NHS Foundation Trust, Floor 23, Tower Wing, Guy's Hospital, Great Maze Pond, London SE1 9RT, UK

Dental Radiology, The Eastman Dental Hospital, University College London Hospitals NHS Foundation Trust, 256 Gray's Inn Road, London WC1X 8LD, UK
e-mail: bethan.thomas@kcl.ac.uk



G. Carpenter (ed.), *Dry Mouth: A Clinical Guide on Causes, Effects and Treatments*, DOI 10.1007/978-3-642-55154-3_9

syndrome primarily involves an ultrasound examination of the major salivary glands. If the ultrasound findings are suggestive of Sjogren's syndrome, few will proceed to sialography. In Guy's Hospital's Dental and Maxillofacial Imaging Department, sialography tends to be reserved primarily for cases with suspected ductal obstruction as a means of identifying the obstruction and its position. This is not the case in other centres, and the emphasis on different imaging modalities varies between countries.

In all clinical scenarios, imaging is almost exclusively limited to the major salivary glands, with limited options currently available to assess the minor salivary glands. Intraoral ultrasound examination, using a small high-frequency transducer, may help to identify a mucocoele or minor salivary gland tumour if an intraoral lump is present, but more generalized minor salivary gland imaging is not currently possible. Therefore imaging in the assessment of dry mouth focuses on examination of the major salivary glands.

Most patients experiencing loss of function of one major salivary gland, for example, due to surgical excision or duct obstruction, do not generally have symptoms of dry mouth as the other salivary glands compensate. An important part of imaging of patients with hyposalivation, however, is to exclude ductal obstruction to ensure this is not a component of the symptoms. When imaging does not reveal any abnormality of the salivary glands, but rather a normal appearance in a patient with a dry mouth, it is much less likely that the patient has a disease such as Sjogren's syndrome as the cause of their dry mouth. Such a finding is useful to support a clinical diagnosis of dry mouth as a result of the side effects of drugs or possibly age-related changes, dehydration, anxiety, etc. The role of imaging is therefore primarily to differentiate disease-related structural changes in the glands from patients with structurally normal glands.

Each of the imaging modalities will be discussed in turn, emphasizing their advantages and disadvantages.

## Ultrasonography

Ultrasound examination has become the main imaging modality of salivary glands in many clinics specializing in salivary gland disease. The equipment is relatively inexpensive in comparison to MRI and CT, providing good quality images of the superficial lobe of the parotid gland and also the submandibular gland (SMG). The limitation of ultrasonography is its inability to access the deep lobe of the parotid gland, thus precluding assessment of any deep lobe disease.

Ultrasonography involves the transmission of ultrasound waves from a transducer, through the skin or mucous membrane, with a coupling gel used to allow good transmission. Sound waves are reflected at junctions where tissues have differing acoustic impedance. The reflected sound waves are detected by the transducer, and the variation in intensity and the depth of reflection of the waves are displayed as a 2D image on a screen. Most ultrasonography of the head and neck uses a linear 7.5–10 MHz transducer [1]. The size of the transducer is important to allow

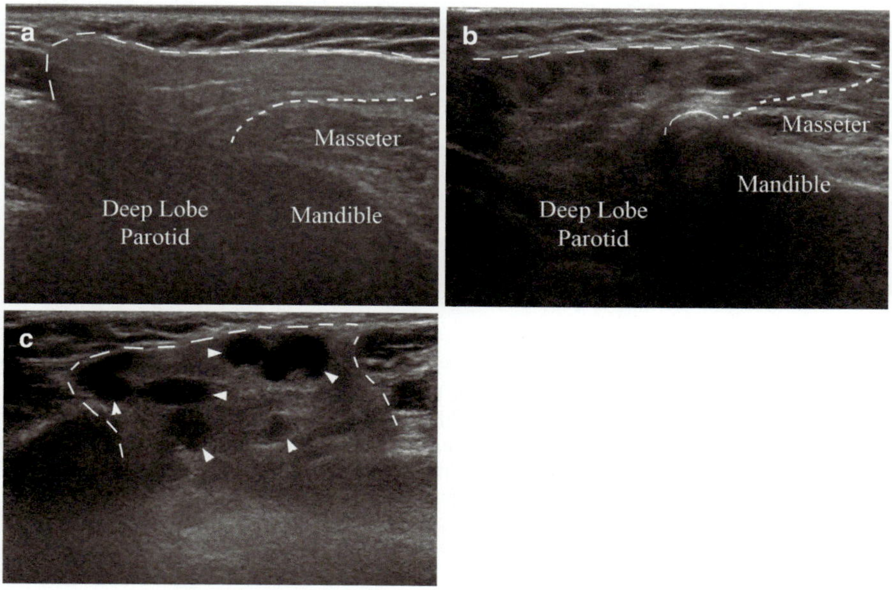


**Fig. 9.1** Ultrasonography of the major salivary glands. (**a**) demonstrates the appearance of a normal right parotid gland (anterior to the *right*, posterior to the *left* of the image). The tissue in the upper part of the image is the skin and dermal layers. The *dashed line* represents the superficial edge of the parotid gland. The shorter *dashed line* indicates the boundary of the parotid and the masseter muscle. Sound waves do not penetrate the mandible, and the white line inferior to the masseter is the buccal (lateral) corticated border of the right ascending ramus. The parotid tissue extends into the deep lobe posterior to the ascending ramus, but its full extent is not visualized. (**b**) demonstrates a right parotid gland at a similar position within the gland. Note the more heterogeneous appearance to the echotexture of the gland, with intermittent hypoechoic (*darker*) areas, particularly within the superficial layers in this case. This is termed a mild honeycomb appearance. (**c**) demonstrates a right parotid gland with more severe changes associated with Sjogren's syndrome. The distinct foci (marked by *white arrowheads*) are darker (hypoechoic) and larger

angulation for adequate imaging around the facial area. Very small transducers are available that can allow ultrasound examination of parts of the mouth.

Normal healthy salivary glands have a homogeneous, smooth, grey appearance on ultrasound appearing lighter than adjacent muscle; this relative increase in brightness is described as hyperechoic [2] (Fig. 9.1a). The ducts are not always visible in a healthy gland, and dilatation of the ducts is an important feature of relevance in cases of ductal obstruction (Fig. 9.2). The use of a sialogogue during an ultrasound examination can allow dynamic assessment of the function of the gland. Mild dilation of the salivary duct would be seen in a normal gland as a result of the rapid production of saliva in response to the sialogogue. In the presence of ductal obstruction, more marked dilation of the duct can occur and can identify the position of the more distally placed obstruction, usually a stone or a stricture, but occasionally obstruction may be due to a mucus plug.

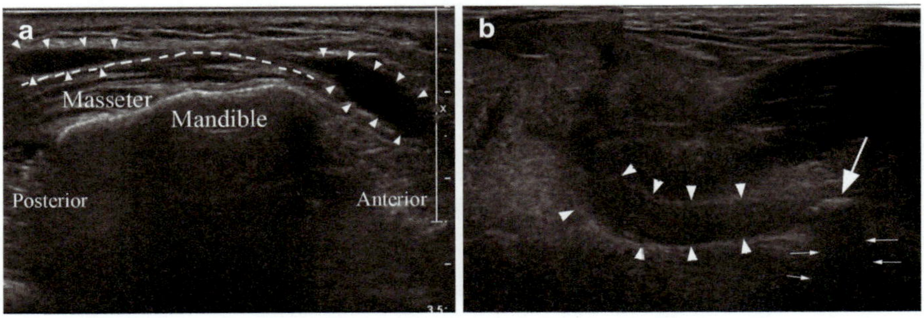


**Fig. 9.2** Ultrasonography of obstructive salivary gland disease. (**a**) shows a right submandibular gland (outlined with *dashes*) with two merged ultrasound images demonstrating the gland and also the dilated duct (outlined with *arrowheads*). Note the dilated duct extending proximally back to the hilum from a calculus located in the mid-third of the main duct (*large arrow*). The stone is calcified and has produced a post-acoustic shadow extending away from the ultrasound source (marked by the small *white arrows*). (**b**) demonstrates a right parotid gland duct with strictures present in the mid-third of the main duct, as it passes over the masseter muscle. The dilated duct is outlined with *arrowheads*

The submandibular glands usually have a slightly heterogeneous appearance in comparison to the parotid glands, a feature thought to relate to the different structure and cellular composition of the two glands.

The current American and European consensus guidelines on the diagnosis of Sjogren's syndrome do not include ultrasound as an accepted imaging modality in the diagnosis, whereas sialography and scintigraphy are accepted [3]. However, ultrasonography has proved particularly useful in the assessment and monitoring of Sjogren's syndrome [4–8]. The ultrasound features noted in early Sjogren's syndrome are mild heterogeneous changes to the echotexture, particularly affecting the parotid glands. As the disease progresses the parenchyma demonstrates more marked heterogeneity, leading to a clear honeycomb appearance (Fig. 9.1), with hypoechoic foci spread throughout the gland. With further progression of the disease, a markedly heterogeneous pattern is seen. The ultrasound changes are usually present bilaterally, but may be much more prominent in a single pair of major salivary glands than the other, for example, the submandibular glands may demonstrate a reasonably normal echotexture, while the parotid glands demonstrate a honeycomb appearance.

Of particular importance to the imaging of dry mouth is the sensitivity and specificity (75–90 % and 84–98 %) of ultrasound examination which has been shown to produce very similar levels to those of MRI (94–96 % and 97–100 %), and both ultrasound and MRI may perform better than both sialography and scintigraphy [7, 8]. Interestingly different groups have used differing scoring systems in their studies on the efficacy of ultrasound in diagnosing Sjogren's syndrome. A future study to compare these individual scoring systems and devise a more sensitive and specific system may assist in driving a move from sialography and scintigraphy as the imaging modalities accepted for the diagnosis of Sjogren's syndrome to the acceptance of ultrasonography, particularly given its relative ease of use, relative costs involved, and with no radiation required.

While ultrasonography is not yet accepted as an imaging modality in the formal diagnosis of Sjogren's syndrome, it is a very valuable tool in monitoring the status of the salivary glands in Sjogren's syndrome without involving a radiation dose. This role in monitoring disease progression becomes significant in managing the small but important group of Sjogren's patients who develop mucosa-associated lymphoid tissue (MALT) lymphoma. The diagnosis of MALT lymphoma is difficult; on ultrasound the features of concern are the development of larger hypoechoic areas (Fig. 9.1), and an important advantage of ultrasound examination is the ability to assess the vascularity in and around these hypoechoic areas which can be suggestive of lymphomatous change.

While ultrasonography is developing as a tool for assessing Sjogren's syndrome, it is important to bear in mind that the changes described in the ultrasound features including the echotexture and the echogenicity seen in Sjogren's syndrome are not specific to Sjogren's syndrome. The interpretation of the ultrasound findings must always be considered in the wider clinical picture. This is not only true for ultrasonography but relevant to the other imaging modalities as well. Similar ultrasound appearances to those seen in Sjogren's syndrome can also be seen in other diseases such as chronic sialadenitis, sarcoidosis, and HIV-associated salivary gland disease. The role of imaging is therefore an adjuvant to support a clinical diagnosis where the findings must be interpreted within the clinical picture.

## Sialography

Conventional sialography is a technique used to image the ductal system of the major salivary glands. An iodine-based water-soluble contrast medium is used. The duct orifice is located and gently dilated with lacrimal dilators, and a sialography catheter is inserted into the duct orifice. The parotid duct orifice can usually be readily located in the buccal mucosa and, in the absence of a stricture at the duct orifice, is often readily cannulated. The submandibular duct orifice by comparison is routinely much smaller; as an indication of the size difference, we routinely use a 20-G cannula for the parotid duct, but require a 27-G cannula for the submandibular duct. The need to cannulate the duct can preclude conventional sialography as a mode of imaging if it is not possible due to a particularly small duct orifice or if there is a lack of specialist experience in a clinical centre.

Once cannulated the contrast can be administered by hand pressure, hydrostatic pressure, or a continuous infusion pressure-monitored pump [9, 10]. Approximately 1 ml of contrast is required, but the volume is tailored to the patient's response. If an obstruction is present, the patient may experience discomfort or pain. With time the pressure in the gland/duct usually reduces allowing further infusion of contrast to permit adequate coating of the ducts; this is important to produce a good image of the ductal system which is seen as a 'river delta' or 'branches of a tree' in the case of a healthy gland. In the presence of ductal dilatation, a significantly larger volume of contrast may be required, but this must be balanced with the desire to avoid overfilling and resultant extravasation of contrast through the gland acini with a resultant radiographic appearance referred to as parenchymal 'blushing' (Fig. 9.2a).

Imaging of the ductal system may involve static images performed following administration of the contrast, using plain radiographs which include lateral views, oblique lateral views (Fig. 9.2b), and anterior-posterior radiographs or alternatively with cross-sectional imaging either as a CT scan or a cone beam CT scan [11, 12]. Cross-sectional imaging studies can provide more information on the course and morphology of the duct than plain radiographic sialography which should suggest it may be the imaging modality of choice for sialography. Personal experience suggests that the added complication of performing sialography in the confines of a cone beam CT scanner may override the benefit of the technique, but published data suggests it is a feasible and useful method [11, 12].

An alternative to a static sialogram is a dynamic study which can be performed with the infusion of contrast occurring under fluoroscopy imaging (Fig. 9.2c) and also allows the possibility of digital subtraction fluoroscopy. Digital subtraction involves initial capture of a mask image that is digitally subtracted from all subsequent images in that imaging sequence run. Digital subtraction imaging provides high definition of an obstruction but requires a patient to remain completely still during infusion of the contrast which is not always possible.

Dynamic imaging with or without digital subtraction involves rapid repeated bursts of radiation which is captured as a sequence and can be played back on a monitor. It offers a significant advantage over static imaging, particularly in cases with salivary gland obstruction. Dynamic imaging allows the observation of flow up to, around, and beyond an obstruction thus not only localizing the position of the obstruction as seen with static imaging but in addition providing information on expansion of the surrounding duct and, if a salivary stone is present, demonstrating the extent of mobility of the stone (Fig. 9.3).

The final stages of a sialogram involve reimaging following removal of the sialography cannula. Clearance of contrast usually occurs in less than 1 min in a normal healthy gland. Delay in emptying can be a direct consequence of an obstruction, but can also give an indirect indication of the function of the gland, such as poor saliva production meaning contrast is not flushed from the ductal system, therefore providing important additional information on gland status in cases without obstruction such as in a case of dry mouth. Whether imaging has indicated the presence of Sjogren's syndrome or not, the lack of clearance of contrast is a useful indicator that a gland is functioning poorly and adds to other clinical tests such as assessment of volume of saliva production.

The use of sialography continues as a main imaging modality in the diagnosis of Sjogren's syndrome. The sialographic changes described in Sjogren's syndrome are sialectasis, with contrast filling areas of breakdown within the acini. Four levels or grades have been described, firstly punctate, with small radiopacities (less than 1 mm) appearing in the terminal branches widely spread through the gland. The next stage is globular with slightly larger radiopacities (1–2 mm) present. The later

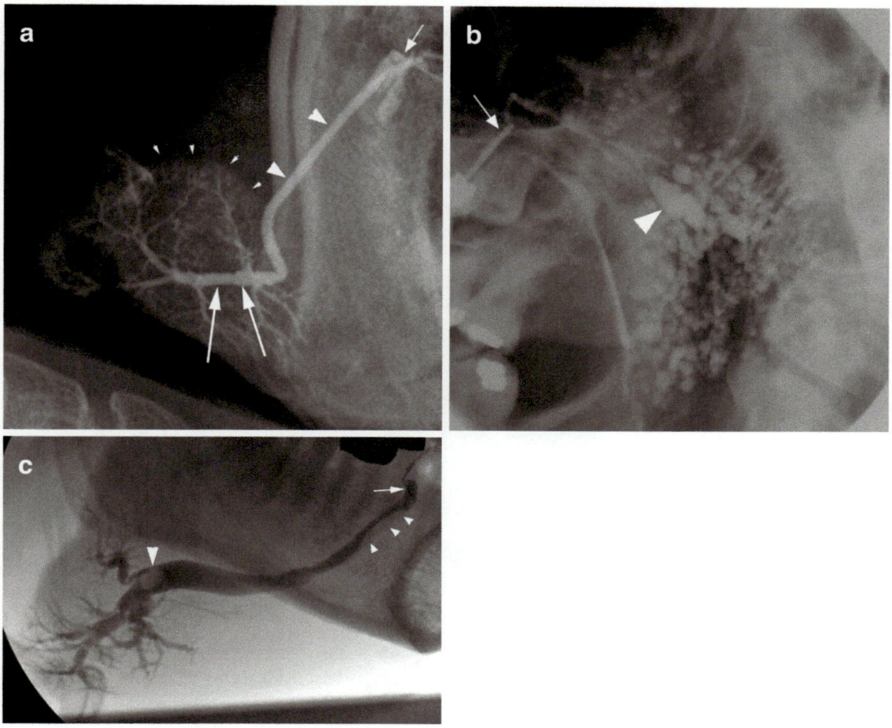


**Fig. 9.3** Sialography. (**a**) demonstrates the sialography appearance of a normal right submandibular gland. The sialography cannula is indicated by the small *white arrow* at the duct orifice. The main duct is marked with *two large arrowheads*. The hilum is marked with *two larger arrows*. Note the extensive branching pattern with clearly visualized secondary and tertiary branches. The *small arrowheads* indicate the anterior limit to the gland; slight overfilling of the ducts has occurred with resultant 'blushing' of the parenchyma. (**b**) demonstrates a right parotid gland with marked sialectasis. The position of the cannula is indicated by the *small arrow* at the duct orifice. The *arrowhead* indicates the hilum in which the duct is dilated. Note the difference to (**a**) with multiple rounded pockets of contrast spread throughout the gland; this is sialectasis with contrast filling dilated acini and pockets within the gland with areas of more severe cavitatory sialectasis and areas of globular sialectasis. (**c**) demonstrates a right submandibular gland sialogram. The position of the cannula is marked with a *small arrow*. The *large arrowhead* indicates a filling defect close to the hilum which represents a calculus that had been identified on ultrasound examination. Note the dilated ducts extending proximally from the hilum indicating a history of obstruction. The sialogram was performed with fluoroscopy that demonstrated movement of the stone from the hilar region to the mid-third of the duct. The *small arrowheads* indicate the true position of the lower border of the main duct; the irregular appearance in this region is due to a mucus plug lying on the floor of the duct. Emptying views demonstrated passage of this mucus plug from the duct

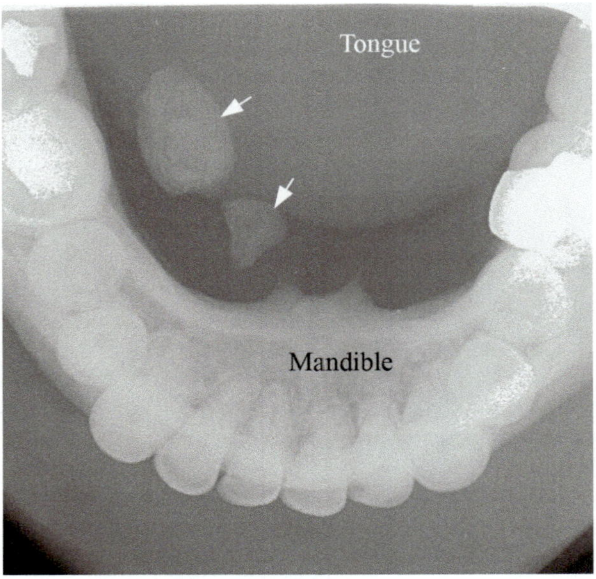


**Fig. 9.4** Plain radiographs. The image demonstrates a lower occlusal radiograph, with two stones (*small arrows*) present in the right sublingual space in the area that would correspond to the position of the submandibular duct. These stones are relatively large and may have been visible on ultrasound. This type of radiograph can also identify much smaller stones which are much more difficult to identify with ultrasound

stages are called cavitary and destructive. The diagnosis of Sjogren's syndrome based on sialography is still complicated and requires specialist analysis to ensure adequate sensitivity and specificity [13]. The radiological appearance can also mimic other diseases including acute and chronic sialadenitis of bacterial origin and granulomatous infections, and the late stages with cavitation can mimic the multiple parotid cysts that can occur with HIV infection [9, 10].

## Plain Radiographs

Plain radiographs have a very limited role in imaging patients with dry mouth. Their main value is to confirm the presence of a stone/calculus. The use of a dental panoramic radiograph may demonstrate a calculus within either the parotid gland or the submandibular gland, but the stone would need to be of significant size to be visible.

Intraoral radiographs are of value, particularly the mandibular occlusal radiographs to image stones located in the main duct of the submandibular gland. Stones in the anterior third of the submandibular duct, located within a few centimetres of the duct orifice in the sublingual space, can be difficult to demonstrate with extraoral ultrasound directed from the submental area, and this region is not always amenable to intraoral ultrasound, particularly if the mandibular incisor teeth are retroclined. Similarly sialography occasionally fails to identify small stones in the anterior third of the submandibular gland duct. In such cases a lower occlusal radiograph is a useful low-dose examination (Fig. 9.4) to avoid recourse to a much higher radiation dose from a CT scan or a cone beam CT scan. It is important to note that not all stones are heavily calcified and if so may not be visible on plain radiographs [9, 10].

## MRI and MRI Sialography

MRI can be very helpful in the assessment of salivary glands, particularly useful when concern is raised of a tumour. MRI provides cross-sectional information of the gland and any pathology present, including the deep lobe as well as the superficial lobe, a significant advantage over ultrasound imaging. Differing sequences will be preferred in different clinical centres, but as a general rule the images acquired will include T1-weighted, T2-weighted, and T1-weighted post-contrast, with fat suppression in the axial plane, with additional views selected dependent on local policy; these are likely to include a selection of coronal images and may include fast-spin echo T2-weighted images.

The best resolution of the images in an MRI salivary gland study is obtained by the use of a 3 T scanner and head coils. Some centres in addition use surface coils over the region of interest. Many centres produce good MR salivary gland studies with a 1.5 T scanner. The use of this equipment can be prohibitive for patients with claustrophobia or difficulty lying horizontally for a period of time, and this must be considered in deciding the imaging modality for a given patient.

More recently MRI sialography has become commonly used in parts of the world as the preferred choice for sialography. It uses the patient's own saliva as the contrast medium to demarcate the salivary ducts and as such avoids all the risks associated with the use of contrast media be it intravenous or the occasional reaction to conventional sialography contrast reagents. It is a technique that has been developed allowing a static form of sialography and more recently a more dynamic version. The plane of imaging is generally adapted including an oblique sagittal plane parallel to the main duct of interest. Maximum intensity projection (MIP) reconstructions are created after the scan to provide a 3D image of the duct that can be used for the diagnosis of strictures, calculi, and other ductal anomalies [13–16].

The difference in dynamic MRI sialography is that rather than relying solely on the quiescent saliva present within the ducts, imaging is performed before and after administration of citric acid, which is used as a sialogogue. MRI imaging is a long process, but to allow more rapid acquisition of images in a time frame to enable any changes in the duct calibre to be identified, the image capture technique is modified. Single thick sections are captured using two-dimensional fast asymmetric spin-echo sequencing which is repeated every 30 s around the time of administering the sialogogue. This is not as rapid as the imaging captured with fluoroscopic sialography, but it does offer advantages over static MRI sialography [17, 18].

MRI sialography has proved successful in the diagnosis of salivary gland obstructive disease [14]. In dry mouth patients, including those with Sjogren's syndrome, this technique can demonstrate poor function as indicated by decreased ductal fill following a sialogogue. The lack of saliva, and therefore inability to fill the ducts with contrast in patients with markedly reduced gland function, results in the lack of detail of the duct morphology and architecture.

The high demand for MRI examinations in comparison to the number of scanners available has largely precluded the use of MRI as the routine examination of choice for imaging dry mouth within the UK. The relative ease of ultrasonography and the comparatively low cost of the examination in comparison to an MRI study results in global variation in the uptake of this imaging modality to assess dry mouth. Nonetheless in many centres with good access to MRI facilities, this is a preferred imaging modality.

## Scintigraphy

Scintigraphy is the only direct imaging method of assessing gland function. The technique involves the use of $^{99m}$technetium-pertechnetate which is administered as an intravenous infusion. The $^{99m}$Tc is concentrated in the salivary glands, as well as the thyroid gland. Maximal uptake usually occurs within 1 h [10]. Measurement of uptake is performed using a gamma camera; however, the images are of low resolution. The use of a sialogogue results in excretion from a healthy functioning gland, but there may be reduced uptake and limited discharge following a sialogogue in glands with reduced function, such as those with a dry mouth.

Assessment of the levels of uptake initially can indicate whether healthy salivary gland tissue is present within the major salivary glands. Rapid excretion and thus reduced signal from the glands can similarly be interpreted as healthy functioning glands. In contrast a gland with less uptake and decreased excretion can be indicative of poor saliva production by the gland, the poor initial uptake indicative of an atrophic gland. The technique has low specificity for Sjogren's syndrome, that is, it cannot provide any distinction between poor gland function due to drug side effects, for example, and decreased saliva production due to Sjogren's syndrome.

## Endoscopy

Endoscopy can be a useful technique to assess duct morphology and the presence of obstruction. It is limited by the calibre of the ducts and distance of an obstruction into the ductal system from the duct orifice. Its role in assessment of dry mouth is limited, but the technique requires irrigation of the duct, and saline is often used. There may be a therapeutic benefit to this irrigation, rather than having a diagnostic value.

## Summary

The assessment of dry mouth can and does involve a combination of imaging modalities. The choice of modality may be governed by local availability, but several have a role to play in assessing the major salivary glands, their status, and function to aid in the management of dry mouth.

While the current guidance on diagnosis of Sjogren's syndrome only includes sialography and scintigraphy, there is significant evidence amassing that supports ultrasonography and MRI sialography as valid imaging modalities in the assessment of Sjogren's syndrome and other causes of dry mouth. Future refinements of the consensus for Sjogren's diagnosis will hopefully consider these modalities to avoid the need for the more invasive techniques currently included, both of which rely on radiation.

## References

1. Evans RM. Anatomy and technique. In: Ahuja A, Evans R, editors. Practical head and neck ultrasound. Cambridge: Cambridge University Press; 2000. p. 1–16.
2. Bradley MJ. Salivary glands. In: Ahuja A, Evans R, editors. Practical head and neck ultrasound. Cambridge: Cambridge University Press; 2000. p. 19–33.
3. Vitali C, Bombardieri S, Jonsson R, et al. Classification criteria for Sjogren's syndrome: a revised version of the European criteria proposed by the American-European Consensus Group. Ann Rheum Dis. 2002;61:554–8.
4. Brown J, Ngu R, Whaites E, et al. Ultrasound in the diagnosis of Sjogren's syndrome and correlation with systemic markers. Conference: 10th Biennial Conference of the European Association of Oral Medicine, EAOM 2010 London United Kingdom. Oral Dis. 2010;16:538.
5. Brown J. Imaging in the patient with hyposalivation. Oral diseases. Conference: 10th Biennial Conference of the European Association of Oral Medicine, EAOM 2010 London United Kingdom. Oral Dis. 2010;16:503–4.
6. Poul JH, Brown JE, Davies J. Retrospective study of the effectiveness of high-resolution ultrasound compared with sialography in the diagnosis of Sjogren's syndrome. Dentomaxillofac Radiol. 2008;37:392–7.
7. Salaffi F, Carotti M, Iagnocco A, et al. Ultrasonography of salivary glands in primary Sjögren's syndrome: a comparison with contrast sialography and scintigraphy. J Rheumatol. 2000;27:1229–36.
8. El Miedany YM, Ahmed I, Mourad HG, et al. Quantitative ultrasonography and magnetic resonance imaging of the parotid gland: can they replace the histopathologic studies in patients with Sjogren's syndrome? Joint Bone Spine. 2004;71:29–38.
9. Whaites E, Drage N. The salivary glands. In: Whaites E, Drage N, editors. Essentials of dental radiography and radiology. 5th ed. Edinburgh: Churchill Livingstone/Elsevier; 2013. p. 447–60.
10. Benson B. Salivary gland radiology. In: White SC, Pharoah MJ, editors. Oral radiology: principles and interpretation. 6th ed. St. Louis: Mosby/Elsevier; 2009. p. 478–596.
11. Drage NA, Brown JE. Cone beam computed sialography of sialoliths. Dentomaxillofac Radiol. 2009;38:301–5.
12. Abdel-Wahed N, Amer ME, Abo-Taleb NSM. Assessment of the role of cone beam computed sialography in diagnosing salivary gland lesions. Imaging Sci Dent. 2013;43:17–23.
13. Kalk WWI, Vissink A, Spijkervet FKL, Bootsma H, Kallenberg CGM, Roodenburg JLN. Parotid sialography for diagnosing Sjogren syndrome. Oral Surg Oral Med Oral Pathol Oral Radiol Endod. 2002;94:131–7.
14. Becker M, Marchal F, Becker C, et al. Sialolithiasis and salivary ductal stenosis: diagnostic accuracy of MR sialography with a three-dimensional extended-phase conjugate-symmetry rapid spin-echo sequence. Radiology. 2000;216:347–58.
15. Astreinidou E, Roesink J, Raaijmakers CPJ, et al. 3D MR sialography as a tool to investigate radiation-induced xerostomia: feasibility study. Int J Radiat Oncol Biol Phys. 2007;68:1310–9.
16. Kalinowski M, Heverhagen J, Rehberg E, et al. Comparative study of MR sialography and digital subtraction sialography for benign salivary gland disorders. Am J Neuroradiol. 2002; 23:1485–92.

17. Tanaka T, Ono K, Ansai T, et al. Dynamic magnetic resonance sialography for patients with xerostomia. Oral Surg Oral Med Oral Pathol Oral Radiol Endod. 2008;106:115–23.
18. Habu M, Tanaka T, Tomoyose T, et al. Significance of dynamic magnetic resonance sialography in prognostic evaluation of saline solution irrigation of the parotid gland for the treatment of xerostomia. J Oral Maxillofac Surg. 2010;68:768–76.

# Part V

# Treatment

# New Radiotherapy Techniques for the Prevention of Radiotherapy-Induced Xerostomia

10

Thomas M. Richards and Christopher M. Nutting

**Abstract**

External beam radiotherapy is a commonly used treatment for the primary and post-operative treatment of head and neck cancer (HNC). The effects of ionising radiation on the parotid and submandibular glands have been investigated in pre-clinical studies and to a limited extent in human studies. These indicate acinar cells are more radiosensitive compared to ductal or adipose cells with post-radiotherapy recovery originating from the ductal cell region. The sequential development of radiotherapy (RT) delivery techniques, most recently with intensity-modulated radiotherapy (IMRT), has allowed increasing conformality of the dose delivered to the primary tumour in HNC patients. This has resulted in a significant reduction in the radiation dose to the parotid gland (PG) and thus better recovery of parotid and whole mouth saliva flow, with improved patient-reported xerostomia compared to conventional RT. The benefit of PG-sparing IMRT is now confirmed in four randomised controlled trials and a systematic review. Implementation of IMRT is a meticulous stepwise process for precise and safe treatment delivery. An associated quality assurance programme is also mandatory. A sizeable minority of HNC patients treated with IMRT still have persistent late xerostomia; therefore, further approaches to spare other salivary tissues may be of benefit. Further optimisation of IMRT delivery combined with complementary pharmacological strategies should continue to improve salivary gland function and reduce xerostomia rates following IMRT treatment for HNC.

T.M. Richards, BSc, MBBS, MRCP, FRCR
C.M. Nutting, MBBS, BSc, MD, PhD, MRCP, FRCR (✉)
Head and Neck Unit, The Royal Marsden Hospital,
Fulham Road, Chelsea, London SW3 6JJ, UK
e-mail: Chris.Nutting@rmh.nhs.uk



G. Carpenter (ed.), *Dry Mouth: A Clinical Guide on Causes, Effects and Treatments*, DOI 10.1007/978-3-642-55154-3_10

## Abbreviations

| | |
|---|---|
| 2D-RT | Two-dimensional radiotherapy |
| 3D-CRT | Three-dimensional conformal radiotherapy |
| ACR | American College of Radiology |
| ASTRO | American Society of Radiation Oncology |
| CTCAE | Common Terminology Criteria for Adverse Effects |
| EORTC | European Organisation for Research and Treatment of Cancer |
| IMRT | Intensity-modulated radiotherapy |
| LENT-SOMA | Late effects on normal tissues, subjective, objective, management, analytical |
| MLC | Multi-leaf collimator |
| NPC | Nasopharyngeal carcinoma |
| OM | Oral mucosa |
| PG | Parotid gland |
| RCT | Randomised controlled trial |
| RTOG | Radiotherapy Oncology Group |
| SG | Salivary gland |
| SMG | Submandibular gland |
| SS | Sticky saliva |
| WMS | Whole mouth saliva |
| XQ | Xerostomia questionnaire |

## Introduction

External beam radiotherapy is a commonly used treatment for the primary and adjuvant (post-operative) treatment of head and neck cancer (HNC), where no distant metastases are present.

HNC including thyroid cancer comprises more than 15 primary tumour subsites above the clavicles, excluding brain tumours. It is the fifth commonest cancer diagnosis with approximately 10,000 new cases in England in 2009 [1].

Despite the benefit from ionising radiation of killing tumour cells, it can also have a deleterious effect on the normal tissues. These normal tissues such as salivary glands (SGs), spinal cord and optic nerves are frequently in close proximity to the site of primary tumour or regions of local lymph node metastases; therefore, the head and neck region is an ideal site to develop and apply improved radiotherapy (RT) delivery techniques.

The radiobiology of the SGs and historical development, current treatments and potential future approaches to using RT techniques to reduce SG toxicity will be discussed in this chapter.

## Radiotherapy-Induced Pathology, Atrophy and Xerostomia

The SGs, particularly the acinar cells, are considered to be one of the most radiosensitive tissues in the body. This is in contrast to the logical assumption that a well-differentiated organ, with very low or no mitotic activity, should be relatively radioresistant, as is seen with central and peripheral nerves.

The understanding of how RT causes SG dysfunction is crucial to formulate a preventative or treatment strategy. Histopathological studies provide an insight into the structural changes caused by RT. Most studies have been in preclinical animal models; however, a few have been performed in humans. A summary of the data is presented below.

*Preclinical* – A recent comprehensive review provides a detailed summary of the preclinical data [2]. In most of the studies, a single large fraction of ionising radiation, 15–40 Gy, was delivered to the SGs of a variety of mammalian animal models. The most common acute changes were a significant reduction in saliva flow, decreased gland weight and reduced acinar cell volume. The association between acinar cell loss and a reduction in salivary flow would be expected as fluid and proteins are predominantly secreted from acinar cells, and these cells constitute ~80 % of the SG volume. Fractionated RT regimens have been less frequently investigated, but several studies, administering 2 Gy per fraction over 6 or 7 weeks (total dose 60–70 Gy), have reported the same acute changes associated with a single fraction.

Konings et al. [3] presented the hypothesis for four phases of radiation damage expression in the rat submandibular gland (SMG). Phase 1, the acute phase (0–10 days), is characterised by a rapid reduction in water excretion, but no cell loss and protein secretion are maintained. In phase 2 (10–60 days), there is a steady loss of damaged acinar cells with an associated reduction in the secretion of amylase. Phase 3 (60–120 days) is a plateau period with stable gland architecture and function, no change in cell number or fluid excretion. Finally phase 4 (120–240 days) is characterised by a late deterioration in function due to lack of stem cells and progenitor cells. Regenerated acinar cells exhibit poor function due to abnormal nerve, vascular and ductal structures.

*Human* – No prospective human studies have been performed to assess the histopathological changes in SGs induced by ionising radiation. Two retrospective reports of changes seen in the major SGs are published.

Sullivan et al. [4] identified ten patients who had received sequential induction chemotherapy then RT with concomitant chemotherapy followed by therapeutic neck dissection (ND). The ND was performed at a median of 10 weeks (range 42–123 days) after completion of RT. A control group of age- and sex-matched oral cancer patients (ND alone, no RT) was selected for comparison. The mean radiation dose to the irradiated SMG was between 50 and 72 Gy. Analysis of the SG morphology indicated pronounced acinar cell loss with ductal cell proliferation after treatment. This was confirmed on immunohistochemistry with an increase in ki-67 and p63 staining suggesting that ductal cells were attempting to proliferate and regenerate.

In a more recent study by Teshima and colleagues [5], parotid gland (PG) and SMG specimens were analysed from six patients, who had received low-dose, preoperative conventional 2D-RT with concomitant chemotherapy (30 Gy in 2 Gy per fraction over 3 weeks). The concomitant chemotherapy was S-1, a novel 5-fluorouracil analogue. All patients had a diagnosis of oral cavity squamous cell carcinoma, and histological specimens were compared to a control cohort ($n=10$, ND alone, no RT). A homogenous radiation dose was delivered to both the PG and SMG (range 29.2–31.1 Gy). Functionally the median whole mouth saliva flow rate (ml/min) was reduced to ~60 % after RT (0.65 vs. 1.5). The ipsilateral whole SMG and part of the ipsilateral PG were resected at ND 3–4 weeks after RT for histology assessment.

The morphological appearance showed a significant decrease in the percentage of acinar cells between control and RT groups for the PG (31.5 % vs. 1.1 %, $p=0.001$) and SMG (43.3 % vs. 19.0 %, $p=0.002$). No significant difference in other SG cell types was noted, but interestingly a nonsignificant increase in the proportion of ductal cells was seen with no difference in the proportion of adipose cells. It was concluded that the loss of salivary flow was related to acinar cell loss.

A limitation of these studies is that they are retrospective and only assess SGs in the early period median of 3.5 and 10 weeks after RT; however, the lack of data in this field is testament to the ethical and logistical difficulties of collecting normal tissue samples in RT-treated HNC patients.

## Dose-Response Relationship and PG Tolerance to Radiation

Several studies have investigated the dose-response relationship of the PG to radiation. Most have compared the PG mean dose to either WMS or individual ductal flow rates. The recent QUANTEC report presented SG dose constraint guidelines based on a detailed review of published literature [6]. The recommendations were that if one whole PG is spared with a mean dose of ~20 Gy or if both are spared with a mean dose of ~25 Gy, then severe PG hypofunction (PG flow rate <25 % of baseline) can be avoided in most cases. This is supported by estimates from combined multicentre databases [7] which indicate that a mean whole PG dose limit of 25–30 Gy is associated with 17–26 % normal tissue complication probability (PG flow rate <25 % of baseline) at 1 year (Fig. 10.1). In addition, there is a 50 % probability of PG flow reduction to <25 % of the pre-RT flow rate with a mean PG dose of 40 Gy. The QUANTEC guidelines have recently been validated in an independent patient cohort [8].

Van Luijk et al. [9] have suggested, in a preclinical study, that there is a differential PG dose response dependent on the distribution of RT dose across the PG. Irradiation of the whole PG, with what is regarded as a sub-tolerance dose of

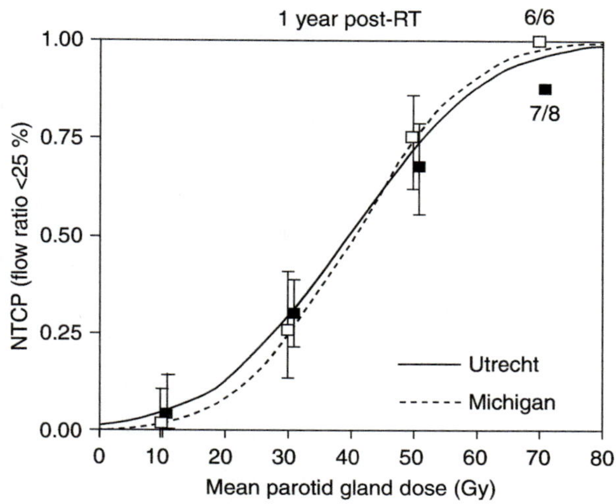


**Fig. 10.1** Normal tissue complication probability curves (*NTCP*) as a function of the mean PG dose for Michigan (*dashed line*) and Utrecht (*solid line*). Clinical NTCP values (using mean dose bins of 20 Gy) are shown for Michigan (*open squares*) and Utrecht (*black squares*), including 95 % confidence intervals (Reproduced with permission from Dijkema et al. [7])

10 Gy, did not result in functional loss (recovery of salivary function). However, when 10 Gy is delivered to the entire PG ("bath dose") and an additional 30 Gy is delivered to a smaller sub-volume ("shower dose"), specifically to the caudal half of the gland, then this resulted in greater functional loss. Conversely the administration of the shower dose (30 Gy) to the cranial half of the gland was shown to not cause additional functional impairment [10]. Buettner et al. [11] showed that a radiobiological model describing the distribution of dose across the PG was better than a mean whole gland dose parameter alone for predicting physician-graded late xerostomia (LENT-SOMA).

## How IMRT Improves Radiation Dose Delivery

The delivery of therapeutic radiation for HNC has changed significantly over the last two decades. The original technique of conventional 2D radiotherapy (2D-RT) delivered a homogenous dose to both the malignant and normal tissues using paired, opposed radiation beams with limited ability to shape the dose distribution (Fig. 10.2). This led to a very high frequency of early and late normal tissue toxicity [12]. The first RT technique that was investigated to reduce SG toxicity, specifically PG dysfunction, was 3D conformal RT (3D-CRT). This technique uses a multi-leaf collimator (MLC) comprising many narrow, mobile lead leaves, to shape the radiation beam and produce convexities in the dose distribution; however, it is not possible to produce concavities.

Intensity-modulated radiotherapy (IMRT), first described in 1997 [13], is an advanced form of 3D-CRT with the MLC used to define the radiation dose intensity independently for different regions of the target volume. This is achieved by using multiple beam directions, commonly five or seven equi-spaced fields. The shape

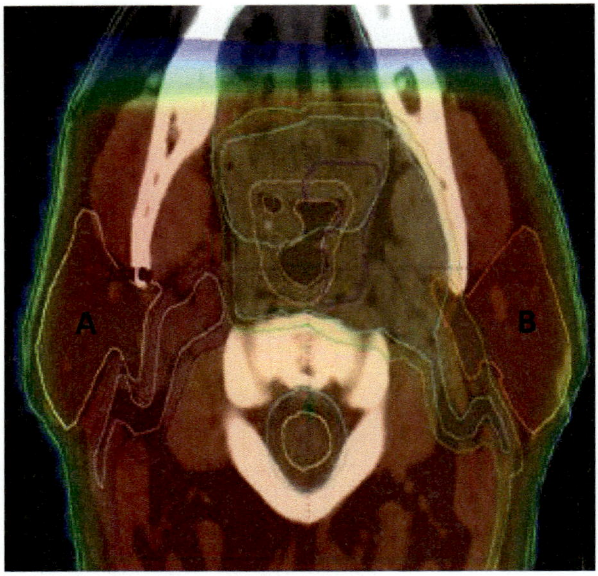


**Fig. 10.2** Dose distribution with a 2D-RT treatment plan for oropharyngeal carcinoma. *A* right PG, *B* Left PG, *red shading* region receiving >95 % of prescribed radiation dose

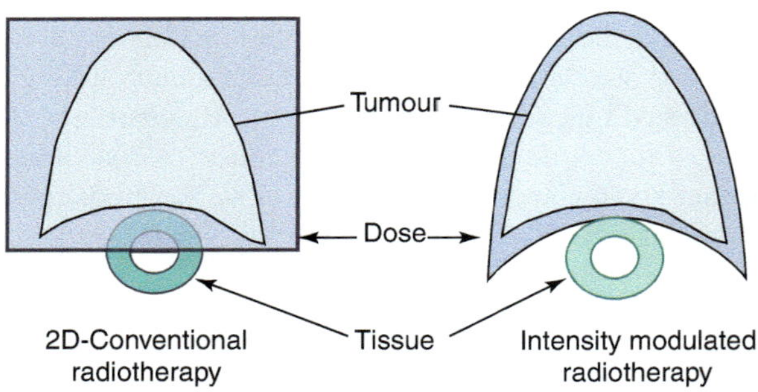


**Fig. 10.3** Schematic diagram showing the improvement in conformality achieved with IMRT (*right*) vs. 2D-RT (*left*)

defined by the MLC is then varied over time. The most frequent methods used are step and shoot, with multiple static fields of different shapes or dynamic MLC with continuous, automated movement of MLCs without treatment interruption. IMRT may also be delivered using arc therapy delivering IMRT with one (360°) or two (720°) continuous rotations of the radiation source around the patient. Examples such as VMAT (Elekta), RapidArc or tomotherapy have the main benefit of a reduction in treatment time [14].

IMRT will therefore define concave and convex shapes (Fig. 10.3) thus allowing high-dose treatment of tumour sites but avoidance of adjacent nontarget normal tissues. The use of IMRT means that delineation of the target and nontarget tissues, patient immobilisation and verification of patient and tumour positions during a course of treatment become even more important. This is to avoid missing the edge of the tumour, which may lead to an increase in recurrence rates (see section "Local disease control with PG-or SMG-sparing IMRT") with possible overdose of normal tissues.

In addition to the reduced normal tissue toxicity, IMRT has the potential to allow dose escalation to the tumour which will increase cell kill and may improve recurrence and cure rates. Dose escalation has been studied recently in a number of phase I/II studies [15–18], and a multicentre phase III RCT is currently recruiting in the UK [19].

## Non-randomised Studies of PG-Sparing RT and IMRT for the Treatment of Head and Neck Cancer

In an early planning study where patients were treated with unilateral irradiation of the neck lymph nodes, 3D-CRT was shown to be superior to 2D-RT for both target volume coverage and contralateral PG sparing [20]. In addition, when treating the bilateral neck, a reduction in the mean radiation dose delivered to the contralateral PG (21 Gy vs. 58 Gy) was reported in a study by Eisbruch et al. [21] using 3D-CRT.

Eisbruch et al. subsequently pioneered the implementation of IMRT for the routine treatment in HNC. Their initial case series of 88 patients treated with IMRT reported that the PG mean dose should be limited to 26 Gy or 24 Gy, for stimulated or unstimulated flow, respectively, to maintain a substantial fraction of pre-IMRT PG saliva flow [22]. Furthermore they showed that patient-reported xerostomia significantly improved over time with the use of IMRT [23].

Further single-arm phase I and II prospective studies have shown that PG-sparing IMRT produces favourable xerostomia rates for several common subsites of HNC (Table 10.1).

## RCTs of PG-Sparing IMRT

### RCT of Conventional RT Versus IMRT

Four phase III randomised controlled trials (RCTs), one multicentre and three single institution, have compared conventional 2D-RT with IMRT.

The PARSPORT trial [32] is the largest study to investigate PG-sparing IMRT in non-nasopharyngeal carcinoma (NPC) patients; it is also the only multicentre IMRT RCT for squamous cell HNC. Ninety-four patients from six UK centres were randomised to IMRT vs. 2D-RT. The primary end point was patient-reported high-grade (≥G2) xerostomia by the LENT-SOMA scale at 12 months after RT. The secondary end points were global and xerostomia-specific quality of life scores, acute and other late radiation side effects, measurable PG and floor of mouth salivary flow and progression-free and overall survival. The salivary function outcomes at 12 months for contralateral measurable PG salivary flow were 47 % for IMRT compared to 0 % for conventional RT ($p<0.0001$). The frequency of high-grade xerostomia was 38 % for IMRT and 74 % for conventional RT ($p=0.0027$) (Fig. 10.4). In addition, the EORTC-HN35 subscale score for dry mouth showed deterioration from baseline (increased mean score) at all time points after

**Table 10.1** Summary of prospective single-arm studies (by subsite), with xerostomia end points where PG-sparing IMRT is used for the treatment of head and neck cancer

| Author (year) | Disease site | Total (*n*) | Months follow-up | Xerostomia end point | Frequency (%) or grade of end point |
|---|---|---|---|---|---|
| Lee et al. (2009) [24] | Nasopharynx | 68 | 31 | ≥grade 2 (RTOG) | 13.5 %[a] |
| Marucci et al. (2012) [25] | Nasopharynx | 31 | 24 | ≥grade 2 (RTOG) | 75 %[b] (5-field plan)<br>44 %[b] (7-field plan) |
| | | | | Mean total XQ score | 20.5[b] (5-field plan)<br>18.5[b] (7-field plan) |
| Hunter et al. [26] | Oropharynx | 72 | 24 | Mean xerostomia score (CTCAE) | 1.0[a] |
| Eisbruch et al. [27] | Oropharynx | 69 | 24 | ≥grade 2 (RTOG) | 67 % (6 m)<br>25 % (12 m)<br>15 % (18 m)<br>16 % (24 m) |
| Richards et al. [28] | Unknown primary | 19 | 23.7 | ≥grade 2 (LENT-SOMA) | 29.4 % (6 m)<br>14.3 % (12 m) |
| Miah et al. (2010) [15] | Larynx and hypopharynx | 60 | 51.2 (DL 1) | ≥grade 2 (LENT-SOMA) | 9 %[a] (DL 1) |
| | | | 36.2 (DL 2) | | 8 %[a] (DL 2) |
| Toledano et al. (2012) [29] | Mixed SCCHN | 208 | 25.3 | ≥grade 2 (RTOG) | 16 % (18 m) |
| Scrimger et al. (2007) [30] | Mixed SCCHN | 64 | 48 | Mean total RTOG score | 1.1[a] |
| Munter et al. (2004) [31] | Mixed SCCHN | 18 | 23 | ≥grade 2 (RTOG) | 17 % (>3 m) |
| Zaidi et al. (2011) [17] | Thyroid | 45 | 12 | ≥grade 2 (LENT-SOMA) | 35 % (DL 1, 0–3 m)<br>65 % (DL 2, 0–3 m) |

*SCCHN* squamous cell carcinoma of the head and neck, *DL 1* dose level 1, *DL 2* dose level 2, *RTOG* radiotherapy oncology group, *CTCAE* common toxicity criteria for adverse events, *XQ* xerostomia questionnaire, *LENT-SOMA* late effects normal tissue subjective, objective, management, analytical
[a]12 months
[b]24 months

RT. At 12 months the mean increases were 56.6 (2D-RT) and 48 (IMRT), and at 24 months the mean increases were 59.3 (2D-RT) and 34.8 (IMRT). Despite numerical improvement in the IMRT arm when compared with the 2D-RT arm, the result was not statistically significant ($p>0.01$) (Fig. 10.5).

Peng et al. [33] published the most recent and largest RCT investigating PG-sparing RT techniques. Patients with NPC and no distant metastases were randomised to IMRT ($n=315$) or 2D-RT ($n=325$). Administration of induction, concomitant and/or adjuvant CT was similar between treatment groups. The 6-month rate of xerostomia (any CTCAE grade) showed a significant benefit for IMRT vs. 2D-RT, 39.5 % vs. 99.4 % ($p<0.001$).

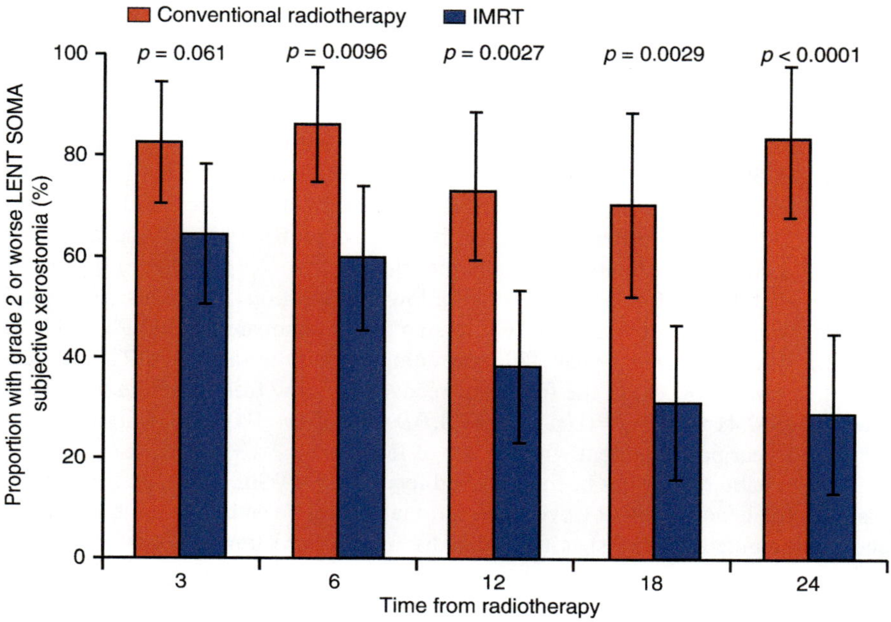


**Fig. 10.4** Proportion of patients reporting grade 2 or worse LENT-SOMA subjective xerostomia salivary gland side effects (primary trial end point ≥ grade 2 subjective xerostomia at 12 months) (Reproduced with permission from PARSPORT trial [32])

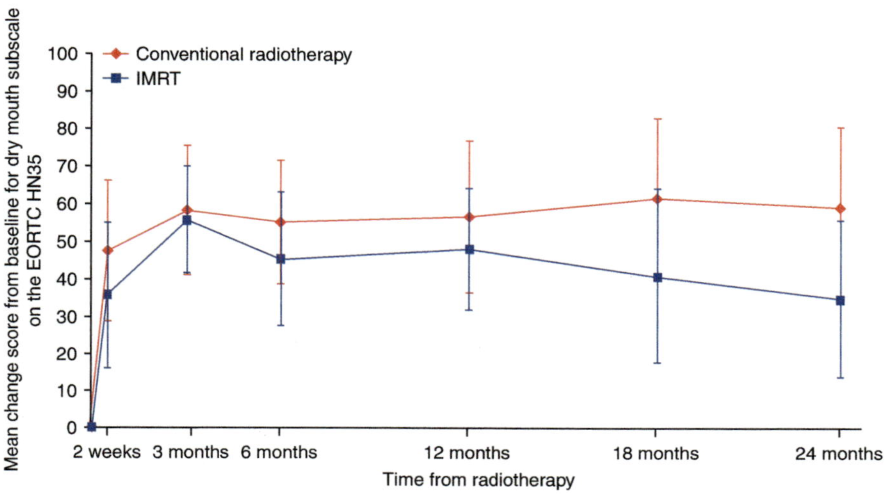


**Fig. 10.5** Mean EORTC QOL HN35 dry mouth subscale score changes from baseline (Reproduced with permission from PARSPORT trial [32])

Two smaller, single institution RCTs are reported for patients with early-stage NPC [34,35]. Pow et al. [34] (45 patients) reported stimulated whole mouth saliva (WMS) and unilateral stimulated parotid saliva (SPS) flow rates. At 12 months post-RT, the proportion of patients with stimulated WMS and SPS flow recovery to >25 % of the pre-RT level was significantly higher with IMRT vs. 2D-RT (stimulated WMS 50 % vs. 4.8 % and SPS 83.3 % vs. 9.5 %). Despite this finding, patient-reported oral quality of life (EORTC-HN35) scores for sticky saliva and dry mouth were not significantly different between the two techniques; this may be related to the small number of patients enrolled in the trial.

Kam et al. [35] (60 patients) reported a lower proportion of patients with ≥ G2 physician-reported xerostomia (RTOG) using IMRT compared to 2D-RT (39.3 % vs. 82.1 %, $p=0.001$) at 1 year. This was comparable to the PARSPORT trial outcomes. As with Pow et al., the fractional recovery of flow from baseline for stimulated WMS, 0.41 vs. 0.2 ($p=0.01$), and SPS, 0.9 vs. 0.05 ($p<0.001$), was significantly better at 1 year posttreatment with the use of IMRT.

A systematic review has been published recently by O'Sullivan et al. [36] which assessed the benefit of IMRT over conventional 2D-RT for multiple adverse effects and disease outcomes and specific to this discussion, xerostomia.

They retrieved seven prospective, retrospective and case-controlled studies with xerostomia as an end point, which enrolled 567 patients between them. Five of the studies reported a statistically significant reduction in xerostomia at 6 months [37], 1 year [32,34,35] or 20 months [38] after RT. However, two other studies [39,40] showed no significant difference in xerostomia outcomes.

The authors concluded that if a reduction of xerostomia and an improvement in quality of life are the main outcomes of interest, then IMRT is the recommended treatment for all nasopharyngeal, oropharyngeal, hypopharyngeal, laryngeal, oral cavity and unknown primary cancers when delivery of RT to lymph node regions, requiring inclusion in the treatment volume, would result in irreparable damage to SG function, if a less conformal RT technique is used due to their inability to maintain SG doses within their tolerance limits.

## RCT of 3D-CRT Versus IMRT

Gupta and colleagues [41] report the only RCT of PG-sparing IMRT vs. 3D-CRT. Sixty patients were assessed for radiation dosimetry and physician-reported SG toxicity (RTOG, acute and late). The ≥ G2 acute SG toxicity using IMRT was lower, 59 % vs. 89 % ($p=0.03$) and for late toxicity ~30 % vs. ~75 % ($p=0.001$, data in histogram figure only). IMRT plans achieved higher dose conformality and PG sparing. The mean (95 % CI) contralateral PG dose for 3D-CRT vs. IMRT plans was 49.8 Gy (46.5–53.1 Gy) and 28.8 Gy (27–30.7 Gy), respectively.

## Implementation of IMRT: National and International Experience

The implementation of IMRT into routine practice is a meticulous process requiring multidisciplinary teamwork to provide the safe and precise delivery of this highly conformal RT technique [42]. For implementation and ongoing routine treatment, the clinical/radiation oncologist, physicist, dosimetrist and therapy radiographer must work closely together. Once the primary tumour site of interest has been determined, a stepwise implementation plan should be developed [42].

Firstly, treatment planning requires reproducible immobilisation of the patient, commonly using a thermoplastic shell. IMRT no longer necessitates a straight cervical spine therefore allowing extension of the neck which can reduce dose to critical normal tissues. The departmental set-up errors and patient movements in the treatment position should be audited to determine margins that should be added to the outlined regions of tumour and normal tissue. Patients should be imaged in the treatment position with axial scans, currently CT+/−MRI or PET, and the tumour and normal tissues delineated using computerised planning software performed by an oncologist. Alongside this a quality assurance programme should be maintained to confirm the accuracy of IMRT treatment delivery, planning systems and software. Guidelines for the roles of each team member in the delivery of IMRT are outlined in a recent joint ACR and ASTRO publication [43].

*UK* – A survey of the use of IMRT in the UK was performed in 2008 [44]. Fifty of 58 UK centres responded (~89 % of all patients treated) with 46 of 50 centres having at least 2 IMRT-capable treatment machines but only 18 centres treating patients with it. Despite HNC and thyroid cancer being the fifth commonest cancer diagnosis, it was the third most common cancer to be treated radically with IMRT in the UK, behind breast and prostate cancer. This indicates the important role it has in HNC treatment.

In 2008, 1,237 of 7,219 patients (17.1 %) eligible for a radical course of RT received IMRT. The same study estimated that 57 % of these patients would benefit from IMRT. The relatively low utilisation of IMRT in 2008 has been addressed over the last 5 years. Improved funding and direct Department of Health guidelines that are in place to bridge the gap between the current and optimal use of IMRT have accelerated this process of IMRT implementation [45]. Such that recently updated data from 2012 show that 68 % of UK centres are now offering IMRT with 83.9 % of all UK HNC patients receiving their radical treatment using an IMRT technique [46].

*Worldwide* – IMRT was developed in the USA and due to the differences in health care funding has been implemented at a faster rate compared to the UK. Between 2002 and 2004, the proportion of radiation oncologists treating with IMRT was reported to increase from 40 % to 73 % [47]. As seen in the UK, the introduction of IMRT in Canada for HNC was slightly slower compared to the USA but has rapidly increased recently with 80 % of centres using IMRT for treatment of HNC in 2010 and 37 % of all centres using IMRT for "virtually all" HNC patients [48]. The reported barriers to IMRT use in Canada are now most frequently the lack of trained IMRT planners or oncologist and no longer the lack of technical capability or support staff to deliver IMRT. Other countries such as India are developing IMRT-capable facilities rapidly and recently reported that 60 of 280 centres in India are delivering IMRT treatment [49].

## Potential Strategies to Improve IMRT-Induced Xerostomia

PG-sparing IMRT is now the standard treatment for HNC. However, residual xerostomia remains a clinical problem for a sizeable minority, and further improvements may be gained through avoidance of the SGs or by the further reduction in dose to the PG with the use of novel RT delivery techniques.

### Submandibular Gland-Sparing IMRT

IMRT for PG sparing has now been extensively studied, but few trials have assessed the possibility of PG and SMG sparing. It is becoming apparent that the SMGs and the minor SGs may have an important role in the prevention of xerostomia as they are the sole source of salivary mucins for the oral cavity [50].

A prospective study [51] which investigated the dose response of the SMG also showed that for a subgroup, 8 of 148 recruited patients, using IMRT and applying a contralateral SMG (cSMG) dose constraint, the mean cSMG dose can be significantly reduced from 48 to 36 Gy ($p=0.001$).

Saarilahti et al. [52] assessed the role of IMRT to spare the PG and the cSMG in 36 patients. Half the patients were treated with cSMG sparing, and a mean cSMG dose of 25.9 Gy (range 18–32 Gy) was achieved. At 12 months the $\geq$ grade 2 subjective xerostomia (LENT-SOMA) frequency was improved with cSMG sparing, 22 % vs. 61 % ($p=0.018$). cSMG sparing significantly improved unstimulated but not stimulated relative-fractional WMS flow at 12 months, 0.6 vs. 0.25 ($p=0.006$). Six-month flow was also significantly improved ($p<0.05$).

Wang and colleagues [53] treated 52 patients with PG-sparing IMRT; 26 patients also had cSMG sparing. Mean unstimulated WMS flow was better with the addition of cSMG sparing compared to PG sparing alone, at all time points from 2 to 18 months ($p<0.0001$ for all). However, any grade xerostomia (RTOG) was only significantly better in the cSMG-sparing group at 2 and 6 months ($p=0.036$ and 0.046) but not at 12 and 18 months. No difference in late xerostomia score might be expected as the RTOG scale assesses xerostomia symptoms predominantly under stimulated conditions, whereas the most likely benefit of cSMG sparing would be found under unstimulated (resting) conditions.

More recently Little et al. [54] reported a study of PG-, cSMG- and oral mucosa-sparing IMRT in 78 patients with stage III or IV HNC. Significant sparing of the cSMG was not possible; mean cSMG dose was 62 Gy (range 29–75 Gy). The proportion of patients with >25 % of baseline flow at 12 months was 17 % (unstimulated) and 14 % (stimulated). When compared to the preceding two studies [52,53], patients in the study by Little et al. were not selected on their suitability for cSMG sparing, hence the high SMG dose of 62 Gy [54] vs. 25.9 Gy [52] or 20.4 Gy [53] and resultant poor, long-term SMG flow rates.

These reports make it apparent that careful selection of patients for cSMG sparing is needed, where the risk of contralateral level 1 lymph node disease is low. However, in a selected cohort good recovery of SG function can be achieved with this approach.

## Oral Mucosa-Sparing IMRT

Within the oral mucosa (OM) are 600–1,000 minor SGs, and until recently there was no option to spare them; also the clinical relevance of these secretions was unclear. Despite contributing <10 % WMS they contribute the majority of mucins [50] which are associated with mucosal moisture retention and xerostomia at rest and at night.

The dosimetric and clinical benefits of IMRT for OM sparing, when compared to 3D-CRT, have been shown in a planning study of oropharyngeal carcinoma patients [55]. IMRT provides a reduction in the maximum OM dose, defined as the OM outside the target tumour volume, but significantly this is only possible when a dose constraint is applied to the OM. In this study a clinically relevant maximum OM dose was defined as 30 Gy (2 Gy per fraction, 6 weeks) to the spared region. When IMRT treatment was replanned for the same patient with no dose constraint applied, a significantly increased dose to the OM was seen, with significantly larger volume of OM receiving ≤39.3 Gy vs. 3D-CRT. This study also reported clinical correlation in 19 IMRT-treated patients by comparing RTOG acute mucositis score, in the spared region of the OM with the region within the PTV. This was significantly reduced from week 2 of treatment onwards ($p<0.01$) compared to the unspared regions. Though not reporting on minor SG function or xerostomia, it is promising that OM may be spared with no significant impact on PG mean dose, target volume coverage or increase in other OAR doses.

A prospective RCT [56] ($n=48$) of OM-sparing IMRT for post-operative treatment of oral tongue SCC showed a significant reduction in grade 2 and 3 acute oral mucositis (0 % and 25 % vs. 45.8 % and 54.2 %, respectively; $p<0.0001$) and reduced mean dose to the OM (41.8±7.4 Gy vs. 58.8±2.2 Gy; $p<0.0001$). Again no xerostomia end points were used in this study, but it shows that it is feasible to spare OM, and no increase in tumour recurrence rate was noted.

Two other prospective studies have examined the relationship of OM dose to patient-reported xerostomia. The first with no SG radiation dose constraints [57] and the second with pre-specified PG, SMG and OM radiation dose constraints [54].

The study by Jellema et al. [57], although treating with 2D-RT only, is the largest to date with 156 patients. It assessed for a correlation between the patient-reported symptoms of dry mouth (DM) and sticky saliva (SS) (EORTC HN35) in relation to mean RT dose to SMGs, PGs and OM. All tumours were squamous cell HNC, and the majority had a primary site in the hypopharynx or larynx (74 %). Seventy-six per cent received primary RT, and no chemotherapy was administered. The 6- and 12-month DM scores were associated with both SMG (OR 1.08, $p = 0.02$) and PG (OR 1.17, $p = 0.002$) mean doses. The rate of the 6-month moderate to severe DM was found to be reversible, dependant on SMG and PG mean dose such that if the mean SMG dose is 30 Gy or 40 Gy, the mean PG dose must be limited to 16 Gy or 10 Gy, respectively, for <20 % probability of moderate to severe DM. This was not seen at 12 months. The 6- and 12-month SS scores were only associated with SMG mean dose (OR 1.03, $p < 0.001$). The dose to the OM did not affect the probability of patient-reported xerostomia or sticky saliva at either time point in this patient cohort. Of note the majority of patients were on early-stage disease T1–2 ~ 85 % and N0 ~ 90 %, and the median radiation dose to bilateral SMG and the OM was low (46.7 and 9.1 Gy, respectively). This was despite no SMG or OM dose constraint. Much higher mean RT doses have been reported [55] when treating with IMRT and no SMG or OM constraint and also when treating more advanced disease stage.

The second prospective study by Little et al. [54], which addresses the limitations of the previous study specifically a cohort with more advanced disease stage and treated using IMRT, has been described earlier. In this study a multivariate analysis indicated that when bilateral PG and partial contralateral SMG-sparing IMRTs were used, then the OM dose was found to significantly correlate with late patient (XQ)-and physician-reported (CTCAE) xerostomia, such that if the mean OM dose <40 Gy, there were no cases of ≥ grade 2 xerostomia (CTCAE).

## Local Disease Control with PG- or SMG-Sparing IMRT

With the increase in dose conformality, concerns have been raised that the risk of geographical miss of the tumour may increase local recurrence rates [58]. Treating the tumour must always remain the priority, and therefore this specific question has been assessed in a number of case series. The largest and most contemporary was Garden et al. [59] reporting the MD Anderson experience of PG-sparing IMRT for oropharyngeal carcinoma ($n = 776$). Promisingly only 12 patients (2 %) had a locoregional recurrence outside the high-radiation dose region, and no patients had a recurrence either within the PG or in the adjacent region of steep dose gradient between the spared PG and the treated nodal region. Smaller trials of SMG-sparing IMRT [52,53] have also shown no recurrences adjacent to the SMG, within the contralateral nodal level 1b region. However, this should be viewed with caution due to a limited number of patients treated with this technique, relatively short follow-up and the site of the SMG within the level 1b nodal region.

## Novel Radiotherapy Techniques

Arc therapies (RapidArc, VMAT and helical tomotherapy) deliver IMRT with one (360°) or two (720°) continuous rotations of the RT source around the patient. Early data indicates they retain the good target tissue dose coverage with possibly better normal tissue sparing compared to static IMRT systems [14]. Arc therapy also benefits from significantly reduced treatment times which may improve patient QOL and increase patient throughput with the associated economic benefit.

Particle therapy with carbon ions or protons both have the benefit of minimal exit dose beyond the target tissue, unlike photons. A few small trials [60,61] in squamous cell HNC patients have been performed; however, the current role remains unclear, but it may have benefit as a focal boost dose when combined with IMRT. The routine use of carbon ions or protons is limited by very high set-up cost and a lack of facilities.

No data for particle therapies is available regarding their effect on SG dysfunction and oral symptoms, but with the extremely precise nature of the dose deposition, it would be hoped that no additional normal tissue toxicity would occur.

### Conclusions

Major advances have been achieved over the last 15 years due to a better understanding of SG radiobiology, a clearer definition of PG tolerance to radiation and the development and implementation of IMRT for routine clinical use.

Despite the significant advances achieved with the reduction in PG radiation dose and hence long-term toxicity, with no reported detrimental effect on tumour control rates, a sizable minority of patients treated with IMRT for HNC continue to be affected by persistent, late xerostomia.

Future strategies for the use of IMRT to spare other SGs and the continued development of novel RT delivery techniques as outlined in this chapter show promise. Further optimisation for the delivery of RT and improving the therapeutic ratio are among several complementary approaches which when combined should continue to improve patient quality of life after RT for HNC over the coming years.

## References

1. ONS. Cancer statistics – registrations, England, 2009. In: Office for National Statistics, Series MB1 no.40. London: Office for National Statistics; 2010.
2. Grundmann O, Mitchell GC, Limesand KH. Sensitivity of salivary glands to radiation: from animal models to therapies. J Dent Res. 2009;88(10):894–903.
3. Konings AWT, Coppes RP, Vissink A. On the mechanism of salivary gland radiosensitivity. Int J Radiat Oncol Biol Phys. 2005;62(4):1187–94.
4. Sullivan CA, Haddad RI, Tishler RB, Mahadevan A, Krane JF. Chemoradiation-induced cell loss in human submandibular glands. Laryngoscope. 2005;115(6):958–64.

5. Teshima K, Murakami R, Yoshida R, et al. Histopathological changes in parotid and submandibular glands of patients treated with preoperative chemoradiation therapy for oral cancer. J Radiat Res. 2012;53(3):492–6.
6. Deasy JO, Moiseenko V, Marks L, Chao KSC, Nam J, Eisbruch A. Radiotherapy dose-volume effects on salivary gland function. Int J Radiat Oncol Biol Phys. 2010;76(3):S58–63.
7. Dijkema T, Raaijmakers CPJ, Ten Haken RK, et al. Parotid gland function after radiotherapy: the combined Michigan and Utrecht experience. Int J Radiat Oncol Biol Phys. 2010;78(2): 449–53.
8. Moiseenko V, Wu J, Hovan A, et al. Treatment planning constraints to avoid xerostomia in head and neck cancer radiotherapy: an independent test of the QUANTEC criteria using a prospectively collected dataset. Int J Radiat Oncol Biol Phys. 2012;82(3):1108–14.
9. van Luijk P, Faber H, Schippers JM, et al. Bath and shower effects in rat parotid gland explain increased relative risk of parotid gland dysfunction after IMRT. Int J Radiat Oncol Biol Phys. 2009;74(4):1002–5.
10. Konings AWT, Faber H, Cotteleer F, Vissink A, Coppes RP. Secondary radiation damage as the main cause for unexpected volume effects: a histopathologic study of the parotid gland. Int J Radiat Oncol Biol Phys. 2006;64(1):98–105.
11. Buettner F, Miah AB, Gulliford SL, et al. Novel approaches to improve the therapeutic index of head and neck radiotherapy: an analysis of data from the PARSPORT randomised phase III trial. Radiother Oncol. 2012;103(1):82–7.
12. Vissink A, Jansma J, Spijkervet FKL, Burlage FR, Coppes RP. Oral sequelae of head and neck radiotherapy. Crit Rev Oral Biol Med. 2003;14(3):199–212.
13. Boyer AL, Geis P, Grant W, Carol M. Modulated beam conformal therapy for head and neck tumors. Int J Radiat Oncol Biol Phys. 1997;39(1):227–36.
14. Van Gestel D, van Vliet-Vroegindeweij C, Van den Heuvel F, et al. RapidArc, SmartArc and TomoHD compared with classical step and shoot and sliding window intensity modulated radiotherapy in an oropharyngeal cancer treatment plan comparison. Radiat Oncol. 2013;8:37.
15. Miah AB, Bhide SA, Guerrero-Urbano MT, et al. Dose-escalated intensity-modulated radiotherapy is feasible and may improve loco-regional control and laryngeal preservation in laryngo-hypopharyngeal cancers. Int J Radiat Oncol Biol Phys. 2012;82(2):539–47.
16. Leclerc M, Maingon P, Hamoir M, et al. A dose escalation study with intensity modulated radiation therapy (IMRT) in T2N0, T2N1, T3N0 squamous cell carcinomas (SCC) of the oropharynx, larynx and hypopharynx using a simultaneous integrated boost (SIB) approach. Radiother Oncol. 2013;106(3):333–40.
17. Zaidi SH, Miah AB, Bhide SA, et al. Radiotherapy for high-risk thyroid malignancies – report of acute toxicities of a phase I sequential cohort dose-escalation IMRT study. Eur J Cancer. 2011;47:S560–S.
18. Cvek J, Kubes J, Skacelikova E, et al. Hyperfractionated accelerated radiotherapy with concomitant integrated boost of 70–75 Gy in 5 weeks for advanced head and neck cancer a phase I dose escalation study. Strahlentherapie Und Onkologie. 2012;188(8):666–70.
19. ARTDECO trial (ISRCTN 01483375). Accessed 20 May 2013, at http://www.controlled-trials.com/ISRCTN01483375/artdeco.
20. Hazuka MB, Martel MK, Marsh L, Lichter AS, Wolf GT. Preservation of parotid function after external-beam irradiation in head and neck cancer patients – a feasibility study using 3-dimensional treatment planning. Int J Radiat Oncol Biol Phys. 1993;27(3):731–7.
21. Eisbruch A, Ship JA, Martel MK, et al. Parotid gland sparing in patients undergoing bilateral head and neck irradiation: techniques and early results. Int J Radiat Oncol Biol Phys. 1996;36(2):469–80.
22. Eisbruch A, Ten Haken RK, Kim HM, Marsh LH, Ship JA. Dose, volume, and function relationships in parotid salivary glands following conformal and intensity-modulated irradiation of head and neck cancer. Int J Radiat Oncol Biol Phys. 1999;45(3):577–87.
23. Eisbruch A, Kim HM, Terrell JE, Marsh LH, Dawson LA, Ship JA. Xerostomia and its predictors following parotid-sparing irradiation of head-and-neck cancer. Int J Radiat Oncol Biol Phys. 2001;50(3):695–704.

24. Lee N, Harris J, Garden AS, et al. Intensity-modulated radiation therapy with or without chemotherapy for nasopharyngeal carcinoma: radiation therapy oncology group phase II trial 0225. J Clin Oncol. 2009;27(22):3684–90.
25. Marucci L, Marzi S, Sperduti I, et al. Influence of intensity-modulated radiation therapy technique on xerostomia and related quality of life in patients treated with intensity-modulated radiation therapy for nasopharyngeal cancer. Head Neck. 2012;34(3):328–35.
26. Hunter KU, Schipper M, Feng FY, et al. Toxicities affecting quality of life after chemo-IMRT of oropharyngeal cancer: prospective study of patient-reported, observer-rated, and objective outcomes. Int J Radiat Oncol Biol Phys. 2012;85(4):935–40.
27. Eisbruch A, Harris J, Garden AS, et al. Multi-institution trial of accelerated hypofractionated intensity-modulated radiation therapy for early stage oropharyngeal cancer (RTOG 00-22). Int J Radiat Oncol Biol Phys. 2010;76(5):1333–8.
28. Richards TM, Bhide SA, Miah AB, et al. Phase 2 trial of total mucosal and bilateral neck intensity modulated radiotherapy in squamous cell cancer of unknown primary. Eur J Cancer. 2011;47:S559.
29. Toledano I, Graff P, Serre A, et al. Intensity-modulated radiotherapy in head and neck cancer: results of the prospective study GORTEC 2004-03. Radiother Oncol. 2012;103(1):57–62.
30. Scrimger R, Kanji A, Parliament M, et al. Correlation between saliva production and quality of life measurements in head and neck cancer patients treated with intensity-modulated radiotherapy. Am J Clin Oncol Cancer Clin Trials. 2007;30(3):271–7.
31. Munter MW, Karger CP, Hoffner SG, et al. Evaluation of salivary gland function after treatment of head-and-neck tumors with intensity-modulated radiotherapy by quantitative pertechnetate scintigraphy. Int J Radiat Oncol Biol Phys. 2004;58(1):175–84.
32. Nutting CM, Morden JP, Harrington KJ, et al. Parotid-sparing intensity modulated versus conventional radiotherapy in head and neck cancer (PARSPORT): a phase 3 multicentre randomised controlled trial. Lancet Oncol. 2011;12(2):127–36.
33. Peng G, Wang T, Yang K-Y, et al. A prospective, randomized study comparing outcomes and toxicities of intensity-modulated radiotherapy vs. conventional two-dimensional radiotherapy for the treatment of nasopharyngeal carcinoma. Radiother Oncol. 2012;104(3):286–93.
34. Pow EHN, Kwong DLW, McMillan AS, et al. Xerostomia and quality of life after intensity-modulated radiotherapy vs. conventional radiotherapy for early-stage nasopharyngeal carcinoma: Initial report on a randomized controlled clinical trial. Int J Radiat Oncol Biol Phys. 2006;66(4):981–91.
35. Kam MKM, Leung S-F, Zee B, et al. Prospective randomized study of intensity-modulated radiotherapy on salivary gland function in early-stage nasopharyngeal carcinoma patients. J Clin Oncol. 2007;25(31):4873–9.
36. O'Sullivan B, Rumble RB, Warde P. Intensity-modulated radiotherapy in the treatment of head and neck cancer. Clin Oncol. 2012;24(7):474–87.
37. Braam PM, Terhaard CHJ, Roesink JM, Raaijmakers CPJ. Intensity-modulated radiotherapy significantly reduces xerostomia compared with conventional radiotherapy. Int J Radiat Oncol Biol Phys. 2006;66(4):975–80.
38. Lee NY, de Arruda FF, Puri DR, et al. A comparison of intensity-modulated radiation therapy and concomitant boost radiotherapy in the setting of concurrent chemotherapy for locally advanced oropharyngeal carcinoma. Int J Radiat Oncol Biol Phys. 2006;66(4):966–74.
39. Jabbari S, Kim HM, Feng M, et al. Matched case-control study of quality of life and xerostomia after intensity-modulated radiotherapy or standard radiotherapy for head-and-neck cancer: initial report. Int J Radiat Oncol Biol Phys. 2005;63(3):725–31.
40. Chen AM, Daly ME, Bucci MK, et al. Carcinomas of the paranasal sinuses and nasal cavity treated with radiotherapy at a single institution over five decades: are we making improvement? Int J Radiat Oncol Biol Phys. 2007;69(1):141–7.
41. Gupta T, Agarwal J, Jain S, et al. Three-dimensional conformal radiotherapy (3D-CRT) versus intensity modulated radiation therapy (IMRT) in squamous cell carcinoma of the head and neck: a randomized controlled trial. Radiother Oncol. 2012;104(3):343–8.
42. McNair HA, Adams EJ, Clark CH, Miles EA, Nutting CM. Implementation of IMRT in the radiotherapy department. Br J Radiol. 2003;76(912):850–6.

43. Hartford AC, Galvin JM, Beyer DC, et al. American College of Radiology (ACR) and American Society for Radiation Oncology (ASTRO) Practice Guideline for Intensity-Modulated Radiation Therapy (IMRT). Am J Clin Oncol Cancer Clin Trials. 2012;35(6):612–7.
44. Mayles WPM. Survey of the availability and use of advanced radiotherapy technology in the UK. Clin Oncol. 2010;22(8):636–42.
45. Radiotherapy Services in England 2012. 2012. Accessed 17 Aug 2013, at https://www.gov.uk/government/publications/radiotherapy-services-in-england-2012.
46. Mayles WPM, Cooper T, Mackay R, Staffurth J, Williams M. Progress with intensity-modulated radiotherapy implementation in the UK. Clin Oncol. 2012;24(8):543–4.
47. Mell LK, Mehrotra AK, Mundt AJ. Intensity-modulated radiation therapy use in the U.S, 2004. Cancer. 2005;104(6):1296–303.
48. AlDuhaiby EZ, Breen S, Bissonnette J-P, et al. A national survey of the availability of intensity-modulated radiation therapy and stereotactic radiosurgery in Canada. Radiat Oncol. 2012;7. Article 18.
49. Kumar R, Sharma SD, Amols HI, Mayya YS, Kushwaha HS. A survey on the quality assurance procedures used in Intensity Modulated Radiation Therapy (IMRT) at Indian hospitals. J Cancer Sci Ther. 2010;2(6):166–70.
50. Tabak LA. In defense of the oral cavity – structure, biosynthesis and function of salivary mucins. Annu Rev Physiol. 1995;57:547–64.
51. Murdoch-Kinch C-A, Kim HM, Vineberg KA, Ship JA, Eisbruch A. Dose-effect relationships for the submandibular salivary glands and implications for their sparing by intensity modulated radiotherapy. Int J Radiat Oncol Biol Phys. 2008;72(2):373–82.
52. Saarilahti K, Kouri M, Collan J, et al. Sparing of the submandibular glands by intensity modulated radiotherapy in the treatment of head and neck cancer. Radiother Oncol. 2006;78(3):270–5.
53. Wang Z-H, Yan C, Zhang Z-Y, et al. Impact of salivary gland dosimetry on post-IMRT recovery of saliva output and xerostomia grade for head and neck cancer patients treated with or without contralateral submandibular sparing: a longitudinal study. Int J Radiat Oncol Biol Phys. 2011;81(5):1479–87.
54. Little M, Schipper M, Feng FY, et al. Reducing xerostomia after chemo-IMRT for head-and-neck cancer: beyond sparing the parotid glands. Int J Radiat Oncol Biol Phys. 2012;83(3):1007–14.
55. Sanguineti G, Endres EJ, Gunn BG, Parker B. Is there a "mucosa-sparing" benefit of IMRT for head-and-neck cancer? Int J Radiat Oncol Biol Phys. 2006;66(3):931–8.
56. Wang Z-H, Zhang S-Z, Zhang Z-Y, et al. Protecting the oral mucosa in patients with oral tongue squamous cell carcinoma treated postoperatively with intensity-modulated radiotherapy: a randomized study. Laryngoscope. 2012;122(2):291–8.
57. Jellema AP, Doornaert P, Slotman BJ, Leemans CR, Langendijk JA. Does radiation dose to the salivary glands and oral cavity predict patient-rated xerostomia and sticky saliva in head and neck cancer patients treated with curative radiotherapy? Radiother Oncol. 2005;77(2):164–71.
58. Cannon DM, Lee NY. Recurrence in region of spared parotid gland after definitive intensity-modulated radiotherapy for head and neck cancer. Int J Radiat Oncol Biol Phys. 2008;70(3):660–5.
59. Garden AS, Dong L, Morrison WH, et al. Patterns of disease recurrence following treatment of oropharyngeal cancer with intensity modulated radiation therapy. Int J Radiat Oncol Biol Phys. 2013;85(4):941–7.
60. Mizoe J-E, Tsujii H, Kamada T, et al. Dose escalation study of carbon ion radiotherapy for locally advanced head-and-neck cancer. Int J Radiat Oncol Biol Phys. 2004;60(2):358–64.
61. Slater JD, Yonemoto LT, Mantik DW, et al. Proton radiation for treatment of cancer of the oropharynx: early experience at Loma Linda University Medical Center using a concomitant boost technique. Int J Radiat Oncol Biol Phys. 2005;62(2):494–500.

# Artificial Salivas: Why Are They Not More Useful?

11

Guy Carpenter

**Abstract**
The potential market for artificial salivas is huge, yet the actual usage is relatively low. One reason may be the lack of effectiveness of current brands. At best they only mimic the viscous nature of saliva but not the other physical properties, such as elasticity. This leads to a poor retention of the product in the mouth which then requires frequent application to provide any kind of relief. Since most dry mouth sufferers have some residual secretory activity, it makes sense to formulate artificial salivas to supplement any pre-existing saliva. Due to their very low surface tension, artificial salivas may displace the pre-existing saliva. This chapter explores the components of some leading brands, examines their physical properties – both neat and when mixed with saliva – and suggests some potential future directions for new product development.

## Introduction

A large number of conditions cause dry mouth, yet the quality of artificial salivas is insufficient to provide sustained relief for any substantial period of time. The physical properties of saliva are as complex and diverse as its components, yet the artificial salivas only mimic one aspect of real saliva – the viscosity. They do not mimic the elastic component of real saliva that has an important function of helping to retain saliva in the mouth. Another deficiency is that most artificial salivas displace, rather than supplement, the existing natural saliva. Few xerostomic patients are completely dry [5], so it makes sense to formulate an artificial saliva that will enhance the

G. Carpenter
Salivary Research, King's College London Dental Institute,
Floor 17, Tower wing, London SE1 9RT, UK
e-mail: guy.carpenter@kcl.ac.uk





G. Carpenter (ed.), *Dry Mouth: A Clinical Guide on Causes, Effects and Treatments*, DOI 10.1007/978-3-642-55154-3_11

properties of pre-existing saliva. Most artificial salivas have such low surface tension that it destroys the properties of any existing saliva – even saliva from a normal healthy person. The recent innovation of hydrogels holds promise for new developments in artificial salivas, but a significant change in the benefits of artificial salivas will only come about if they mimic more closely the real saliva. This may require the use of peptides and other bioactives rather than chemical actives and new delivery systems that formulate the product in the mouth (from two or more separate containers) rather than applying a preformulated product to the mouth. In this chapter, the author will review some of the artificial salivas currently prescribed to patients, analyse their components and present some data on their physical properties in comparison to natural saliva and their retention in the mouth. It should be realised that no single artificial saliva will suit all patients, and indeed few studies compare more than two artificial salivas in any one study. Thus the author will refrain from naming the "best" artificial saliva.

## Clinical Studies and Trials

The gold standard for clinical efficacy is the randomised controlled trial (RCT) in which large groups of patients are either given the drug treatment or a suitable placebo, but both the patient and the administering clinician are blinded so that neither knows which patient gets which treatment. The study should use objective outcome measures to determine efficacy, and the code determining which patient received which treatment should only be broken at the end of the study. These studies are usually large and costly which may account for the low number of studies that have been conducted using artificial saliva. Despite some studies showing a beneficial effect [12], a recent Cochrane review [9] concluded that there was insufficient evidence that artificial salivas have any proven effect. Partly this was due to poorly designed studies but also because the main outcome measure is the subjective feeling of oral dryness. Another review suggested that although no clinical benefit was seen, several studies revealed a patient-reported improvement in symptoms [23] suggesting that we may not be able to measure the right parameters. A more objective measure might be bacterial counts adhered to the mucosa [26] or the whole mouth salivary flow rates, but there is no rationale for the flow rates to change. Unlike the eye, we do not make saliva if we perceive dryness. An interesting study in mice found that the size of filiform papillae on the tongue, swallowing and resistance to bacterial infections could be useful indicators of salivary function since they all improved after salivary flow was increased by transplantation [19]. These objective and functional measures of salivary function are preferable to subjective awareness of oral dryness; however, they are very rarely reported in human studies mostly because they are time-intensive.

Another problem with studies assessing the subjective feeling of dryness is the large placebo effect. For subjective measures such as dry mouth, the placebo effect is particularly powerful. In addition, choosing a suitable comparator is also difficult. Water is often used but is not inert and can, to a degree, reduce oral dryness even if only temporarily.

## How Frequently Are Artificial Salivas Used?

As noted in several chapters in this book, the incidence of a dry mouth is relatively high and certainly higher than the diagnosis of hyposalivation, whether one uses the Sjogren's diagnostic criteria of 0.1 ml/min or the more pragmatic limit of 0.2 ml/min as abnormal. Most studies define the incidence rates of dry mouth specifically for one patient group, but estimates of dry mouth for the whole population are harder to find. For the recent UK Biobank study of half a million 40–69-year-olds, saliva samples were collected from 120, 000 subjects. Although the samples were not timed, it is interesting to note that around a third of subjects (40,000) were unable to provide a sufficient saliva sample – suggesting salivary hypofunction may be as high as 30 % in this age range. Unfortunately no oral dryness questions were added to the questionnaire of all participants although possibly a follow-up study could still be conducted. Smaller cohort studies show a range of between 20 % and 50 % incidence of dry mouth. A recent study of 1,148 community-dwelling adults (20–80 years old) in Japan found a high incidence of 50 % [27], whereas a larger study of Swedes found an incidence around 24 % [18]. Thus determining the incidence of dry mouth in general populations appears to be quite difficult but it is even harder to estimate the usage of artificial salivas. Sales from a leading pharmaceutical company in the UK suggest around 50–100,000 units are sold each year. This is rather small when compared to even the lowest estimates of dry mouth prevalence in the UK of around 10 % (roughly six million). By way of comparison, the incidence of dry eye is around 20–30 % in the UK with most (40 %) self-treating with eye drops from the pharmacy rather than consulting the ophthalmologists [6]. Clearly then there is a mismatch between incidence of dry mouth and the use of artificial salivas to relieve symptoms. The obvious answer is that the artificial salivas are both too expensive and ineffective. Eye drops work because they replace the aqueous component of tear film on the eye – the oil film is relatively intact. In contrast, the mouth has no oil film but relies on lubricating properties of salivary proteins to maintain a normal-feeling mouth. Artificial salivas are potentially ineffective because they do not lubricate oral surfaces in the same way that natural saliva does.

## Intraoral Lubrication and Hydration

The mouth has a large surface area, between 200 and 400 $cm^2$, which needs to be hydrated and lubricated so that it can both resist mechanical abrasion from the eating of foods and resist the drying action of air flowing across it. Mouth breathing is particularly effective at drying the mouth and occurs during speaking, sleep, and exercise or if the nose becomes blocked. The salivary glands maintain a hydrated mucosa by the continuous flow of watery saliva over the mucosa and lubricates mostly by the selective adhesion of salivary proteins onto the mucosa. Although saliva is mostly water (approx. 99 %), it does not act like water. For example, it has a much lower surface tension than water created by the presence of surface active proteins. The lower surface tension of saliva aids the spreading of a thin film over

**Table 11.1** The surface tension of saliva is affected by the addition of artificial salivas as measured by the hanging drop technique

| Surface tension (mN/m) | WMS | 1:14 | 1:6 | 1:1 | Artificial saliva |
|---|---|---|---|---|---|
| BioXtra | 50 | 55 | 50 | 35 | 45 |
| Saliveze | 50 | 50 | 55 | 55 | 60 |
| Saliva Orthana | 50 | 50 | 45 | 45 | 45 |
| Biotene | 50 | n/a[a] | n/a[a] | n/a[a] | 30 |

[a]For Biotene mixed with WMS, no values could be obtained as the sample constantly wicked – implying a very low surface tension

the mucosa. Artificial salivas also have a very low surface tension (see Table 11.1 and [22]), but this is created mostly by the addition of volatiles such as menthol, presumably to provide a minty taste, but this can lead to a faster evaporation rate and therefore drying of the mucosa.

Most salivary lubrication of surfaces is provided by salivary mucins which act in solution to provide hydrodynamic lubrication in the mixed regime [25] but also absorbs to mucosa [10] to provide a boundary-type lubrication. Other proteins in saliva such as statherin [14], cystatin [3] and albumin [15] may also provide a boundary or close contact-type lubrication. Although most artificial salivas are viscous which will contribute to hydrodynamic lubrication, none of the current artificial salivas mimic the pellicle-forming properties of salivas by binding to the mucosa. The lack of binding also increases the speed at which the artificial salivas are cleared from the mouth by swallowing. This could be a major reason why artificial salivas are not perceived to have a lasting beneficial effect. The lack of substantivity may be addressed by the use of hydrogels which can adhere to the mucosa as reviewed recently [28].

## Systems to Model the Efficacy of Artificial Salivas

One problem in developing artificial salivas is the lack of a suitable in vitro model; most salivas have to be tested in vivo using expensive, time-consuming human studies that often only measure the perception of dryness. Whilst these studies directly address the key symptom of oral dryness, they give no information on the mechanism of symptom alleviation and so are highly susceptible to the placebo effect. For dry mouth patients putting any liquid into the mouth probably has a beneficial effect. Consequently the correct control using a double crossover study should be used, but these are costly and do not allow many artificial salivas to be tested. However there are not many useful in vitro systems that can mimic the oral mucosa. Ex vivo pig's tongue has been used [24] but obviously has some differences compared to the human tongue. Cell models of the oral mucosa are becoming available [7] although they are expensive and may not resemble all the structural qualities of the oral mucosa. Instead investigators have used synthetic mimetics to model the oral surface including glass/silica [1] and PDMS [31].

## Composition of Artificial Salivas

For the artificial salivas commonly available via the NHS (see www.medicinesresources.nhs.uk) in the UK or over the counter in most countries, the main polymer is either carboxymethylcellulose or xanthan gum. Only Saliva Orthana uses a biological base – purified mucin extracted from pig gastric mucosa (see Table 11.2). All these polymers are present at high concentrations to create a solution which is quite viscous [30]. The viscosity of the solutions is beneficial and reflects the viscosity of whole mouth saliva, aids the lubrication of tissues and slows its removal from the mouth by swallowing. In addition, to these thickening agents, all artificial salivas need to have preservatives added, so the product can be stored on the shelf. The potentially harmful effects of swallowing large amounts of these preservatives are discussed in an earlier chapter by Prof Ligtenberg. This appears to be an unavoidable effect of taking artificial salivas; however, it has to be noted that adverse side effects of artificial salivas are very uncommon. Most patients seem to stop using these products because of the cost (the same as a prescription charge in the UK) and/or because they do not provide sufficient relief rather than any perceived side effect from the consumption of the product.

As noted in Table 11.2 some artificial salivas also contain bioactives – components extracted from natural sources (animals or plants) that are added to replicate some of the bacteriostatic or antibacterial effects of natural saliva. The benefits of these added bioactives are largely unproven or at least difficult to distinguish from placebo effects [11]. However the addition of bioactives certainly warrants further attention and is likely to be the area in which greatest innovation of artificial salivas occurs. For example, non-salivary proteins could be added to improve the lubricating properties of saliva [16]. Indeed the inclusion of supercharged polypeptides [29] has already shown beneficial effects although their safety in humans has yet to be proven. The addition of calcium and fluoride should be a regular inclusion in artificial salivas to aid in the protection of teeth. Several chapters have already detailed

**Table 11.2** The components of artificial salivas

| Name | Bulk polymer | Actives | Preservatives | Others |
|---|---|---|---|---|
| BioXtra | Hydroxyethylcellulose | Lactoferrin, lactoperoxidase lysozyme | Potassium thiocyanate | *Aloe barbadensis* |
| Saliveze | Carboxymethylcellulose | Calcium chloride | Methylparaben | |
| GC Dry Mouth Gel | Cellulose gum/carrageenan | | Ethylparaben | |
| Saliva Orthana | Pig gastric mucin | Potassium fluoride | Benzoate | EDTA |
| Biotene | Xanthan gum/glycerine | Cetylpyridinium chloride | Benzoate, methylparaben | |
| Glandosane | Sodium carboxymethylcellulose | Calcium chloride | Sodium chloride | |

**Table 11.3** The pH of artificial salivas and when mixed with whole mouth saliva (single subject)

| pH | WMS | 1:14 | 1:6 | 1:1 | Artificial saliva |
|---|---|---|---|---|---|
| Saliveze | 6.7 | 6.7 | 6.7 | 7.0 | 7.0 |
| Saliva Orthana | 6.7 | 6.6 | 6.6 | 6.6 | 6.5 |
| Biotene | 6.7 | 6.8 | 6.6 | 6.6 | 5.9 |
| BioXtra | 6.7 | 6.9 | 6.8 | 7.4 | 7.5 |

Even at high dilutions such as 1:14, saliva effectively neutralises acidic artificial salivas

the deleterious effects of a lack of saliva on tooth integrity. Since saliva is already naturally high in calcium, the addition of this ion would seem obvious; however, maintaining its solubility for long periods may be a problem for manufacturers. Likewise the addition of fluoride often requires an acidic medium to maintain its solubility. Usually an acidic saliva would not be recommended because it may lead to the accelerated dissolution of teeth. However as shown in Table 11.3, if there is any saliva present in the mouth – which will be true for most patients – the acidic pH of the artificial salivas will quickly be neutralised by saliva's buffering system (bicarbonate, carbonic anhydrase and proteins). Hence the benefits of including calcium and fluoride probably outweigh the potential danger from the acidic pH, for most patients.

## Physical Properties of Artificial and Natural Salivas

In addition to the viscosity mentioned earlier, natural saliva has many unique physical properties. One aspect that our group is particularly interested in is the elasticity or spinnbarkeit properties. Saliva when pulled between opposing surfaces such as the fingers or metal plates exhibits a terrific ability to form strings, quite often with beads (beads on a string morphology), which probably represents the heterogenous nature of saliva [2]. Some preliminary data from the author suggests this property is particularly important for saliva's ability to bind onto the surfaces such as the oral mucosa. It would seem useful then that any artificial saliva would aim to enhance this property. However as shown in Table 11.4, the addition of moderate amounts of artificial saliva (as shown by the 1:6 dilution) affects the elastic properties of natural saliva and destroys it if even greater amounts are added. Although not proven in vivo, this data would suggest that using artificial saliva may reduce the effectiveness of the natural saliva that is already present. One could argue that a major deficit of all artificial salivas is that they do not complement existing salivary properties but instead replace it with a different solution. There is little evidence to support this theory except for the preliminary data presented in this chapter. For most patients it is understandable to believe that some treatment is better than nothing, but some considerable progress in formulating improved artificial salivas could be made by trying to complement the existing saliva properties rather than destroying it.

**Table 11.4** The elasticity of saliva is reduced as more of the artificial saliva is mixed in

| Elasticity (Pa) | WMS | 1:14 | 1:6 | 1:1 | Artificial saliva |
|---|---|---|---|---|---|
| Water | 50 | 40 | 60 | 0.00 | 0 |
| Saliveze | 50 | 30 | 40 | 0.00 | 0 |
| Saliva Orthana | 50 | 50 | 30 | 0.00 | 0 |
| Biotene | 50 | 50 | 50 | 0.00 | 0 |
| BioXtra | 50 | 30 | 0.00 | 0.00 | 0 |

Even at one part artificial saliva to 14 parts of saliva, there is a noticeable effect

## Future Directions of Artificial Salivas

It is understandable that few patients would want a "saliva transplant" from someone else although the recent studies on faecal transplants for the treatment of inflammatory bowel disease may be paving the way for this to happen in the future. A more immediate potential therapy is the transplantation into the salivary glands of stem cells (detailed in Chap. 10) or the transplantation of whole glands using bioengineered glands [19] although the challenge to use adult rather than embryonic tissue source is considerable. In the meantime, the development of alternative artificial salivas would appear to provide the best alternative to salivary gland transplants. The major problem for the manufacturer is sourcing cheap bioactives to add to polymer solutions. It is increasingly possible to either use purified proteins from a biological source (as BioXtra and Biotene have done) or to synthesise them from new. A recent report has suggested that an extract of yam tuber may confer similar properties as saliva [20] although only the viscosity and surface tension was considered. The use of plant materials has many possible benefits – scalability, reduced infectious agents, etc. – and may be a good first step. The mucilage often surrounding seeds is an interesting area that several groups have already considered for ocular drug delivery systems [21]. Another likely source of bioactives is food proteins. Many food proteins have strong rheological activity that may well complement saliva's properties. A recent example is lecithin – the emulsifier used in chocolate. Emulsions using this food protein exhibit both viscosity at low shear rates and elasticity at higher shear rates, which mimics human saliva [13].

A rather unusual approach is being taken in the author's lab to produce a novel artificial saliva. Cuckoo spit is the product of the froghopper insect (Cercopoidea) during its initial larval stage and is commonly seen on plants in spring (when the cuckoo arrives/sings). Initial analysis by the author has revealed that it is both calcium rich and mucinous. The mucin-like components create both elasticity and viscosity (as human saliva does). Potentially it mimics saliva very well. Since the froth is created by the insect, adding proteins to the plant sap, we have tested to see if we can enhance the cuckoo spit by feeding the insects on tobacco plants expressing human proteins (courtesy of Prof Ma, St George's Hospital, London). These plants have been engineered to express antibodies both IgG and secretory

IgA [8]. Surprisingly the insects were effective at enhancing the cuckoo spit with plant-derived proteins including the human antibodies. Molecular pharming is the use of plant-based pharmaceuticals and has great promise in delivering cheap pharmaceutics [17].

**Acknowledgements** The data shown in this chapter was produced by Amandeep Bains as part of a summer project during her BDS programme. The author is very grateful for her helpful comments in preparing this chapter.

## References

1. Berg CH, Lindh L, Arnebrant T. Intraoral lubrication of PRP-1, statherin and mucin as studied by AFM. Biofouling. 2004;20(1):65–70.
2. Bhat PP, Appathurai S, Harris MT, Pasquali M, McKinley GH, Basaran OA. Formation of beads on a string structures during break-up of viscoelastic filaments. Nat Phys. 2010;6(8):625–31.
3. Bradway SD, Bergey EJ, Scannapieco FA, Ramasubbu N, Zawacki S, Levine MJ. Formation of salivary-mucosal pellicle – the role of transglutaminase. Biochem J. 1992;284:557–64.
4. Cardenas M, Elofsson U, Lindh L. Salivary mucin MUC5B could be an important component of in vitro pellicles of human saliva: an in situ ellipsometry and atomic force microscopy study. Biomacromolecules. 2007;8(4):1149–56.
5. Castro I, Sepulveda D, Cortes J, Quest AFG, Barrera MJ, Bahamondes V, Aguilera S, Urzua U, Alliende C, Molina C, Gonzalez S, Hermoso MA, Leyton C, Gonzalez MJ. Oral dryness in Sjogren's syndrome patients. Not just a question of water. Autoimmun Rev. 2013;12(5):567–74.
6. Clegg JP, Guest JF, Lehman A, Smith AF. The annual cost of dry eye syndrome in France, Germany, Italy, Spain, Sweden and the United Kingdom among patients managed by ophthalmologists. Ophthalmic Epidemiol. 2006;13(4):263–74.
7. Dongari-Bagtzoglou A, Kashleva H. Development of a highly reproducible three-dimensional organotypic model of the oral mucosa. Nat Protoc. 2006;1(4):2012–8.
8. Frigerio L, Vine ND, Pedrazzini E, Hein MB, Wang F, Ma JKC, Vitale A. Assembly, secretion, and vacuolar delivery of a hybrid immunoglobulin in plants. Plant Physiol. 2000;123(4): 1483–93.
9. Furness S, Worthington HV, Bryan G, Birchenough S, McMillan R. Interventions for the management of dry mouth: topical therapies Cochrane Database Syst Rev. 2011;(12):106.
10. Gibbins HL, Yakubov GE, Wilson S, Carpenter GH. Concentration of salivary protective proteins in the bound oral mucosal pellicle. Oral Dis. 2013. doi:10.1111/odi.12194.
11. Gil-Montoya JA, Guardia-Lopez I, Gonzalez-Moles MA. Evaluation of the clinical efficacy containing the antimicrobial of a mouthwash and oral gel proteins lactoperoxidase, lysozyme and lactoferrin in elderly patients with dry mouth a pilot study. Gerodontology. 2008;25(1):3–9.
12. Gomez-Moreno G, Aguilar-Salvatierra A, Guardia J, Uribe-Marioni A, Cabrera-Ayala M, Delgado-Ruiz RA, Calvo-Guirado JL. The efficacy of a topical sialogogue spray containing 1% malic acid in patients with antidepressant-induced dry mouth: a double-blind, randomized clinical trial. Depress Anxiety. 2013;30(2):137–42.
13. Hanning SM, Yu T, Jones DS, Andrews GP, Kieser JA, Medlicott NJ. Lecithin-based emulsions for potential use as saliva substitutes in patients with xerostomia – viscoelastic properties. Int J Pharm. 2013;456(2):560–8.
14. Harvey NM, Carpenter GH, Proctor GB, Klein J. Normal and frictional interactions of purified human statherin adsorbed on molecularly-smooth solid substrata. Biofouling. 2011;27(8): 823–35.
15. Hatton MN, Loomis RE, Levine MJ, Tabak LA. Masticatory lubrication – the role of carbohydrate in the lubricating property of a salivary glycoprotein albumin complex. Biochem J. 1985;230(3):817–20.

16. Klein J. Polymers in living systems: from biological lubrication to tissue engineering and biomedical devices. Polym Adv Technol. 2012;23(4):729–35.
17. Ma JKC, Christou P, Chikwamba R, Haydon H, Paul M, Ferrer MP, Ramalingam S, Rech E, Rybicki E, Wigdorowitz A, Yang DC, Thangaraj H. Realising the value of plant molecular pharming to benefit the poor in developing countries and emerging economies. Plant Biotechnol J. 2013;11(9):1029–33.
18. Nederfors T, Isaksson R, Mornstad H, Dahlof C. Prevalence of perceived symptoms of dry mouth in an adult Swedish population – relation to age, sex and pharmacotherapy. Community Dent Oral Epidemiol. 1997;25(3):211–6.
19. Ogawa M, Oshima M, Imamura A, Sekine Y, Ishida K, Yamashita K, Nakajima K, Hirayama M, Tachikawa T, Tsuji T. Functional salivary gland regeneration by transplantation of a bioengineered organ germ. Nat Commun. 2013;4:2498.
20. Park MS, Chang JY, Kim YY, Kang JH, Kho HS. Physical and biological properties of yam as a saliva substitute. Arch Oral Biol. 2010;55(2):177–83.
21. Pathak D, Kumar P, Kuppusamy G, Gupta A, Kamble B, Wadhwani A. Physicochemical characterization and toxicological evaluation of plant-based anionic polymers and their nanoparticulated system for ocular delivery. Nanotoxicology. 2014;8(8):843–55.
22. Proctor GB, Hamdan S, Carpenter GH, Wilde P. A statherin and calcium enriched layer at the air interface of human parotid saliva. Biochem J. 2005;389:111–6.
23. Ramos-Casals M, Brito-Zeron P, Siso-Almirall A, Bosch X, Tzioufas AG. Topical and systemic medications for the treatment of primary Sjogren's syndrome. Nat Rev Rheumatol. 2012;8(7):399–411.
24. Ranc H, Elkhyat A, Servais C, Mac-Mary S, Launay B, Humbert P. Friction coefficient and wettability of oral mucosal tissue: changes induced by a salivary layer. Colloids Surf Physicochem Eng Asp. 2006;276(1–3):155–61.
25. Stokes JR, Davies GA. Viscoelasticity of human whole saliva collected after acid and mechanical stimulation. Biorheology. 2007;44(3):141–60.
26. Sugiura Y, Soga Y, Yamabe K, Tsutani S, Tanimoto I, Maeda H, Kokeguchi S, Fujii N, Ishimaru F, Tanimoto M, Nishimura F, Takashiba S. Total bacterial counts on oral mucosa after using a commercial saliva substitute in patients undergoing hematopoietic cell transplantation. Support Care Cancer. 2010;18(3):395–8.
27. Toida M, Nanya Y, Takeda-Kawaguchi T, Baba S, Iida K, Kato K, Hatakeyama D, Makita H, Yamashita T, Shibata T. Oral complaints and stimulated salivary flow rate in 1188 adults. J Oral Pathol Med. 2010;39(5):407–19.
28. Tsibouklis J, Middleton AM, Patel N, Pratten J. Toward mucoadhesive hydrogel formulations for the management of xerostomia: the physicochemical, biological, and pharmacological considerations. J Biomed Mater Res A. 2013;101(11):3327–38.
29. Veeregowda DH, Kolbe A, van der Mei HC, Busscher HJ, Herrmann A, Sharma PK. Recombinant supercharged polypeptides restore and improve biolubrication. Adv Mater. 2013;25(25):3426–31.
30. Vissink A, Waterman HA, Sgravenmade EJ, Panders AK, Vermey A. Rheological properties of saliva substitutes containing mucin, carboxymethylcellulose or polyethylenoxide. J Oral Pathol Med. 1984;13(1):22–8.
31. Yakubov GE, McColl J, Bongaerts JHH, Ramsden JJ. Viscous boundary lubrication of hydrophobic surfaces by mucin. Langmuir. 2009;25(4):2313–21.

# The Beneficial Effects of Regular Chewing

# 12

Taichi Inui

**Abstract**

Saliva stimulation relieves dry mouth symptoms for those who have functioning salivary glands. Chewing gum and lozenges are the two major forms of saliva stimuli for dry mouth patients. Their mechanism of action is a combination of two oral stimuli, that is, taste and mastication. Taste stimulation provides an acute increase of saliva and thus instant relief, whereas masticatory stimulation is long lasting, keeping the relief prolonged. Comparative studies suggest that chewing gum, lozenges, and also artificial saliva work equally effectively against self-perceived dry mouth symptoms. Individual conditions as well as etiology influence the effect of these products and thus the preference for use. Patients' preference is an important factor for improving long-term compliance. Acid-free and sugar-free products should be recommended in order to maximize the saliva's protective properties for the dentition. In addition to stimulated saliva, unstimulated (resting) saliva is also of importance in the management of dry mouth because it functions for maintenance of oral lubrication and is present in the oral cavity for a much longer period than stimulated saliva. Unstimulated salivary flow is influenced by an individual's masticatory functions, particularly by bite force. Maintaining good functional occlusal areas and jaw-closing muscle strength is critical for keeping an adequate bite force level, especially in the elderly. The working hypothesis is that mastication, saliva, and oral health are interdependent factors to maintain oral functions that are compromised when the mouth is dry. Good oral hygiene practice, in addition to regular exercise of the muscles of mastications, is important for maintaining the unstimulated salivary flow rate and therefore preventing dry mouth.

T. Inui, PhD
Department of R & D, Wm. Wrigley Jr. Company,
1132 W. Blackhawk St., Chicago, IL 60642, USA
e-mail: taichi.inui@wrigley.com



G. Carpenter (ed.), *Dry Mouth: A Clinical Guide on Causes, Effects and Treatments*, DOI 10.1007/978-3-642-55154-3_12

## Introduction

As described throughout this book, there are a number of conditions that can cause dry mouth. Thus, it is critical to have proper diagnosis in order to determine appropriate treatment options. Diagnosis of dry mouth can consist of multiple medical and oral exams along with subjective responses and questionnaires. In many cases, the process of dry mouth diagnostics begins with the patient's complaints around oral functions and discomforts. These complaints typically include the lack of salivary flow, self-perceived discomfort, and difficulties in oral functions such as food ingestion and speech. Lower salivary flow rate is a risk factor for many oral ailments, for example, caries and yeast infection.

Hyposalivation is more prevalent with aging. Although dry mouth is not an issue only for the elderly, the percentage of the population who suffer from dry mouth increases to 25 % for those above 50 years old, whereas the rate is 6–10 % for the whole population [1]. This does not mean that aging itself is a risk factor. However, the prevalence of dry mouth is associated with age-related ailments and the number of prescription drugs. The accumulation of damage to the dentition over years is also associated with dry mouth [2]. Among the known causes, polypharmacy is considered a leading cause of dry mouth especially for the aging population (Chap. 3). The impact from prescribed medicine is proportional to the number of drugs a patient takes. Salivary flow rate, both unstimulated and stimulated, is negatively correlated with age and the number of medications taken, for both male and female patients [3, 4]. Other causes include medical treatment that results in damage to the salivary glands as a side effect, for example, radiation therapy for head and neck cancer. While salivary flow rate is not the only variable to determine the dry mouth symptom, all causes that contribute to dry mouth negatively impact on saliva secretion.

If there is a viable salivary gland remaining, such as is the case with polypharmacy, oral and masticatory stimuli are an option to alleviate the dry mouth symptoms. Needless to say, replacing the prescription drugs by those with less risk for dry mouth should always be considered while seeking a remedy in sialogogues. A number of studies have tested the efficacy of oral stimuli for relief of dry mouth symptoms. The efficacy of the treatments is measured in multiple ways including subjective response and salivary flow rate. Dry mouth, manifested as lack of saliva protection of the oral cavity, leads to various oral diseases. It also suppresses oral functions including the ability to process food and swallow. Mastication and gustatory stimuli increase salivary secretion, which in turn alleviates dry mouth symptoms (Fig. 12.1). Figure 12.1 illustrates the cyclic relation among chewing, saliva, and oral health around dry mouth. Increase in salivary secretion also promotes oral health by removing food debris and neutralizing plaque acids. In addition, maintenance of good oral health facilitates good masticatory ability with longer occlusal arches and a higher bite force. These factors are associated with unstimulated saliva, which coats and protects the oral mucosal surfaces and thus helps prevent dry mouth. There are two main topics in this chapter. The first is how mastication promotes salivation and thus provides relief from dry mouth. The second topic is

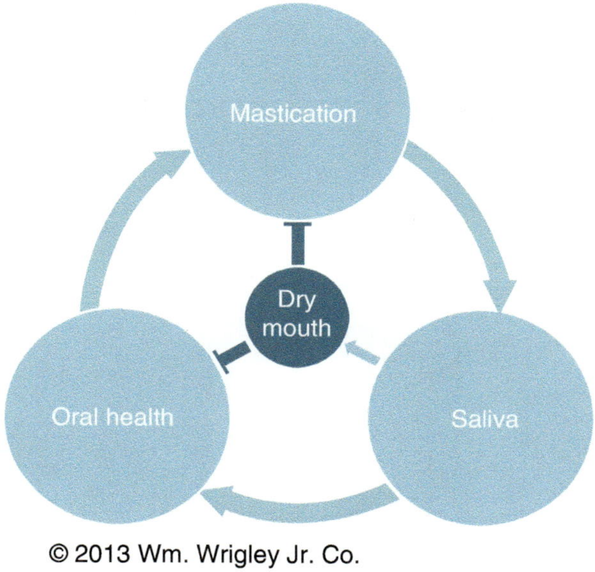


**Fig. 12.1** Schematic diagram to show how saliva stimulation contributes to the management of dry mouth and also participates in a positive cycle in maintenance of oral health. Saliva coverage of oral mucosa is key to preventing dry mouth. Dry mouth compromises oral health and mastication abilities, including patients' ability to chew and swallow. Mastication stimulates saliva flow and helps maintain oral health. Good oral health and a preserved dentition lead to good occlusion. This translates to sufficient mastication, thereby creating positive 360° feedbacks. A healthy and functional mouth plays an integral role in saliva secretion

how a regular chewing habit, in conjunction with good oral hygiene practices, helps salivary secretion in the prevention of dry mouth.

## Nonprescriptive Sialogogues as Dry Mouth Treatment

Saliva stimulants, or sialogogues, are treatment options for dry mouth as long as the salivary glands remain functional. Prescription sialogogues, such as pilocarpine and cevimeline, stimulate saliva via muscarinic receptors and the parasympathetic nervous system (Chap. 3). Excess sweating is a common side effect of these drugs because their efficacy is not localized to the oral cavity.

By definition, food is also a sialogogue and can be used as a functional natural stimulant. Chewing gum and lozenges are the two major food products used for this self-care purpose. The mechanism by which chewing gum and lozenges stimulate saliva is also by the autonomic nerve system (ANS). It is indeed the same mechanism by which food stimulates saliva production. While sialogogue drugs stimulate muscarinic cholinergic receptors, nondrug sialogogues stimulate the ANS via taste receptors and periodontal mechanoreceptors. Among the five basic tastes, sourness,

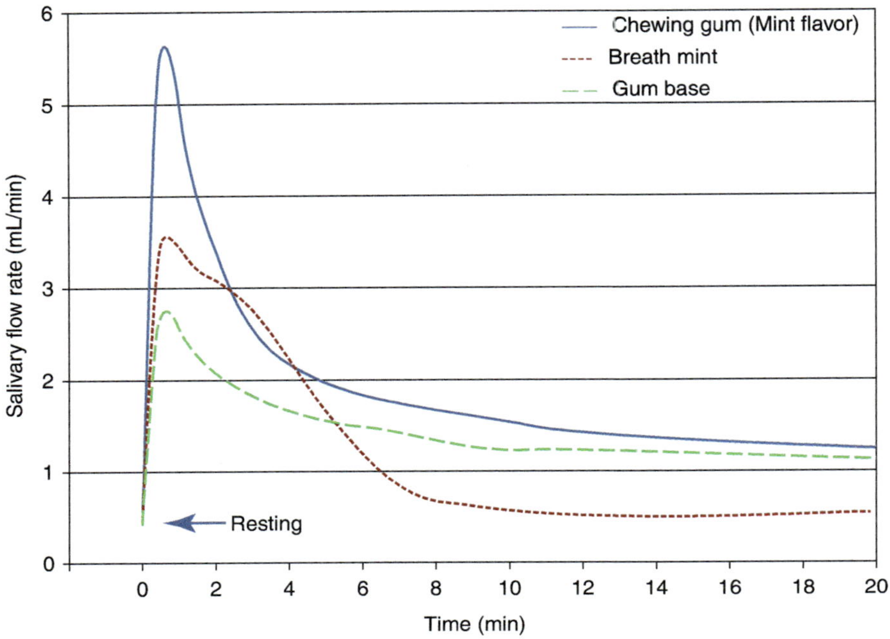


**Fig. 12.2** Salivary flow rate stimulated by different oral compositions

saltiness, and sweetness are the most potent drivers for salivation in that order. Mechanical stimuli are derived from the physical properties of the food bolus, such as hardness, elasticity, and bolus size. Large cohort studies on normal salivators found the average unstimulated salivary flow rate to be 0.3–0.4 mL/min [5]. This value increases about tenfold with oral stimuli. The taste stimulus diminishes as subjects swallow the dissolved tastants in saliva, while the magnitude of stimulation is greater than with mechanical stimulation. The taste receptors are adaptive to gustatory stimuli [6]. The halftime for adaptation, measured by salivary flow rate, is about 11 s if the source of the stimuli is not moved around in the mouth. The adaptation for taste stimuli falls exponentially and is not dependent on the type of stimulus. In contrast, mechanical stimuli usually cause a lower magnitude of saliva secretion, but it lasts as long as the subject keeps chewing the oral composition in their mouth.

Figure 12.2 illustrates salivary secretion by three types of food substances, that is, chewing gum, lozenge, and gum base, the latter being the elastic substance of chewing gum without sweetener or flavor. Saliva stimulation by chewing gum peaks in the first 1–2 min, reaching about a tenfold increase from the unstimulated salivary flow rate, and then gradually declines to about twice the unstimulated salivary flow rate [7, 8]. This is because the combination of gustatory and masticatory stimuli takes place at the beginning of chewing and the stimuli from sweeteners or acids decrease as they are extracted from chewing gum and then swallowed. The lozenge stimulates saliva via taste receptors. Its effect diminishes as it dissolves and the tastants are swallowed; therefore, the salivary flow rate goes down to the unstimulated level. Gum base stimulates saliva via mechanical stimulation when it is chewed. The magnitude of its stimulation is not as potent as with taste stimuli. However, the effect lasts as long as the patient keeps chewing the gum base. The combination of flavor and sweetener, and also the presence of organic acids, influences the flow rate and pH level of chewing gum-stimulated saliva [9, 10]. The size of bolus is also a factor in salivary stimulation, for example, chewing 1 g of taste-free and flavor-free gum base leads to about a fourfold increase in flow rate, whereas a 9 g piece leads to a 13-fold increase [11].

The increase in the amount of saliva is not the only mechanism by which these food products work against dry mouth symptoms. Saliva is composed of 99.5 % water with 0.2 % protein and 0.3 % inorganic substances. These relatively small fractions of constituents are critical for saliva's functions. For example, rinsing the mouth with pure water does not provide the same level of dryness relief as saliva stimulants [12]. The main mechanism is the increase in salivary components that deliver protective functions for the oral cavity. Saliva contains mucins and other glycoproteins that maintain the homeostasis of the mouth, including lubrication and coating of the oral mucosa.

Saliva covers oral surfaces as a thin film which has a higher protein content than the secreted whole saliva. MUC5B, a large-molecular-weight mucin, has been found to be present at a lower concentration in the salivary films of dry mouth patients compared with those from normal salivators [13]. Minor gland saliva, which is rich in mucin content, is considered to play a critical role in coating oral surfaces. In fact, minor salivary gland secretion has a higher correlation with dry mouth symptoms than that of chewing-stimulated whole saliva [14]. Both saliva substitutes and sialogogues focus on maintaining lubrication in the oral cavity to reduce discomfort as well as the dryness of the mouth. The shared advantages of these treatments are the ease of use and localized effect. Artificial saliva contains lubricating macromolecules as substitutes for these glycoproteins. By increasing salivary flow rate, sialogogues also increase specific protein output, that is, the amount of protein secreted per minute increases. Artificial saliva (Chap. 11), in the form of an oral spray, is often presented as a treatment option along with chewing gum. As such, many studies have looked into the efficacy of chewing gum, sucking hard candy, or using artificial saliva, not only for the effectiveness of the treatments but also for patients' preferences.

Multiple studies have shown consistently that chewing flavored and sweetened gum increases salivary flow rate and provides relief from dry mouth symptoms, as long as the subjects keep chewing. Chewing the sugar-free gum promoted the saliva's protective function and prevented the fall in cemental plaque pH in response to a sucrose challenge [15, 16]. These effects were consistent for patients with various etiologies of dry mouth [3, 5, 17–24]. For example, patients who suffer from end-stage renal disease have higher risk of dry mouth. This is because patients receiving hemodialysis need to restrict fluid intake, which reduces salivary flow and thus causes chronic thirst and dry mouth. Bots et al. conducted a crossover clinical trial using two chewing gum formulae and also artificial saliva. The results suggested that both chewing gums and artificial saliva were effective in the reduction of dry mouth as well as thirst [23].

Some studies compared multiple chewing gum formulae for their efficacy and saliva stimulation. The majority of gum products used in the dry mouth studies were sugar-free and formulated with active ingredients such as xylitol, chlorhexidine, or urea for dental benefits. One study compared the efficacy of two chewing gums with one formulated with mucin and the other with urea. The mucin gum was perceived more effective for self-perceived dry mouth symptoms compared with urea gum. The subjects also liked the mucin gum better and used it more frequently than urea-containing gum upon ad libitum administration in a 2-week-long crossover trial [22]. No study reported statistical difference among multiple chewing gum formulations compared in terms of salivary flow rate. This was not surprising as these active ingredients were not expected to stimulate salivary secretion. There was a trend that gum containing actives, for example, chlorhexidine, showed additional dental benefits such as lower plaque and gingival indices. To our best knowledge, there has been no dry mouth study conducted using a chewing gum product specifically formulated to maximize salivary flow rate. Organic acids are potent salivary stimulants commonly used in fruit-flavored chewing gums. Organic acids, such as citric and malic acids, are also naturally present in fruits and other foods. Fruit-flavored gums have shown to increase salivary secretion more than mint-flavored gum [25]. However, there appears to be no study using fruit-flavored chewing gum for dry mouth. On the other hand, the same organic acids are formulated in lozenges and citrus candies. These confections are also effective in stimulating saliva and thus relieving dry mouth symptoms although for a shorter duration than chewing gum (see Fig. 12.2) [12, 26, 27]. When consuming acidic food, it is important to maintain the hydrogen ion concentration in saliva in order to minimize the risk for acid enamel loss. This is particularly critical for hyposalivators as the rate of acid clearance by saliva is lower than in normosalivators. Salivary flow rate is positively correlated with acid clearance rate and also the bicarbonate ion concentration. Patients' ability to secrete stimulated saliva needs to be taken into account when recommending a nonprescriptive sialogogue. It is also recommended to focus on acid clearance and refrain from brushing teeth for at least half an hour after consuming acidic food, including fruits.

## Patients' Preferences on Products

For all three nonprescription treatments (i.e., chewing gum, lozenges, and artificial saliva), their mode of action is to lubricate the oral mucosa.

All products in these three categories are acceptable forms of treatment, although there may be a preference for one treatment over another based on individual patient's conditions [28]. The drivers for the preference include (1) ease of use, (2) effect in relieving dry mouth symptoms, and (3) taste acceptability (Table 12.1). Side effects also influence the preference of patients (Table 12.2).

**Table 12.1** Reasons to prefer one product over the other

| Chewing gum | Artificial saliva |
|---|---|
| More effective | More effective |
| Liking of taste | Did not like chewing |
| Easier to use | Liking of taste |
| Fewer side effects | Easier to use |

**Table 12.2** Common complaints and side effects associated with nonprescription remedies

| Chewing gum | Artificial saliva |
|---|---|
| Irritation of mouth | Unpleasant taste |
| Nausea | Nausea |
| Unpleasant taste | Irritation of mouth |
| Jaw discomfort | Vomiting |
| Biting cheek or tongue | Diarrhea |
| Sensitive teeth | |
| Flatus | |

Some studies evaluated subjects' liking of the flavor or the taste of the tested products. While liking may not provide a short-term clinical advantage for alleviating dry mouth symptoms, the long-term benefit may be that subjects who use sialogogues with higher liking may (1) be more compliant with the treatment procedure and thus more likely to increase the chance of successful treatment and (2) use the product for longer periods, resulting in prolonged stimulation time [17]. There is a reported trend that the more unstimulated salivary flow the patient has, the more likely that they are to prefer chewing gum over artificial saliva. For example, 60 % of tested subjects expressed their preference for chewing gum over artificial saliva in a study with patients on hemodialysis therapy [23]. These patients have several oral complications, including dry mouth, while having functional salivary glands but impairment in renal functions.

## Specific Advantages of Different Treatment Options

In addition to the shared advantages, artificial saliva has a distinct advantage in that it may be used by those who do not have sufficient salivary gland function for stimulation of saliva flow (see Chap. 11 for more details about artificial saliva). On the other hand, there are two unique advantages in using sugar-free chewing gum as a sialogogue: (1) It increases salivary pH as well as buffer capacity. It also neutralizes plaque acid created by starchy food, thus enhancing the remineralization potential of dental plaque. (2) The effect lasts much longer because the masticatory stimuli remain effective as long as one keeps chewing the gum cud. To be more precise, this effect lasts as long as the bolus maintains sufficient textural properties to stimulate saliva flow. One study showed the stimulated salivary flow being significantly higher than that of unstimulated throughout a 2 h chewing period using chewing gum with 2.7 g starting weight [7]. Another study found the stimulated salivary flow rate was significantly higher than that of unstimulated for the first 55 min of 90 min chewing, using a smaller gum pellet of 1.5 g [8]. Obviously, this increase in salivary flow rate disappeared when subjects stopped chewing. However, the level of salivary flow just after chewing is stopped is equivalent to the unstimulated flow rate but not lower [29]. In addition, the initial increase in salivary flow rate can be reproduced at least every 90 min if subjects start chewing a fresh piece of gum.

## The Importance of Unstimulated Saliva

Although the stimulated salivary flow rate is significantly higher than that of the unstimulated, the oral cavity is mostly exposed to unstimulated saliva, both in terms of the amount and duration. The total volume of saliva for a normal salivator adds up to 500–600 mL/day, of which unstimulated saliva contributes about 340 mL. This comes from 300 mL during the waking period at 0.3 mL/min for 16 h and about 40 mL during sleep at less than 0.1 mL/min for 7 h. The total amount of daily stimulated saliva is estimated to be about 200 mL. The average time spent eating each day has been estimated as 54 min, and the average stimulated flow rate during a meal is estimated to be about 4 mL/min [5].

There are characteristic differences between stimulated saliva and unstimulated saliva. The ratio of the contributions from the different glands changes when saliva is stimulated. In unstimulated saliva, the contribution from amylase-rich serous parotid glands is about 25 %, about 70 % is from mucin-rich viscous submandibular and sublingual gland secretions, and 7–8 % is from mucin-rich minor glands. On the other hand, stimulated saliva is composed of about 50 % parotid saliva, 45 % submandibular-sublingual saliva, and 7–8 % minor gland saliva. This aligns with the main functions of both saliva types, that is, the digestive function of stimulated saliva and the lubricating and protective function of unstimulated saliva. Saliva from minor glands should also be considered, as these viscous secretions have a high impact on dry mouth.

Another reason why unstimulated saliva is important is because saliva lubricates and coats oral mucosal surfaces. As mentioned earlier, the protective property of saliva is exhibited as the thin film layer coating the mucosal surface. Hyposalivators whose unstimulated salivary flow rate <0.1 mL/min had significantly lower mucosal thickness of saliva compared with normosalivators. Normosalivators with dry mouth symptoms also showed thinner salivary film compared with the saliva sampled from normosalivators without the symptoms. The differences among three groups were most prominent at specific sites, namely, the tongue, lips, vestibule, and mouth floor. Considering the flow of saliva in the oral cavity, increasing parotid secretion should contribute to increased wetness of the cheeks, whereas an increase in submandibular-sublingual secretions should contribute to wetness at the floor of the mouth (Fig. 12.3) [30]. The flow schematic also infers that lubrication of lips and vestibule is more dependent on the minor salivary glands, rather than, for example, the parotid glands.

The fact that unstimulated saliva bathes the floor of the mouth and tongue has implications for taste perception. Dry mouth patients often notice that their taste

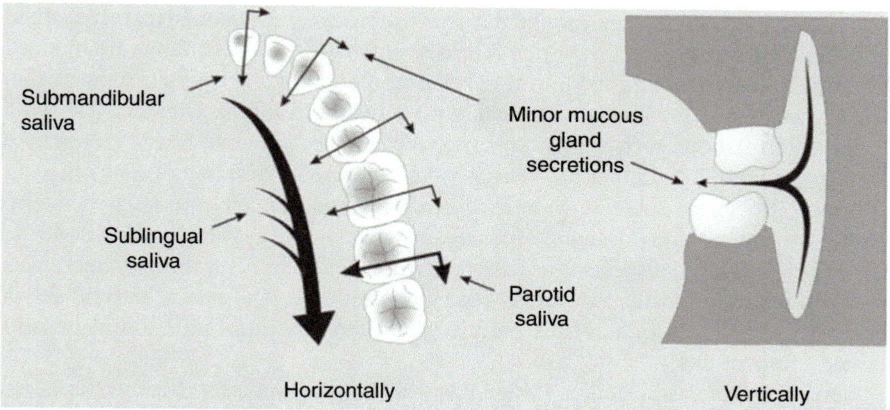


**Fig. 12.3** Schematic of salivary flow in oral cavity (Reprinted with permission from [31]). The saliva film moves in a general direction from the upper anterior buccal side to the lower posterior lingual side and then gets swallowed. The velocity of the film increases while traveling through the oral cavity. The thickness of the film has been calculated to average just less than 0.1 mm in the mouth, and an increase in saliva from various glands results in increasing velocity of the film. Another noteworthy point is that saliva secreted on one side tends to remain on the same side and does not migrate evenly around the whole mouth [32]

perception alters after onset of the symptoms (Chap. 5). Taste receptor cells are regenerated and replaced on average every 10 days [33]. This suggests that without saliva protecting the taste cells, the number of taste receptors may not keep up with the turnover and thus the taste sensitivity may decline. Animal studies support this hypothesis. Rats show a decreased taste nerve response upon the elimination of the submandibular and sublingual glands. The sensitivity improved within the same animals after 1 week of treatment with artificial saliva.

In elderly adults, there was a positive correlation between the flow rate of unstimulated saliva and that of stimulated saliva [32, 34]. This implies that improving the unstimulated salivary level will increase the degree of relief delivered by an oral sialogogue.

Maintaining an unstimulated salivary flow rate sufficiently high to coat the oral cavity is one very important approach to preventing dry mouth. There are relatively few studies which have evaluated the drivers for unstimulated saliva flow aside from cholinergic agonists such as pilocarpine.

## Regular Chewing and Salivary Secretion

While the increase in saliva during chewing is well established, the question remaining to be answered is: "Will a regular chewing habit increase salivary secretion and improve dry mouth symptoms within the same individual?" This question is critical, not because higher salivation means lack of a dry mouth, but because increase of salivation in the same individual is important for an individual's perception of oral dryness. For example, dry mouth patients' subjective symptoms recurred when unstimulated whole saliva flow rate fell to about 40–50 % of the flow rate induced by anticholinergic drugs [35]. Animal and epidemiological studies suggest that masticatory stress positively correlates with salivary secretion. One study showed positive correlations between the unstimulated salivary flow rate and (1) frequency of gum chewing, (2) number of pieces per day, and (3) the duration of each chewing episode [36]. These subjects were stratified with age, gender, and dietary pattern. There are several animal studies on saliva secretion and regular mastication, the latter being altered by changing food texture [35]. Salivary output decreases with reduction in masticatory stress and causes reduced flow rate of parotid saliva in humans. A liquid diet causes parotid gland atrophy and reduction in parotid salivary flow in rats.

Several intervention studies investigated salivary output after the long-term use of chewing gum or lozenges for both dry mouth patients and also normal salivators (Table 12.3). Overall, intervention studies with a planned regular chewing pattern show inconsistent outcomes in whether a regular chewing gum habit increases salivary flow rate. This is possibly due to difference in the output measures between the studies, that is, unstimulated salivary flow or that of mastication stimulated with paraffin or acid. Caution is needed as there is a large variation in the duration and frequency of consumption in the various studies. The subject groups also varied among the studies, from healthy young students to frail institutionalized elderly in whom the masticatory stress would be different when chewing a piece of gum. Other factors, such as compliance rate and saliva sampling timing (see below), further complicate the outcome.

## Factors Influencing Saliva Secretion

There are numerous factors influencing both stimulated and unstimulated salivary secretions. Major factors include hydration level, circadian rhythm, circannual rhythm, body position, exposure to light, and previous stimulation, for example, last meal. These factors should be standardized for saliva collection [4, 39]. Previous intake of food and circadian rhythm are two major confounders that are often overlooked in studies analyzing saliva samples. Salivary flow rate and body temperature follow the same pattern in a 24 h cycle. These parameters reach their peaks (acrophase) in the afternoon and their minimum during sleep. A majority of studies that controlled the time for saliva collection took place between 9 and 11 a.m. Subjects should be instructed to refrain from eating and drinking (except for water) for at least 90 min prior to the saliva collection. Other factors include gender, body weight, salivary gland size, number of natural teeth, and bite force [5].

### Gland Size

Salivary glands acutely adapt to the hardness of the diet. Changing from normal hardness to a soft diet has been shown to decrease salivary output as well as reduce the size of the salivary glands [35]. Changing the diet back to normal hardness

**Table 12.3** The impact of regular chewing on salivary secretion

| Subject group | Intervention | Subject number | Duration | Frequency | Outcomes after intervention | Ref |
|---|---|---|---|---|---|---|
| Community-dwelling elderly | Sugar-free gum vs. no gum | $N=91$ and 95 | 6 months | Twice a day for 15 min | No significant change in paraffin-stimulated salivary flow rate | [19] |
| Average of 20 natural teeth | Parallel, randomized | | | | Gum group showed a reduction in plaque and gingival indices<br>Wide variance in compliance rate | |
| Chronic dry mouth patients | Chewing gum, sour lemon lozenge, and sweetened artificial saliva spray | $N=80$ | 2 weeks | Ad libitum (max 10 lozenges a day) | No significant increase in paraffin-stimulated salivary flow rate for any of the three products<br>No difference in terms of the patients' preference among three options | [27] |
| Subjective and objective dry mouth patients | 4 lozenges, 1 chewing gum, and 3 artificial saliva types<br>Randomized, crossover | $N=106$ | 2 weeks | Not regulated | None of 8 products caused a significant increase in paraffin-stimulated whole saliva secretion<br>Chewing gum and acid-containing lozenge were among the most preferred products, based on patients' ratings | [26] |
| Elderly in retirement homes | Chewing gum vs. no gum<br>Parallel | $N=31–43$ | 1 year | Twice a day for 15 min | Gum group increased paraffin-stimulated salivary flow rate over baseline | [20] |
| Elderly with dry mouth symptoms | 3 types of chewing gum | $N=38–43$ | 2 weeks | Ad libitum, average 5–6 times a day | No changes in either unstimulated or paraffin-stimulated salivary flow rate<br>Significantly higher preference for mucin supplement gum product among patients who had trouble with speech and swallowing | [22] |

(continued)

**Table 12.3** (continued)

| Subject group | Intervention | Subject number | Duration | Frequency | Outcomes after intervention | Ref |
|---|---|---|---|---|---|---|
| Rheumatic patients with dry mouth symptoms | Chewing gum and lozenges | $N=16$ | 2 weeks | Gum: 2–5 times a day for 30 min | Neither gum nor lozenge improved unstimulated or stimulated salivary flow rate | [24] |
| | Crossover | | | Lozenge: 4–8 pieces a day | A third of 18 patients reported their symptoms improved after the treatment | |
| Hemodialysis patients | Chewing gum and artificial saliva | $N=65$ | 2 weeks | >6 times a day for 10 min | No change in unstimulated or paraffin-stimulated saliva flow rates | [37] |
| | Crossover | | | | Chewing gum decreased xerostomia index | |
| Young healthy adults | Sugar-free gum | $N=11$ | 2 weeks | 10 min every waking hour | Increase in acid-stimulated parotid saliva flow rate | [18] |
| | | | | | No significant increase in unstimulated whole saliva flow rate | |
| Young healthy adults | Chewing gum | $N=73$ and 42 at two locations | 8 weeks | 4 sticks a day | Elevation in unstimulated salivary flow rate, particularly for subjects with lower baseline flow rates | [38] |

resulted in an increase in gland weight to the normal level. The parotid gland size, measured by magnetic resonance imaging (MRI), correlated with the flow rate and total protein concentration of unstimulated whole saliva [40]. The parotid salivary gland size was also positively correlated with gum base-stimulated salivary flow rate [41].

## Number of Remaining Teeth

Saliva secretion has been found to correlate with the number of natural teeth. In a study with community-dwelling elderly, participants with ≥21 teeth had significantly higher stimulated salivary flow rates and also lower plaque scores, fewer decayed root surfaces, and lower salivary lactobacillus counts than those with <21 natural teeth [19]. An epidemiological study on elderly Thai subjects showed that subjects in the hyposalivation group had a higher number of decayed teeth and a lower number of teeth present [42]. Of course, these observational data do not justify the assumption of causality. In fact, it is possible that the hyposalivation leads to tooth decay and loss due to the reduced clearance of food debris and plaque acid. A 6-month-long craniofacial exercise program increased both unstimulated saliva and stimulated saliva for elderly with more than 20 natural teeth [43]. The subjects were instructed to perform a daily routine of exercise for expression muscles, tongue, and swallowing, along with craniofacial massages on the areas of major salivary glands. The salivary secretion was measured before and after the exercise regime. The results were dichotomized by the number of remaining teeth. While overall results showed a statistically significant increase of both unstimulated and stimulated salivary flow rates, a subgroup of subjects who had fewer than 20 natural teeth did not show significant change in salivary flow rate after 6 months of exercise, probably due to the smaller occlusal area.

## Bite Force

There is consistent evidence that higher bite force is correlated with higher salivary flow rate. Bite force, or occlusal force, is the pressure generated on occlusal surfaces when subjects bite on a food bolus. Using transducers made of metal or a thin film, the pressure generated between occlusal surfaces of teeth when subjects clench their teeth or dentures as hard as possible can be measured (Fig. 12.4) [44]. A cross-sectional study showed that reduced occlusal force is associated with a decline in stimulated whole saliva flow rate in older adults with varying numbers of teeth and functional occlusions [4]. The positive correlations between bite force and salivary flow rate were found true for unstimulated whole saliva, chewing-stimulated whole

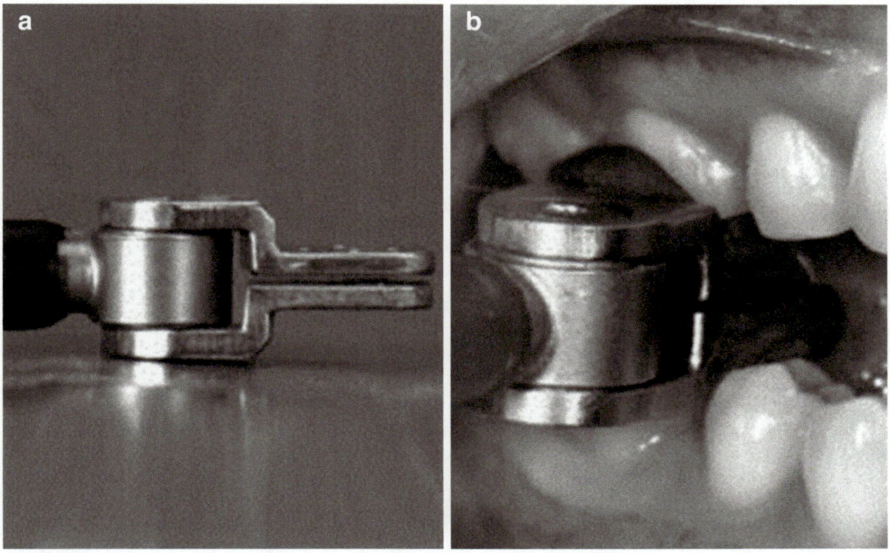


**Fig. 12.4** Bite force measurement using transducer (Reprinted with permission from Farella et al. [44])

saliva, and stimulated submandibular-sublingual saliva [45, 46]. These correlations were independent of age and gender. In addition, they showed that the replacement of complete dentures for edentulous elderly improved not only occlusal force but also unstimulated saliva and chewing-stimulated whole saliva flow rates within the same subject group [47]. The level of occlusal force and both salivary flow rates after the denture replacement was proportional to those levels before the replacement, suggesting that improvement of occlusal force can increase salivary secretion in accordance with the individual's salivary gland capacity.

These reports are in alignment with the mechanism by which the texture of a food bolus stimulates saliva. The response of salivary glands to diet texture is mediated by neural input to the glands from mechanoreceptors located in the periodontal ligament or the gingiva [48]. Higher bite force translates into higher pressure on the periodontal mechanoreceptors, which induces salivary secretion upon masticatory stimulation. Since the stimulation of these mechanoreceptors is based on substantial resistance between opposing teeth, it should not be confused with muscle activity measured by electromyography (EMG). Therefore, empty clenching, that is, clenching with maximum force with nothing between teeth, does not increase salivary flow rate as much as it does with a food bolus [48]. It is also noteworthy that sham chewing, an action mimicking chewing a food bolus with no food in the mouth, similarly does not have the same effect as actually chewing food in increasing salivary flow. These observations are in agreement with the fact that unilateral clenching on bite blocks or rubber disks increases parotid salivary secretion on the same side (ipsilateral) with no comparable increase in the opposite side (contralateral) [49]. Although the muscle activity is not the direct cause of salivary secretion, it is an important factor as it is the muscle movement that puts load on the dentition and thus provides pressure on the mechanoreceptors.

## Masticatory Muscles, Dentition, and Masticatory Function

The current working hypothesis is that the texture of food sensed by periodontal mechanoreceptors via contact between tooth and food plays an important role for the brain to perform oral functions. Specifically, the signals from periodontal mechanoreceptors are used to regulate the craniofacial muscles to create bite force and other manipulative functions required for food processing. The bite force, the total occlusal surface, and the occlusal contact area are the three critical factors that transduce texture of food to pressure on periodontal mechanoreceptors and therefore are the key to maintaining salivation. These factors, along with saliva secretion, influence masticatory function. Indeed, most studies concerning relations between salivary flow rate and bite force or occlusion focused on mastication rather than dry mouth.

Aging is negatively correlated with performance of mastication, as with salivary secretion. However, aging itself does not directly influence masticatory performance within the same dentition, suggesting that the decline in masticatory performance with age is a result of the accumulation of insults to the orofacial structures and the degradation of the dentition over many years [50].

One area of physiology where aging leads to marked systemic changes is skeletal muscles. In general, aging is associated with a decrease in the proportion of slow and fatigue-resistant type I fibers. Human jaw-closing muscles are composed of a relatively homogeneous mixture of slow (type I) and fast (type II) muscles. Like other skeletal muscles, jaw-closing muscles are capable of changing their anatomical characteristics depending on the functional demands. Resistance training, for example, the increased load of isometric contraction and relaxation caused by mastication, can increase the thickness of the muscle and enhances muscular strength. These changes may be expressed in terms of the increase in the cross-sectional areas of the muscle fibers and higher levels of stored glycogen as well as mitochondrial content. These changes contribute to skeletal muscles becoming more fatigue resistant and are fully reversible. In general, overloading and increased muscular activity shift muscle fiber composition to a higher ratio of slow and fatigue-resistant type I muscles [51].

Both human and animal studies suggest that the increase in mastication derived from a harder texture of diet influences both salivary output and also jaw muscle activities. Chronic exposure to a soft diet causes craniofacial muscle to adapt, resulting in the reduction in functions such as myoelectric activity, force output, muscle fiber type, and muscle mass. These influences have been documented for both short- and long-term effects. The acute muscle response to harder food texture has been documented in several human studies. In summary, the harder the food bolus texture, (1) the higher the muscle activity and (2) the more the subjects open their jaws for mastication. The long-term impact of food texture on craniofacial muscle is better studied with animal models. Animals raised on experimental diets with a soft texture showed lower levels of muscle tension after stimulation, lower levels of mitochondrial activity, smaller cross-sectional muscle areas, and a decrease in slow fatigue-resistant type I muscle fiber ratio. These observations suggest that a long-term change in diet texture leads to functional and morphological adaptation which translates into motor unit activity changes [51].

The dentition influences the muscle response to food. Lesser degree of masseter muscle activation has been reported in fully dentate subjects compared with subjects with natural dentition. In an extreme scenario, an increased proportion of fat tissue has been shown among subjects who had been edentulous for a long period of time [51].

Caution is needed when measuring bite force on residual natural teeth of the elderly. The overall bite force tends to decrease with shortening of the dental arch even when the local bite force on the individual dentition may increase because the force is applied on a smaller surface area resulting from the fitting of dentures.

The natural dentition seems to relay the information on food texture more sensitively than dentures. An experimental study on subjects with natural dentition and those with implant-supported prostheses in both jaws showed that the prosthesis group showed weaker adaptation patterns in muscle activity against an increase in food hardness, while both groups showed the adaptation of muscle activity. In addition, while the natural dentition group showed acute adaptation in muscle activity during the processing of the food bolus, the level of muscle activity was not as responsive for the prosthesis group. This impairment in adaptation is probably due to the reduction of somatosensory sensitivity in periodontal mechanoreceptors. Another piece of evidence came from a simple test. Subjects were asked to judge the magnitude of force applied to their teeth mechanically. The force applied was also monitored by acrylic blocks connected with a transducer to record the actual force applied on natural teeth or prosthesis. A higher frequency of incorrect judgment was observed among the prosthesis group compared with the natural dentition group, regardless of age, sex, implant type, or occlusion. This was particularly noticeable with force applied between 1 and 4 N. As the force applied increased, the rate of wrong judgment decreased between both groups, suggesting that receptors in the bone and peri-implant mucosa compensate for the absence of periodontal and pulpal receptors [52].

The best strategy for preserving the natural dentition and dental arches is to maintain good oral hygiene and lifestyle habits (e.g., not smoking) and have regular checkups by dentists. In addition, food choice will influence occlusion for children who are still developing. Impact of food on bite force as well as craniofacial morphology has been an interest for anthropological studies. The human craniofacial morphology has been shown to change from wide and short facial structure to that of long and narrow ones over history as well as over a few generations. This pattern of temporal change is consistent across regions, such as the USA, Europe, and Japan [53]. Relatively recent studies also suggest that indigenous populations, whose diet consists of less processed food, have higher maximal bite force than their regional counterparts whose diet source is more industrialized and thus processed. These data also highlight that the mandibular shape is more closely reflected by the dietary pattern than the maxillary shape. The palatomaxillary region, which forms the occlusal surface with the mandibular region, showed a similar pattern, however to a lesser degree. Overall, it suggests that mastication pressure primarily impacts on the morphological change in the mandibular rather than the maxillary region, while the maxillary region adapts to the mandible to maintain occlusion. This is in agreement with a narrow and longer facial structure and also higher prevalence of dental crowding and malocclusion among industrialized populations [54].

## Masticatory Function and Oral Food Processing

Considering the mouth's function as the starting point of digestion, maintaining masticatory performance has impact beyond salivary secretion to protect and lubricate the mouth. Mastication is a process in which the food bolus is being prepared, with grinding into a fine state and mixing with saliva, for transfer to the stomach. Fragmentation and moistening of food is the main function of mastication, but it also imparts enjoyable sensations related to taste and the pleasure of eating [55]. Taste and flavor perception also act as cues for the digestive system to prepare for the incoming food bolus. The sensory cue for swallowing is mediated by the physical properties of the food bolus, such as size, hydration level (i.e., amount of saliva incorporated), and surface mouthfeel (i.e., degree of lubrication by mucin coating). Subjects with a high masticatory performance will, on average, swallow finer food particles than subjects with a lesser performance. Compromised masticatory performance therefore may induce poor dietary practices and marginal nutritional intakes [56]. Salivary flow rate, bite force, and masticatory ability have not been shown to correlate with dietary selection and the nutritional value of food choice [57]. However, note needs to be taken that these assessments are based on the choice of food and thus do not take into account nutritional uptake or absorption. In an experiment in which subjects chewed meat until they thought that it was ready to be swallowed, older subjects, whose salivary flow rate and bite force were lower than for their younger counterparts, took a larger number of chews before they thought that the meat bolus was ready to be swallowed, and each bolus was less processed than in their younger counterparts. The amount of saliva incorporated into the bolus was lower in hard-texture meat for the older group. Overall, the results suggested that those with lower salivary flow rate and bite force ingested a less digestible bolus [58].

**Conclusion**

Dry mouth is not just a discomfort but impacts on quality of life and overall oral and general health, and a holistic approach is needed to address it. Patients and their physicians should be encouraged to consider substitutions for polypharmacy and also to consider counseling for specific behavioral changes, for example, avoiding tobacco and alcohol. Treatments include the use of oral lubricants (Chap. 11) and cholinergic agonist medications. For those with viable salivary glands, nonprescriptive sialogogues such as lozenges and chewing gum are also options to relieve the symptom of dry mouth. These treatments have advantages in ease of use and portability. Patients' preference is critical in ensuring continued use of the treatment. The consistency in the effect of chewing gum for the relief of dry mouth symptoms is reflected in advice to patients with xerostomia as a self-care step given by the National Institute of Dental and Craniofacial Research and the National Institutes of Health in the USA and the National Health Service in the UK [59, 60].

Unstimulated saliva lubricates the oral cavity for the majority of the day and therefore is the single critical factor for the prevention of dry mouth symptoms. It is unclear whether long-term use of chewing would significantly improve saliva secretion. It is important to have physiological functions related to mastication for the production of sufficient saliva, both unstimulated and stimulated. These functions require healthy salivary glands, neural circuits, and masticatory function [33].

With increasing age, maintaining a sufficient number of healthy natural teeth is the best strategy for retaining masticatory function, salivation, and thus oral comfort. The masticatory system has complex physiological functions that are essential functions of normal daily life, such as speaking, eating, swallowing, and smiling. The keys are to practice good oral hygiene and also dietary choice that requires jaw-closing muscle activity. Preventive measures against dry mouth positively influence the maintenance of oral health. Saliva plays a pivotal role in the overall maintenance of a healthy homeostatic condition in the oral cavity, which from the dental perspective is usually considered to be related to protection of the teeth and mucosal surfaces. This implies that proper care for dental health can contribute to the prevention of dry mouth. Keeping a good occlusion and dentition will help maintain the capacity to secrete saliva, while saliva will help maintain oral health and thus preserve oral function. The oral cavity is also the starting point of the digestive system, and saliva has a critical role in mastication, the maintenance of whose function is critical for both protection of the oral cavity, nutritional intake, and thus efficient digestion.

## References


1. van Nieuw AA, Veerman EC, Vissink A. Saliva: properties and functions. In: Wong DT, editor. Salivary diagnostics. 1st ed. Ames: Wiley-Blackwell; 2008. p. 27–36.
2. Sreebny LM. Saliva in health and disease: an appraisal and update. Int Dent J. 2000;50(3):140–61.
3. van der Putten G-J, Brand HS, de Visschere LMJ, Schols JMGA, Baat C. Saliva secretion rate and acidity in a group of physically disabled older care home residents. Odontology. 2013;101(1):108–15.
4. Ikebe K, Matsuda K, Morii K, Hazeyama T, Kagawa R, Ogawa T, et al. Relationship between bite force and salivary flow in older adults. Oral Surg Oral Med Oral Pathol Oral Radiol Endod. 2007;104(4):510–5.
5. Dawes C. Factors influencing salivary flow rate and composition. In: Edgar M, Dawes C, O'Mullane D, editors. Saliva and oral health. 4th ed. London: Stephen Hancocks Limited; 2012. p. 37–55.
6. Dawes C, Watanabe S. The effect of taste adaptation on salivary flow rate and salivary sugar clearance. J Dent Res. 1987;66(3):740–4.
7. Dawes C, Kubieniec K. The effects of prolonged gum chewing on salivary flow rate and composition. Arch Oral Biol. 2004;49(8):665–9.
8. Polland KE, Higgins F, Orchardson R. Salivary flow rate and pH during prolonged gum chewing in humans. J Oral Rehabil. 2003;30(9):861–5.
9. Bots CP, Brand HS, Veerman EC, van Amerongen BM, Nieuw Amerongen AV. Preferences and saliva stimulation of eight different chewing gums. Int Dent J. 2004;54(3):143–8.
10. Macpherson LM, Chen WY, Dawes C. Effects of salivary bicarbonate content and film velocity on pH changes in an artificial plaque containing Streptococcus oralis, after exposure to sucrose. J Dent Res. 1991;70(9):1235–8.
11. Rosenhek M, Macpherson LM, Dawes C. The effects of chewing-gum stick size and duration of chewing on salivary flow rate and sucrose and bicarbonate concentrations. Arch Oral Biol. 1993;38(10):885–91.
12. Femiano F, Rullo R, di Spirito F, Lanza A, Festa VM, Cirillo N. A comparison of salivary substitutes versus a natural sialogogue (citric acid) in patients complaining of dry mouth as an adverse drug reaction: a clinical, randomized controlled study. Oral Surg Oral Med Oral Pathol Oral Radiol Endod. 2011;112(1):e15–20.
13. Pramanik R, Osailan SM, Challacombe SJ, Urquhart D, Proctor GB. Protein and mucin retention on oral mucosal surfaces in dry mouth patients. Eur J Oral Sci. 2010;118(3): 245–53.
14. Satoh-Kuriwada S, Iikubo M, Shoji N, Sakamoto M, Sasano T. Diagnostic performance of labial minor salivary gland flow measurement for assessment of xerostomia. Arch Oral Biol. 2012;57(8):1121–6.
15. Abelson DC, Barton J, Mandel ID. The effect of chewing sorbitol-sweetened gum on salivary flow and cemental plaque pH in subjects with low salivary flow. J Clin Dent. 1990;2(1):3–5.
16. Edgar WM. Sugar substitutes, chewing gum and dental caries–a review. Br Dent J. 1998;184(1):29–32.
17. Olsson H, Spak CJ, Axell T. The effect of a chewing gum on salivary secretion, oral mucosal friction, and the feeling of dry mouth in xerostomic patients. Acta Odontol Scand. 1991;49(5):273–9.

18. Dodds MW, Hsieh SC, Johnson DA. The effect of increased mastication by daily gum-chewing on salivary gland output and dental plaque acidogenicity. J Dent Res. 1991;70(12):1474–8.
19. Al-Haboubi M, Zoitopoulos L, Beighton D, Gallagher JE. The potential benefits of sugar-free chewing gum on the oral health and quality of life of older people living in the community: a randomized controlled trial. Community Dent Oral Epidemiol. 2012;40(5):415–24.
20. Simons D, Brailsford SR, Kidd EA, Beighton D. The effect of medicated chewing gums on oral health in frail older people: a 1-year clinical trial. J Am Geriatr Soc. 2002;50(8):1348–53.
21. Dawes C, Macpherson LM. Effects of nine different chewing-gums and lozenges on salivary flow rate and pH. Caries Res. 1992;26(3):176–82.
22. Aagaard A, Godiksen S, Teglers PT, Schiødt M, Glenert U. Comparison between new saliva stimulants in patients with dry mouth: a placebo-controlled double-blind crossover study. J Oral Pathol Med. 1992;21(8):376–80.
23. Bots CP, Brand HS, Veerman EC, Valentijn-Benz M, Van Amerongen BM, Nieuw Amerongen AV, et al. The management of xerostomia in patients on haemodialysis: comparison of artificial saliva and chewing gum. Palliat Med. 2005;19(3):202–7.
24. Risheim H, Arneberg P. Salivary stimulation by chewing gum and lozenges in rheumatic patients with xerostomia. Scand J Dent Res. 1993;101(1):40–3.
25. Karami NM, Janghorbani M, Kowsari IR, Hosseini BM. Effects of chewing different flavored gums on salivary flow rate and pH. Int J Dent. 2012. Available from: http://dx.doi.org/10.1155/2012/569327.
26. Bjornstrom M, Axell T, Birkhed D. Comparison between saliva stimulants and saliva substitutes in patients with symptoms related to dry mouth. A multi-centre study. Swed Dent J. 1990;14(4):153–61.
27. Stewart CM, Jones AC, Bates RE, Sandow P, Pink F, Stillwell J. Comparison between saliva stimulants and a saliva substitute in patients with xerostomia and hyposalivation. Spec Care Dentist. 1998;18(4):142–7.
28. Davies AN. A comparison of artificial saliva and chewing gum in the management of xerostomia in patients with advanced cancer. Palliat Med. 2000;14(3):197–203.
29. Dawes C. The unstimulated salivary flow rate after prolonged gum chewing. Arch Oral Biol. 2005;50(6):561–3.
30. Wolff M, Kleinberg I. Oral mucosal wetness in hypo- and normosalivators. Arch Oral Biol. 1998;43(6):455–62.
31. Dawes C. Salivary clearance and its effect on oral health. In: Edgar M, Dawes C, O'Mullane D, editors. Saliva and oral health. 4th ed. London: Stephan Hancocks Limited; 2012. p. 81–96.
32. Hector MP, Sullivan A. Migration of erythrosin-labelled saliva during unilateral chewing in man. Arch Oral Biol. 1992;37(9):757–8.
33. Mese H, Matsuo R. Salivary secretion, taste and hyposalivation. J Oral Rehabil. 2007;34(10): 711–23.
34. Bourdiol P, Mioche L, Monier S. Effect of age on salivary flow obtained under feeding and non-feeding conditions. J Oral Rehabil. 2004;31(5):445–52.
35. Dodds MW, Johnson DA, Yeh CK. Health benefits of saliva: a review. J Dent. 2005;33(3): 223–33.
36. Wang XP, Zhong B, Chen ZK, Stewart ME, Zhang C, Zhang K, et al. History of frequent gum chewing is associated with higher unstimulated salivary flow rate and lower caries severity in healthy Chinese adults. Caries Res. 2012;46(6):513–8.
37. Bots CP, Brand HS, Veerman EC, Korevaar JC, Valentijn-Benz M, Bezemer PD, et al. Chewing gum and a saliva substitute alleviate thirst and xerostomia in patients on haemodialysis. Nephrol Dial Transplant. 2005;20(3):578–84.
38. Jenkins GN, Edgar WM. The effect of daily gum-chewing on salivary flow rates in man. J Dent Res. 1989;68(5):786–90.
39. Vissink A, Wolff A, Veerman EC. Saliva collections. In: Wong DT, editor. Salivary diagnostics. 1st ed. Ames: Wiley-Blackwell; 2008. p. 37–59.
40. Ono K, Morimoto Y, Inoue H, Masuda W, Tanaka T, Inenaga K. Relationship of the unstimulated whole saliva flow rate and salivary gland size estimated by magnetic resonance image in healthy young humans. Arch Oral Biol. 2006;51(4):345–9.

41. Ono K, Inoue H, Masuda W, Morimoto Y, Tanaka T, Yokota M, et al. Relationship of chewing-stimulated whole saliva flow rate and salivary gland size. Arch Oral Biol. 2007;52(5):427–31.
42. Samnieng P, Ueno M, Shinada K, Zaitsu T, Wright FA, Kawaguchi Y. Association of hyposalivation with oral function, nutrition and oral health in community-dwelling elderly Thai. Community Dent Health. 2012;29(1):117–23.
43. Ibayashi H, Fujino Y, Pham T-M, Matsuda S. Intervention study of exercise program for oral function in healthy elderly people. Tohoku J Exp Med. 2008;215(3):237–45.
44. Farella M, De Oliveira ME, Gallo LM, Läubli T, Tomatis L, Müller C, et al. Firing duration of masseter motor units during prolonged low-level contractions. Clin Neurophysiol. 2011;122(12):2433–40.
45. Yeh CK, Johnson DA, Dodds MWJ, Sakai S, Rugh JD, Hatch JP. Association of salivary flow rates with maximal bite force. J Dent Res. 2000;79(8):1560–5.
46. Ikebe K, Matsuda K, Kagawa R, Enoki K, Okada T, Yoshida M, et al. Masticatory performance in older subjects with varying degrees of tooth loss. J Dent. 2012;40(1):71–6.
47. Matsuda K, Ikebe K, Ogawa T, Kagawa R, Maeda Y. Increase of salivary flow rate along with improved occlusal force after the replacement of complete dentures. Oral Surg Oral Med Oral Pathol Oral Radiol Endod. 2009;108(2):211–5.
48. Hector MP, Linden RWA. The possible role of periodontal mechanoreceptors in the control of parotid secretion in man. Exp Physiol. 1987;72(3):285–301.
49. Kerr AC. The effects of chewing on the production of salivary secretions. In: The physiological regulation of salivary secretions in man: a study of the response of human salivary glands to reflex stimulation. Oxford: Pergamon Press; 1961. p. 48–60.
50. Ikebe K, Matsuda K, Kagawa R, Enoki K, Yoshida M, Maeda Y, et al. Association of masticatory performance with age, gender, number of teeth, occlusal force and salivary flow in Japanese older adults: is ageing a risk factor for masticatory dysfunction? Arch Oral Biol. 2011;56(10):991–6.
51. Grünheid T, Langenbach GEJ, Korfage JAM, Zentner A, van Eijden TMGJ. The adaptive response of jaw muscles to varying functional demands. Eur J Orthod. 2009;31(6):596–612.
52. Trulsson M, van der Bilt A, Carlsson GE, Gotfredsen K, Larsson P, Müller F, et al. From brain to bridge: masticatory function and dental implants. J Oral Rehabil. 2012;39(11):858–77.
53. Weisensee KE, Jantz RL. Secular changes in craniofacial morphology of the Portuguese using geometric morphometrics. Am J Phys Anthropol. 2011;145(4):548–59.
54. von Cramon-Taubadel N. Global human mandibular variation reflects differences in agricultural and hunter-gatherer subsistence strategies. Proc Natl Acad Sci U S A. 2011;108(49):19546–51.
55. Pereira LJ, Duarte Gaviao MB, van der Bilt A. Influence of oral characteristics and food products on masticatory function. Acta Odontol Scand. 2006;64(4):193–201.
56. van der Bilt A, Mojet J, Tekamp FA, Abbink JH. Comparing masticatory performance and mixing ability. J Oral Rehabil. 2010;37(2):79–84.
57. Österberg T, Tsuga K, Rothenberg E, Carlsson GE, Steen B. Masticatory ability in 80-year-old subjects and its relation to intake of energy, nutrients and food items. Gerodontology. 2002;19(2):95–101.
58. Mioche L, Bourdiol P, Monier S, Martin J-F, Cormier D. Changes in jaw muscles activity with age: effects on food bolus properties. Physiol Behav. 2004;82(4):621–7.
59. Dry Mouth (Xerostomia) Bethesda: National Institute of Dental and Craniofacial Research; 2013. Updated 18 Jul 2013; cited 30 Aug 2013. Available from: http://www.nidcr.nih.gov/oralhealth/topics/drymouth/.
60. Treating Sjogren's syndrome London: National Health Service; 2013. Updated 10 Sept 2012; cited 30 Aug 2013. Available from: http://www.nhs.uk/Conditions/Sjogrens-syndrome/Pages/Treatment.aspx.

# Future Prevention and Treatment of Radiation-Induced Hyposalivation

# 13

Robert P. Coppes and Tara A. van de Water

**Abstract**

Radiation-induced hyposalivation and consequential xerostomia have devastating effects on the quality of life of patients treated for head and neck cancer. Regretfully, currently there are no adequate or safe treatments. This chapter describes the mechanism of radiation-induced salivary gland damage and current and potential treatments. The reduced function of the salivary gland after irradiation is mainly due to loss of acinar cell function and number. Therefore, future strategies are aimed to restore saliva flow through manipulation of the remaining cells through gene therapy or by stimulation of the generative potential of the glands. The latter can be induced by stimulation of proliferation of remaining cells through the administration of cytokines or transplanted mesenchymal cells. Stem cell therapy seems to have the highest potential as in preclinical studies it has been shown to restore glandular homoeostasis and long-term regenerative capacity. However, less radiation dose as possible with proton therapy may be the best way to prevent hyposalivation.

## Introduction

Yearly worldwide, more than 550,000 new patients are expected to be diagnosed with head and neck cancer (HNC) [1]. The majority of these patients are (co-)treated with radiotherapy which plays a pivotal role in the curative treatment of HNC, either

R.P. Coppes, PhD (✉)
Department of Radiation Oncology and Cell Biology, University Medical Center Groningen, Internal Zipcode DA30, 30001, Groningen 9700 RB, The Netherlands
e-mail: r.p.coppes@umcg.nl

T.A. van de Water, PhD
Department of Radiation Oncology, University Medical Center Groningen, Groningen, The Netherlands



G. Carpenter (ed.), *Dry Mouth: A Clinical Guide on Causes, Effects and Treatments*, DOI 10.1007/978-3-642-55154-3_13

as a single modality or in combination with surgery and/or chemotherapy [2]. The overall 5-year survival for squamous cell carcinoma of the head and neck is about 80 % for the early stages of oral cancer and about 35 % for locally advanced stages. Despite the beneficial effects of radiotherapy regarding loco-regional tumour control, damage inflicted to normal tissues surrounding the tumour may cause severe complications. Tissues at risk include the salivary glands, which are generally co-irradiated during the treatment of HNC. Exposure of the salivary gland to radiation results in a progressive loss of gland function (hyposalivation) within the first weeks of radiotherapy [3].

Hyposalivation causes xerostomia and subsequent side effects such as alterations in speech and taste and results in difficulties with mastication and deglutition [3, 4]. Oral mucosal dryness predisposes tissues to fissures and ulcerations and to changes in the composition of the oral flora. The reduced oral clearance in combination with the altered oral flora may lead to severe dental caries and infections. A reduction in salivary flow also contributes to the risk of osteoradionecrosis of the mandible and to oesophageal injury, due to a decrease in the rate of oral clearance. All these adverse effects severely hamper the quality of life (QoL) of affected patients [3, 5, 6].

In a recent clinical trial, we showed that prophylactic administration of pilocarpine improved salivary flow post-irradiation in only a subset of patients treated for HNC and that this effect was dependent on the parotid gland radiation dose and volume irradiated [7]. Intensity-modulated radiation therapy (IMRT) spares the parotid gland and improves the xerostomia-related QoL [8] and general dimensions of QoL, such as social functioning and overall global QoL [9], but still approximately 40 % of these patients will develop hyposalivation and consequential life-long complaints [9]. Thus, even with these modern radiation techniques and currently available preventive measurements aimed to reduce early and late side effects, hyposalivation will remain one of the most frequently occurring side effects after curative radiation [10]. Therefore, an effective approach to protect or regenerate salivary gland function from radiation injury is of great importance to ensure survivors of HNC treatment a more pleasant and healthy life.

To appreciate approaches to improve salivary gland function after irradiation, a thorough knowledge on the mechanisms as mostly derived from preclinical experiments of radiation-induced salivary gland damage is necessary.

Actually, the response of salivary glands to irradiation is rather atypical. Classically, the response to radiation is dependent on the tissue turnover time, meaning that tissues with a rapid cell turnover like the intestine and the hematopoietic system respond quickly in days to weeks to the insult, whereas tissues with a slow turnover time may take months to years to respond (like the kidney and heart). Strangely, although the tissue turnover rate is rather slow (≈60 days) [11], salivary glands respond very rapidly within the first 24 h in experimental animals [12] and to radiotherapy already within the first weeks of treatment [13]. The response of the salivary gland to radiation can be separated into four phases (Fig. 13.1): the acute phase (0–10 days after irradiation), where the decrease of function has been attributed to apoptosis and/or to membrane damage and consequential impaired water excretion [13–20]; the second phase, with loss of acinar cells (10–60 days post-radiation);

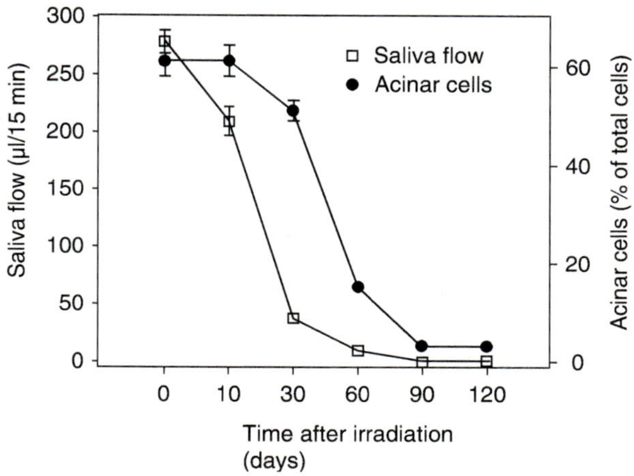


**Fig. 13.1** Salivary gland function is reduced after irradiation before acinar cells disappear probably due to membrane damage (Adapted from [29], data from [14]; see also [15])

the third phase (60–120 days), status quo; and the fourth phase (>120 days), with a further degeneration due to further cells loss [14]. The later phases (phases 3 and 4, from 60–120 to 120–240 days after radiotherapy, respectively), wherein functionally mature acinar cells senesce and are not replenished with new ones, are now suggested to be due to RT-induced sterilization of salivary gland stem/progenitor cells (SSPCs) and vascular damage [14, 15, 21–29]. This eventually results in salivary glands almost devoid of acinar cells, with only ductal tissue and fibrosis left [15].

## Gene Therapy

Gene therapy was recently reviewed by Baum [30]. With the above described knowledge, the group of Baum hypothesized that since irradiated glands are devoid of functioning acinar cells, the remaining duct cells could be changed in function to allow fluid secretion. To achieve this it was proposed to generate an osmotic lumen with a large interstitium gradient over duct cells facilitating water permeability. A serotype 5, adenoviral (Ad5) vector encoding the human water channel protein aquaporin-1 (hAQP1) was constructed. Human aquaporin-1 can facilitate the extremely rapid movement of water over cell layers. Expression of this protein in cells, normally not transporting water, can lead to increases in osmotic gradient-driven water movement. First, retrograde Stensen's duct injection of the AdhAQP1 in rats [31] and minipigs [32] was tested. In both species the dramatically radiation-induced reduction in salivary fluid secretion was restored to almost normal levels, albeit transiently. Indeed, the hAQP1 transgene was expressed only in duct cells, implicating that the increased salivary secretion observed is most likely due to enhanced water permeability in the normally water-impermeable duct cells [32, 33]. Next a large toxicity study in rats was performed which showed that retrograde ductal delivery in submandibular glands of AdhAQP1 to salivary glands appears to induce at most some early toxicity [33]. Now very recently [34], a phase I study was performed to determine whether hAQP1 gene transfer is safe and effective in humans (http://www.clinicaltrials.gov/ct/show/NCT00372320). This trial was performed in individuals previously treated for HNC with salivary hypofunction more than 5 years after radiotherapy. No deaths or serious dose-limiting toxicities and only few mild to moderate adverse events were observed. Most importantly, in about half of the patients, objective responses were seen with even a subjective improvement in xerostomia. Therefore, AdhAQP1 vector delivery to a single parotid gland was considered safe and effective in a subset of subjects [34]. Permanent gene transfer and the use of less immunogenic vectors, however, will be necessary to induce long-lived expression of hAQP1 in salivary glands. Therefore, further studies for the use of gene therapy to relieve xerostomia patients from their burden are warranted.

## Prevention

### Radioprotectors

Many approaches have been pursued to protect normal tissues and specifically the salivary gland from radiation damage. The most obvious one is the reduction of the physical dose to the tissue, as radiation exerts its effect through the generation of free electrons and free radicals, which subsequently damage cellular proteins. Of these cellular proteins, the DNA and, as mentioned above, the membranes are the most important targets, inducing cell death of cell dysfunction [15]. For years radical scavengers have been tested for their efficacy to reduce damage to normal tissues. Radical scavengers oxidize free radicals and peroxides, thereby reducing the radiation dose effect. However, when radical scavengers are being used during cancer treatment, a clear difference should be demonstrated between the protection of the tissue in question and the tumour showing an actual improved therapeutic ratio.

A potential interesting scavenger is Tempol. In a mouse head and neck radiation model, it was shown that Tempol reduced irradiation-induced salivary gland hypofunction [35] without protection of tumour tissue [35]. However, no clear therapeutic ratio has been determined and no clinical data are available yet [36].

More extensively studied is the oxygen radical scavenger amifostine (WR-2721 or Ethyol). Murine studies showed a high and rapid accumulation of amifostine in a selective number of healthy tissues among which the salivary glands [37] and a poor and slow accumulation in tumours [38]. Several animal studies showed radioprotection of parotid glands' function and structure [39]. Currently, amifostine is not widely used due to some toxicity, price and an unclear therapeutic ratio. However, depending on the type of cancer treatment, symptoms can be reduced to some degree [40]. Interestingly, the protective ability of amifostine strongly depends on the irradiated glandular region and is observed for later damage only. The major effect of the drug seems to be the prevention of volume effects caused by secondary damage occurring in shielded parts of the gland [39].

Three decades ago, the acute response of salivary glands to radiation was hypothesized to be due to damage to the granulas inside the acinar cells. These membrane-enclosed organelles are rich in heavy metals (Zn, Mn and Fe) and could be subjected to radiation-induced lipid peroxidation, evoked by a metal catalysation process. As a consequence granulas could leak proteolytic enzymes that would evoke immediate cell lysis and subsequent loss of granula-containing cells [16]. Degranulation prior to irradiation would therefore protect the salivary gland [16, 17]. Although this is an attractive explanation for the acute response and offers means to protect the salivary gland from radiation, it was found not to be the sole cause. Proteolytic enzymes are exclusively present in GCT cells and can therefore not explain protective effects on acinar cells, and actually no significant cell lysis (i.e. cell loss) was observed in rat glands after clinical relevant doses [41]. Interestingly, also drugs that stimulated saliva secretion without degranulation protected against radiation-induced damage [42, 43]. Moreover, recently it was suggested that this at least in part is due to compensatory mechanisms through increased proliferation of undamaged cells.

## Stimulation of Regeneration

Many factors play a role in the response of a tissue to radiation [44]; however, the onset and the severity of the radiation effects are ultimately determined by the (in) ability of stem/progenitor cells to reconstitute functional cells [18, 45]. Recovery and compensatory responses in non-irradiated regions presumably containing stem/progenitor cells have been observed after radiation, indicating the potential of surviving stem/progenitor cells to regenerate the tissue [15, 46].

In every tissue, homoeostasis is maintained by proliferation and differentiation of the tissues's progenitor/stem cells compensating for cell loss due to aging or cytotoxic insults. Progenitor cells are often responsible for the bulk of proliferation and regeneration, whereas the stem cell becomes only active after substantial damage. In the adult salivary gland, nearly all of the differentiated cell types seem to retain the ability to replicate [22, 47]. Although it is still not completely clear what the exact stem and progenitor cells of the salivary gland are, it has been proposed that the intercalated ducts contain progenitor cells [11, 23] and the excretory ducts harbour the stem cells [24, 48, 49]. Immediately after irradiation, all proliferation ceased, where after 3 days of compensatory proliferation is started in the intercalated duct compartment [50]. However, after some months, hardly any proliferation is detected anymore [51], indicative of a strong reduction in regenerative capacity. Strangely, when taken out of the environment, salivary gland stem cells can still be cultured in vitro [52] indicating that radiation-induced anti-proliferative signals are being produced within the irradiated gland. Stimulating the proliferative process of the remaining stem/progenitor cells in the salivary gland (as described above) seems to at least induce some regenerative response. Indeed, stimulation of proliferation and differentiation of radiation surviving stem cells have been shown to be beneficial in salivary glands. Cytokines like EGF [53, 54], insulin growth factor [54, 55] and bFGF [55] have been suggested not only to enhance proliferation, but also inhibit apoptosis. Especially for keratinocyte growth factor (KGF or FGF7), induction of proliferation and expansion of stem/progenitor cells have been suggested to be the mechanism of reduction of radiation-induced salivary gland damage in the mouse submandibular gland [52]. ΔN23-KGF treatment for 4 days prior to irradiation was shown to induce general proliferation including stem/progenitor cells, increasing the stem and progenitor cell pool. As such the absolute higher number of stem/progenitor cells and acinar cells that survived irradiation increased, although the relative radiation sensitivity of the stem/progenitor cells was not affected. Post-irradiation treatment with ΔN23-KGF accelerated the expansion of the pool of progenitor/stem cells that survived the irradiation treatment to further improve gland function [52].

Another cytokine pathway is that of Wnt/β-catenin known to be essential for the maintenance and activation of various adult stem cells. Transient over-expression of Wnt1 in basal epithelia in a Wnt1 transgenic mice activated Wnt/β-catenin pathway in submandibular glands of male mice. This prevented radiation-induced salivary gland dysfunction potentially through the inhibition of apoptosis in stem cells [56], allowing enhanced regeneration. Also, basic fibroblast growth factor (bFGF) was shown to prevent salivary gland dysfunction after irradiation. Again, this effect was attributed to the inhibition of radiation-induced apoptosis in the secretory salivary gland tissue and the paracrine effect of this factor on these tissues [57]. Next to this signalling molecules like roscovitine, which inhibit cyclin-dependent kinase and acts to transiently inhibit cell cycle progression allowing improved DNA repair and suppress apoptosis, has potential to reduce radiation-induced hyposalivation [58].

All these cytokines, growth factors or signalling molecules clearly show some beneficial effect increasing salivary flow after irradiation, either through inhibition of apoptosis or enhanced proliferation of progenitor and/or stem cells. However, whether or not these substances ever make it to the clinic is rather unsure, as potential inhibition of cell death or induction of proliferation of (remaining) tumour cells is a big drawback. First, increases in therapeutic ratio should be shown before such substances can be used. The use of these substances ex vivo, however, could yield promises.

## Mesenchymal Stem Cells

Many attempts have been made to use multipotent stem cells derived from several tissues to induce regeneration of damage salivary glands. Long-term adherent cultures of cells derived from the human submandibular gland have been established [59]. These cells could undergo chondrogenic, osteogenic and adipogenic differentiation, hallmarks for mesenchymal stem cells (MSCs). Although these salivary gland-derived MSCs were shown to be supportive in the regeneration, differentiation into all salivary gland lineages was not shown [47]. Mesenchymal cells from other tissues may also have therapeutic potential for salivary gland disorders. Bone marrow MSCs have been suggested to be able to differentiate into myoepithelial cells or exert a supportive action through the secretion of growth factors and immunosuppression [60]. As such these supportive salivary gland MSCs may offer

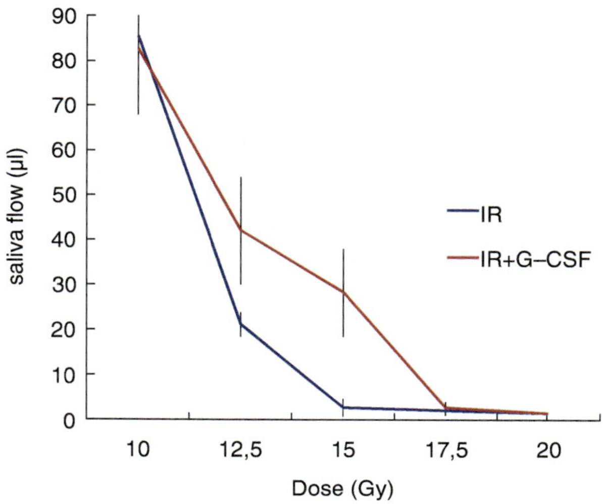


**Fig. 13.2** Window of effect of G-CSF on saliva flow 30 days following different radiation doses (Adapted from [29])

therapeutic potential during recovery and regeneration of damaged salivary glands [47]. Indeed, allogeneic bone marrow-derived MSCs were shown to suppress autoimmunity and restore salivary gland secretory function in both mouse models of Sjögren syndrome (SS) [61] and SS patients [61, 62]. Interestingly, the soluble intracellular content of lysed whole BM cells was shown to be advantageous in the repair of irradiation-damaged salivary glands [63], indicating that indeed probably the supportive action of secreted components is inducing the regeneration and not major transdifferentiation into salivary gland lineages [47]. Regretfully, still viable stem and progenitor cells are necessary for regeneration, since complete sterilization of the progenitor/stem cells of the salivary gland with higher radiation doses abrogates the supportive action of bone marrow-derived cells [29, 64] (Fig. 13.2).

## Stem Cell Therapy

The field of stem cell research has made a huge progress in the last decades indicating exciting possibilities for stem cell-based therapies for regeneration of tissues. Stem cells play a pivotal role in the response of salivary glands to radiotherapy as they play an important role in tissue repair [47]. With the discovery and experimental handling of many different types of stem cells in general, stem cell-based therapies may in the near future be used to protect, accelerate or enhance salivary gland regeneration. A prerequisite is however that the stem cells potentially used for therapy are shown to be able to self-renew (produce more stem cells) and produce more committed progenitor or functional salivary gland cells (differentiation) (Fig. 13.3).

Three different types of stem cells exist; embryonic stem (ES) cells, induced pluripotent stem (iPS) cells and adult stem cells (ASCs). ES cells, derived from the inner cells mass of blastocysts, can easily be cultured for experimental purposes and

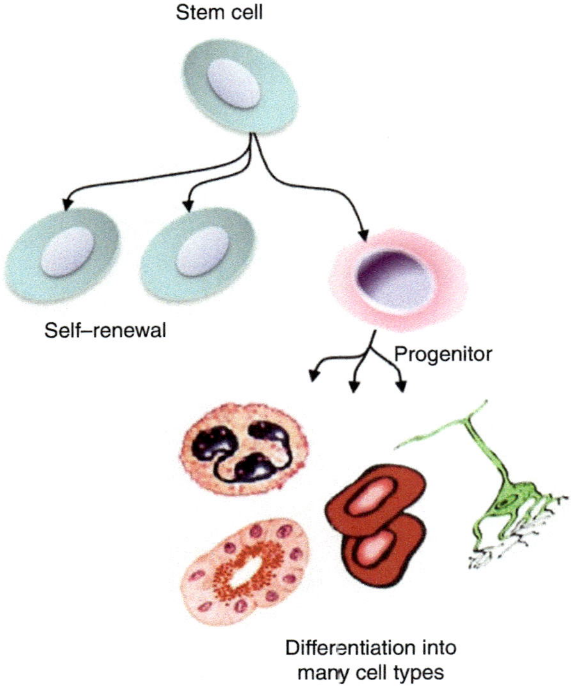


**Fig. 13.3** Tissue stem cells are able to self-renew and differentiate in precursors and functional cells

can form all tissues of the body. In 2006 [65], 2012 Nobel Prize winner Shinya Yamanaka's team at Kyoto University, Japan, managed to culture ES cell-like iPS cells from adult somatic cells, such as fibroblasts, by introduction of pluripotency genes like the transcription factors Oct-3/4, SOX2, c-Myc and Klf4. Similarly to ES cells, these cells can indefinitely self-renew, are pluripotent and able to produce all cell types of the body after injection into blastocysts. iPS cells hold high promises for fundamental and therapeutic applications. Adult stem cells are a population of undifferentiated cells that are maintained through development and into adulthood. Such ASCs are believed to be present in every tissue or organ in the body and are committed to that specific tissue type to repair damage.

So far to the best of our knowledge, no salivary gland cells have been derived from iPS cells nor have iPS cells been transplanted into salivary glands. Murine early ES cells, however, seem to differentiate in three-dimensional structures of the salivary glands after co-culturing with human salivary gland-derived fibroblasts and display some neogenetic ability after transplantation [66]. Regretfully, both ES cells and iPS cells are prone to develop teratoma's and are not ready to use for stem cell therapy until fully differentiated into salivary gland stem/progenitor or differentiated cells. Therefore, for the purpose of stem cell therapy, the focus lies mostly on the ASCs. Currently, salivary gland stem cells have not been fully characterized but some promising results have been obtained so far (reviewed in [49]).

Although adult stem cell therapy for the hematopoietic system has been in use already for many decades, for other tissues, such a therapy is only in its infancies. Several groups have been working on salivary gland stem cells and the potential application in therapy (see, e.g., [47, 49, 67, 68]).

Label retaining, stem cell marker and duct ligation studies (see [49]) have conclusively indicated that the tissues' stem progenitor cell resides in the major ducts of the salivary gland. ASC Isolation prior to radiotherapy culturing during and transplantation after radiotherapy, similar to the bone marrow transplantation protocols could restore tissue homoeostasis and regenerative potential. However, bone marrow-derived stem cells are relatively easy to obtain, whereas ASCs are mostly invisibly integrated in the tissue. Therefore, several techniques have been developed to obtain putative murine salivary gland stem cells. One option is to mince and enzymatically digest the tissue and subsequently use stem cell markers to select the ASCs, either directly after digestion or after some days of culturing [69]. The latter method is based on the idea that only stem progenitor cells are able to proliferate extensively and form spheres (named salispheres) that consist of many cells [48]. From the tissue material and the spheres, several cell types have been selected that have shown to have at least some potential to self-renew and differentiate either in vitro or in vivo (see [49]). As such cells expressing CD24, CD29, CD49f, CD117, ALDH, Sca-1 and Ascl-3 have been isolated from rodent and CD29, CD34, CD49f, CD90, CD117, CD166 and ALDH from human salivary glands. Cells expressing these markers have shown at least some in vitro differentiation potential [49]. Regretfully, only view studies have shown functional restoration after transplantation of marker expressing cells.

In our laboratory, we developed culture method, which allows the growth of salispheres from mouse and human salivary glands [48, 70]. Interestingly, salisphere-derived cells were able to self-renew in vitro and differentiate into salivary gland lineages suggesting that they encompass ASCs. We also showed that murine salispheres express adult stem cell marker proteins CD117, CD24, CD29, CD49f, Sca-1, Mushashi-1, CD44, CD90 and CD34, all of which could be localized to ducts of naïve SGs [49]. Of these, especially CD117 cells were shown to be able to reconstitute homoeostasis in murine salivary gland after irradiation [48, 71]. Interestingly, only 300 CD117+ cells induced recovery to 70 % of the original saliva flow. Cells expressing CD24, CD29, CD49f and potentially combinations of these markers have also shown promising regeneration effects, albeit only after injection of higher cell numbers [72]. Importantly, the transplanted ASCs had functionally integrated within the secretory tissue of the recipient gland, expressed donor-derived markers and displayed ductal and acinar cell-type morphologies.

Cells derived from human salispheres also have shown to express multiple stem cell markers and have been shown to be able to self-renew and differentiate in vitro [70]. The most potent stem cell containing populations however still need to be determined.

The human salivary gland may harbour stem cells that are similar to the mouse; however, it is plausible that they will differ. Potentially it may be better to start with a trial in which all the cells from human salispheres are transplanted. This will contain a cocktail of stem and progenitor cells and may provide optimal gland recovery, otherwise inhibited by the relatively long tissue turnover time. As such, progenitor cells induce short-term recovery, whereas the stem cells take care of the long-term maintenance and homoeostasis. The exact number of stem cells necessary for salivary gland rescue will depend on the patient age, extent of irradiation and potentially on use of medication. Since the stem and progenitor cells seem to reside in the major ducts, this may be the best place to inject the stem cells.

But first the salivary gland culture should be further optimized and translated for compliance to current good manufacturing practice (GMP) regulations, e.g. using MACS- and cGMP-approved antibodies [73]. Furthermore, the culture period should be followed by cryopreservation until the radiotherapy is finished and the patient is ready for transplantation. HNC patients are mostly older, and old age has been suggested to lead to an even more dramatically response to radiation [74]. A reduced salisphere-forming capability of cells from salivary glands of old mice was observed [70] which when combined with a small salivary gland biopsy that may be obtained prior to the radiotherapy makes it probably necessary to increase the number of ASCs before transplantation. It is of eminent importance to find protocols that safely allow this. Recent in vitro culture, self-renewal and differentiation methods for ASCs may be used for screening of novel factors useful for amplification. Adult stem cell therapy in patients after radiotherapy may dramatically reduce the decline in quality of life.

## Head and Neck Cancer and Radiotherapy Treatment

This sub-chapter partly contains quotations from the thesis of T.A. van de Water [75]. Radiotherapy, often applied in combination with surgery or chemotherapy, is an important treatment modality for the management of head and neck cancer. The main objective of radiotherapy is to optimize the dose to the tumour (sterilizing the tumour cells by administering a dose as high as possible) while avoiding the normal surrounding tissues as much as possible.

In head and neck cancer patients, target volumes are often complex shaped, large and surrounded by various critical and vital structures (e.g. the spinal cord, salivary glands, the hearing organ, the optic structures and structures involved in swallowing). Therefore, radiotherapy of the head and neck region is frequently associated with radiation-induced acute and late side effects that adversely affect quality of life [5, 6, 76, 77]. Hence, apart from eradication of the tumour, preservation of organ function is of major clinical importance as well.

More specifically, xerostomia or oral dryness is the most frequently reported side effect occurring after radiotherapy of the head and neck region [5, 78] and has a significant adverse effect on quality of life [5, 6]. The salivary glands that are responsible for a sufficient saliva production and composition are the parotid, submandibular and sublingual glands (the major salivary glands) and the minor salivary glands lining the oral cavity [79, 80]. Radiation results in a progressive loss of salivary gland function and therefore in a decrease in saliva output and a change in saliva composition, resulting in the sense of dry mouth and sticky saliva [10, 81]. Moreover, salivary dysfunction may result in considerable additional problems, including severe oral discomfort, impairment of oral functions (speech, chewing, swallowing) due to insufficient wetting and an increased incidence of caries and mucosal infections [10, 78].

It is important to note that the probability of radiation-induced complications markedly depends on the radiation dose to the organs at risk (OARs). Thus, by conforming the radiation dose to the target and simultaneously limiting the dose to the OARs, the severity and incidence of the radiation-induced side effects can be reduced.

## Clinical Studies

Over the years, radiotherapy treatment techniques have been improved and allow better conformation of the high-dose region to the PTV, while OARs can be spared more adequately.

Clinical studies indicated that compared with more conventional radiotherapy techniques, intensity-modulated radiotherapy with photons (IMRT) significantly reduces the parotid gland dose, resulting in higher flow rates after treatment and/or lower rates of xerostomia contributing to an improved quality of life [82–84] (also see Chap. 10 [Chris Nutting – IMRT as improved irradiation treatment]). However, sufficient sparing of the parotid glands with IMRT below the threshold cannot be achieved in all patients. Furthermore, sparing the parotid glands alone does not always translate into a reduced probability of patient-rated xerostomia [83, 84], reflecting the need to enhance sparing of other salivary glands as well. Consequently, further dose reductions in all relevant salivary glands by using more advanced radiotherapy techniques, like proton therapy, can help to reduce the probability of patient-rated xerostomia and hence improve quality of life during and after radiotherapy treatment.

## Proton Therapy

From a physical point of view, protons have an evident advantage over photons. Whereas photons are highly penetrating with a maximum dose near the patient's surface followed by an exponential reduction of the dose with increasing depth, protons have a finite range with a plateau dose that at first slowly and then rapidly increases with depth, resulting in a maximum dose near to the end of the proton beam range, the so-called Bragg peak, which is followed by a rapid drop to nearly zero dose (Fig. 13.4).

The position of the Bragg peak depends on the proton energy. By varying the individual proton energies in a proton beam, a spreadout Bragg peak (SOBP) can be produced that covers the tumour with a uniform dose while minimizing the dose to the normal tissues distal to the tumour (Fig. 13.4).

Overall, the physical properties of protons allow further improvement of the dose distribution. However, clinical studies concerning head and neck cancer patients

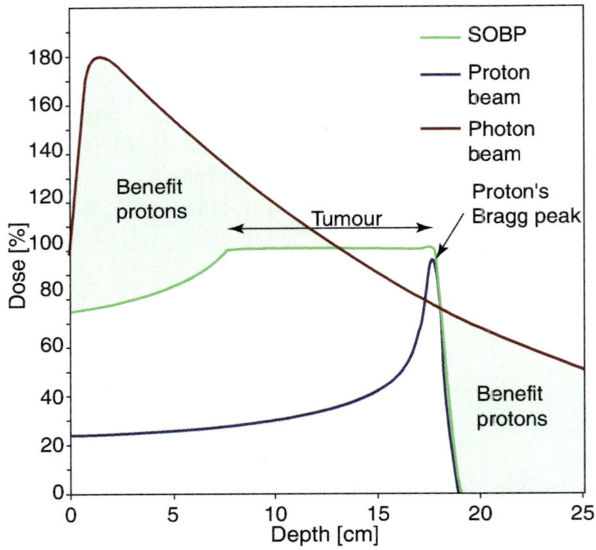


**Fig. 13.4** Schematic comparison between the depth dose profiles of photons and protons in tissue. The photon dose gradually decreases as the photons further penetrate the tissue. The proton dose profile is characterized by the so-called Bragg peak. By varying the individual proton energies in a proton beam, a spreadout Bragg peak (*SOBP*) can be produced that covers the tumour with a uniform dose while minimizing the dose to the normal tissues beyond the tumour. This figure illustrates the benefits of protons in terms of lower dose to the proximal and distal target sides

treated with proton therapy are scarce. Moreover, most clinical studies that use protons to treat head and neck cancers, use mixed photon-proton techniques: protons are only used during part of the radiation treatment course [85, 86]. Besides, reviews on the added value of protons over photons mainly focus on the role of protons in terms of treatment efficiency (by reporting on local tumour control and overall survival), rather than on potential benefits of protons with regard to reduction of radiation-induced side effects [87–89].

The first step in analyzing if a new radiation technique will have the potential to reduce radiation-induced side effects is by comparing dose distributions that can be obtained with the new technique referenced to the current standard technique, also referred to as in silico planning comparative (ISPC) studies. Various ISPC studies that compare photons with protons in head and neck cancer indicate that protons have the potential to significantly reduce the normal tissue dose, including the dose to the parotid salivary glands while keeping similar or better target coverage [90–92]. Most of the ISPC studies only focussed on reducing the dose to the parotid salivary glands and did not consider sparing of the submandibular glands. However, clinical studies that did investigate the feasibility of submandibular gland sparing with radiotherapy showed that sparing of those glands resulted in a reduced probability of xerostomia [93, 94]. Two ISPC studies also focussed on reducing the dose of submandibular glands in addition to parotid gland sparing [90, 91]. Those studies indicated that advanced scanned intensity-modulated proton therapy, as compared

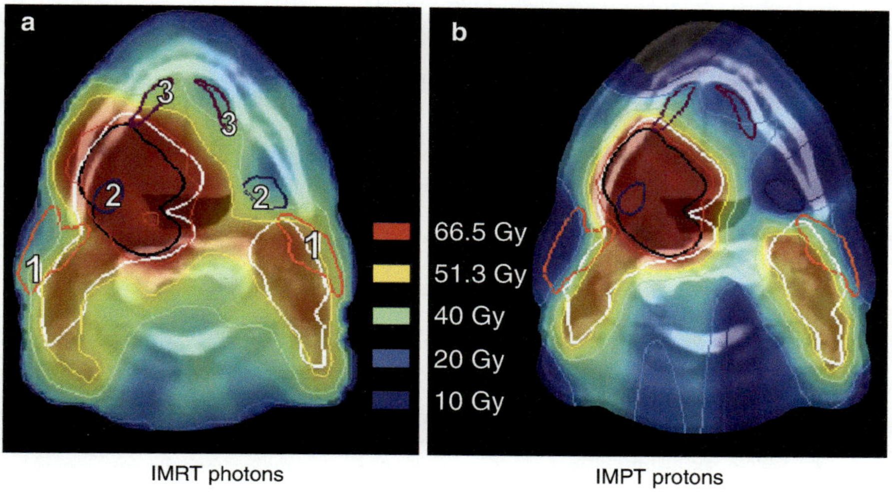


**Fig. 13.5** Dose distribution comparison between intensity-modulated radiotherapy (*IMRT*) with photons and advanced scanned intensity-modulated proton therapy (*IMPT*). Contours of the volumes of interest are thickened: elective nodal areas (*white contour*); boost volume enclosing the primary tumour (*black contour*); parotid glands (*1*); submandibular glands (*2*); sublingual glands (*3*). This figure illustrates the potential benefits of protons regarding sparing of the salivary glands

with photon IMRT (the current standard), significantly reduced the dose to both the submandibular glands and the parotid salivary glands [90]. They furthermore showed that the level of benefit that can be obtained with advanced intensity-modulated proton therapy in terms of less dose to the healthy tissues varies among the individual patients and is case specific. Figure 13.5 displays for one specific case the benefits of the advanced scanned proton therapy technique regarding sparing of the salivary glands. According to existing normal tissue complication probability models for parotid and submandibular salivary flow dysfunction and patient-rated xerostomia, these dose reductions result in significant clinical benefits in most of the cases [90]. Hence, it is expected that advanced scanned intensity-modulated proton therapy, as compared with photon IMRT, improves quality of life during and after radiotherapy treatment.

## Summary

Regretfully many of the current treatments or preventive strategies to treat radiation-induced hyposalivation and consequential xerostomia have not shown sufficient potential to be of general use in the clinic. Regeneration-inducing factors, such as growth factors, have shown to be promising but remain difficult in the use of cancer patient due to their potential effect on tumours. Therefore, most promising for the future prevention and treatment of radiation-induced hyposalivation seems to be gene therapy or stem cell therapy or a combination of both. However, reducing the irradiated gland volume using proton therapy may be the preferred solution.

## References


1. Jemal A, Bray F, Center MM, Ferlay J, Ward E, Forman D. Global cancer statistics. CA Cancer J Clin. 2011;61(2):69–90.
2. Hunter KD, Parkinson EK, Harrison PR. Profiling early head and neck cancer. Nat Rev Cancer. 2005;5(2):127–35.
3. Vissink A, Jansma J, Spijkervet FK, Burlage FR, Coppes RP. Oral sequelae of head and neck radiotherapy. Crit Rev Oral Biol Med. 2003;14(3):199–212.
4. Sciubba JJ, Goldenberg D. Oral complications of radiotherapy. Lancet Oncol. 2006;7(2): 175–83.
5. Jellema AP, Slotman BJ, Doornaert P, Leemans CR, Langendijk JA. Impact of radiation-induced xerostomia on quality of life after primary radiotherapy among patients with head and neck cancer. Int J Radiat Oncol Biol Phys. 2007;69(3):751–60.
6. Langendijk JA, Doornaert P, Verdonck-de Leeuw IM, Leemans CR, Aaronson NK, Slotman BJ. Impact of late treatment-related toxicity on quality of life among patients with head and neck cancer treated with radiotherapy. J Clin Oncol. 2008;26(22):3770–6.
7. Burlage FR, Roesink JM, Kampinga HH, Coppes RP, Terhaard C, Langendijk JA, et al. Protection of salivary function by concomitant pilocarpine during radiotherapy: a double-blind, randomized, placebo-controlled study. Int J Radiat Oncol Biol Phys. 2008;70(1): 14–22.
8. Eisbruch A. Intensity-modulated radiation therapy in the treatment of head and neck cancer. Nat Clin Pract Oncol. 2005;2(1):34–9.
9. Vergeer MR, Doornaert PA, Rietveld DH, Leemans CR, Slotman BJ, Langendijk JA. Intensity-modulated radiotherapy reduces radiation-induced morbidity and improves health-related quality of life: results of a nonrandomized prospective study using a standardized follow-up program. Int J Radiat Oncol Biol Phys. 2009;74(1):1–8.
10. Vissink A, Burlage FR, Spijkervet FK, Jansma J, Coppes RP. Prevention and treatment of the consequences of head and neck radiotherapy. Crit Rev Oral Biol Med. 2003;14(3):213–25.
11. Zajicek G, Yagil C, Michaeli Y. The streaming submandibular gland. Anat Rec. 1985; 213(2):150–8.
12. Nagler RM, Baum BJ, Fox PC. Acute effects of X irradiation on the function of rat salivary glands. Radiat Res. 1993;136(1):42–7.
13. Burlage FR, Coppes RP, Meertens H, Stokman MA, Vissink A. Parotid and submandibular/sublingual salivary flow during high dose radiotherapy. Radiother Oncol. 2001;61(3):271–4.
14. Coppes RP, Zeilstra LJ, Kampinga HH, Konings AW. Early to late sparing of radiation damage to the parotid gland by adrenergic and muscarinic receptor agonists. Br J Cancer. 2001;85(7):1055–63.
15. Konings AW, Coppes RP, Vissink A. On the mechanism of salivary gland radiosensitivity. Int J Radiat Oncol Biol Phys. 2005;62(4):1187–94.
16. Abok K, Brunk U, Jung B, Ericsson J. Morphologic and histochemical studies on the differing radiosensitivity of ductular and acinar cells of the rat submandibular gland. Virchows Arch B Cell Pathol Incl Mol Pathol. 1984;45(4):443–60.
17. Nagler R, Marmary Y, Fox PC, Baum BJ, Har-El R, Chevion M. Irradiation-induced damage to the salivary glands: the role of redox-active iron and copper. Radiat Res. 1997;147(4): 468–76.
18. Zeilstra LJ, Vissink A, Konings AW, Coppes RP. Radiation induced cell loss in rat submandibular gland and its relation to gland function. Int J Radiat Biol. 2000;76(3):419–29.
19. Stephens LC, Schultheiss TE, Price RE, Ang KK, Peters LJ. Radiation apoptosis of serous acinar cells of salivary and lacrimal glands. Cancer. 1991;67(6):1539–43.
20. Stephens LC, Schultheiss TE, Small SM, Ang KK, Peters LJ. Response of parotid gland organ culture to radiation. Radiat Res. 1989;120(1):140–53.
21. Takahashi S, Nakamura S, Shinzato K, Domon T, Yamamoto T, Wakita M. Apoptosis and proliferation of myoepithelial cells in atrophic rat submandibular glands. J Histochem Cytochem. 2001;49(12):1557–64.

22. Denny PC, Chai Y, Klauser DK, Denny PA. Parenchymal cell proliferation and mechanisms for maintenance of granular duct and acinar cell populations in adult male mouse submandibular gland. Anat Rec. 1993;235(3):475–85.
23. Denny PC, Ball WD, Redman RS. Salivary glands: a paradigm for diversity of gland development. Crit Rev Oral Biol Med. 1997;8(1):51–75.
24. Man YG, Ball WD, Marchetti L, Hand AR. Contributions of intercalated duct cells to the normal parenchyma of submandibular glands of adult rats. Anat Rec. 2001;263(2):202–14.
25. Konings AW, Faber H, Cotteleer F, Vissink A, Coppes RP. Secondary radiation damage as the main cause for unexpected volume effects: a histopathologic study of the parotid gland. Int J Radiat Oncol Biol Phys. 2006;64(1):98–105.
26. Ihrler S, Zietz C, Sendelhofert A, Lang S, Blasenbreu-Vogt S, Lohrs U. A morphogenetic concept of salivary duct regeneration and metaplasia. Virchows Arch. 2002;440(5):519–26.
27. Roesink JM, Konings AW, Terhaard CH, Battermann JJ, Kampinga HH, Coppes RP. Preservation of the rat parotid gland function after radiation by prophylactic pilocarpine treatment: radiation dose dependency and compensatory mechanisms. Int J Radiat Oncol Biol Phys. 1999;45(2):483–9.
28. Liu RP, Fleming TJ, Toth BB, Keene HJ. Salivary flow rates in patients with head and neck cancer 0.5 to 25 years after radiotherapy. Oral Surg Oral Med Oral Pathol. 1990;70(6):724–9.
29. Lombaert IM. Regeneration of irradiated salivary glands by stem cell therapy. PhD thesis ed. Groningen: University of Groningen; 2008.
30. Baum BJ. Gene therapy. Oral Dis. 2014;20(2):115–8.
31. Delporte C, O'Connell BC, He X, Lancaster HE, O'Connell AC, Agre P, et al. Increased fluid secretion after adenoviral-mediated transfer of the aquaporin-1 cDNA to irradiated rat salivary glands. Proc Natl Acad Sci U S A. 1997;94(7):3268–73.
32. Shan Z, Li J, Zheng C, Liu X, Fan Z, Zhang C, et al. Increased fluid secretion after adenoviral-mediated transfer of the human aquaporin-1 cDNA to irradiated miniature pig parotid glands. Mol Ther. 2005;11(3):444–51.
33. Zheng C, Goldsmith CM, Mineshiba F, Chiorini JA, Kerr A, Wenk ML, et al. Toxicity and biodistribution of a first-generation recombinant adenoviral vector, encoding aquaporin-1, after retroductal delivery to a single rat submandibular gland. Hum Gene Ther. 2006; 17(11):1122–33.
34. Baum BJ, Alevizos I, Zheng C, Cotrim AP, Liu S, McCullagh L, et al. Early responses to adenoviral-mediated transfer of the aquaporin-1 cDNA for radiation-induced salivary hypofunction. Proc Natl Acad Sci U S A. 2012;109(47):19403–7.
35. Cotrim AP, Hyodo F, Matsumoto K, Sowers AL, Cook JA, Baum BJ, et al. Differential radiation protection of salivary glands versus tumor by Tempol with accompanying tissue assessment of Tempol by magnetic resonance imaging. Clin Cancer Res. 2007;13(16):4928–33.
36. Citrin D, Cotrim AP, Hyodo F, Baum BJ, Krishna MC, Mitchell JB. Radioprotectors and mitigators of radiation-induced normal tissue injury. Oncologist. 2010;15(4):360–71.
37. Utley JF, Marlowe C, Waddell WJ. Distribution of 35S-labeled WR-2721 in normal and malignant tissues of the mouse1,2. Radiat Res. 1976;68(2):284–91.
38. Yuhas JM, Spellman JM, Culo F. The role of WR-2721 in radiotherapy and/or chemotherapy. Cancer Clin Trials. 1980;3(3):211–6.
39. Konings AW, Faber H, Vissink A, Coppes RP. Radioprotective effect of amifostine on parotid gland functioning is region dependent. Int J Radiat Oncol Biol Phys. 2005;63(5):1584–91.
40. Jensen SB, Pedersen AM, Vissink A, Andersen E, Brown CG, Davies AN, et al. A systematic review of salivary gland hypofunction and xerostomia induced by cancer therapies: management strategies and economic impact. Support Care Cancer. 2010;18(8):1061–79.
41. Paardekooper GM, Cammelli S, Zeilstra LJ, Coppes RP, Konings AW. Radiation-induced apoptosis in relation to acute impairment of rat salivary gland function. Int J Radiat Biol. 1998;73(6):641–8.
42. Coppes RP, Vissink A, Zeilstra LJ, Konings AW. Muscarinic receptor stimulation increases tolerance of rat salivary gland function to radiation damage. Int J Radiat Biol. 1997; 72(5):615–25.

43. Coppes RP, Zeilstra LJ, Vissink A, Konings AW. Sialogogue-related radioprotection of salivary gland function: the degranulation concept revisited. Radiat Res. 1997;148(3):240–7.
44. Bentzen SM, Harari PM, Bernier J. Exploitable mechanisms for combining drugs with radiation: concepts, achievements and future directions. Nat Clin Pract Oncol. 2007;4(3):172–80.
45. Coppes RP, van der Goot A, Lombaert IM. Stem cell therapy to reduce radiation-induced normal tissue damage. Semin Radiat Oncol. 2009;19(2):112–21.
46. Braam PM, Roesink JM, Moerland MA, Raaijmakers CP, Schipper M, Terhaard CH. Long-term parotid gland function after radiotherapy. Int J Radiat Oncol Biol Phys. 2005;62(3):659–64.
47. Coppes R, Stokman M. Stem cells and the repair of radiation-induced salivary gland damage. Oral Dis. 2011;17(2):143–53.
48. Lombaert IM, Brunsting JF, Wierenga PK, Faber H, Stokman MA, Kok T, et al. Rescue of salivary gland function after stem cell transplantation in irradiated glands. PLoS One. 2008;3(4):e2063.
49. Pringle S, Van Os R, Coppes RP. Concise review: adult salivary gland stem cells and a potential therapy for xerostomia. Stem Cells. 2013;31(4):613–9.
50. Peter B, Van Waarde MA, Vissink A, 's-Gravenmade EJ, Konings AW. Radiation-induced cell proliferation in the parotid and submandibular glands of the rat. Radiat Res. 1994;140(2):257–65.
51. Coppes RP, Vissink A, Konings AW. Comparison of radiosensitivity of rat parotid and submandibular glands after different radiation schedules. Radiother Oncol. 2002;63(3):321–8.
52. Lombaert IM, Brunsting JF, Wierenga PK, Kampinga HH, de Haan G, Coppes RP. Keratinocyte growth factor prevents radiation damage to salivary glands by expansion of the stem/progenitor pool. Stem Cells. 2008;26(10):2595–601.
53. Ohlsson B, Jansen C, Ihse I, Axelson J. Epidermal growth factor induces cell proliferation in mouse pancreas and salivary glands. Pancreas. 1997;14(1):94–8.
54. Limesand KH, Said S, Anderson SM. Suppression of radiation-induced salivary gland dysfunction by IGF-1. PLoS One. 2009;4(3):e4663.
55. Thula TT, Schultz G, Tran-Son-Tay R, Batich C. Effects of EGF and bFGF on irradiated parotid glands. Ann Biomed Eng. 2005;33(5):685–95.
56. Hai B, Yang Z, Shangguan L, Zhao Y, Boyer A, Liu F. Concurrent transient activation of Wnt/beta-catenin pathway prevents radiation damage to salivary glands. Int J Radiat Oncol Biol Phys. 2012;83(1):e109–16.
57. Kojima T, Kanemaru S, Hirano S, Tateya I, Suehiro A, Kitani Y, et al. The protective efficacy of basic fibroblast growth factor in radiation-induced salivary gland dysfunction in mice. Laryngoscope. 2011;121(9):1870–5.
58. Martin KL, Hill GA, Klein RR, Arnett DG, Burd R, Limesand KH. Prevention of radiation-induced salivary gland dysfunction utilizing a CDK inhibitor in a mouse model. PLoS One. 2012;7(12):e51363.
59. Gorjup E, Danner S, Rotter N, Habermann J, Brassat U, Brummendorf TH, et al. Glandular tissue from human pancreas and salivary gland yields similar stem cell populations. Eur J Cell Biol. 2009;88(7):409–21.
60. Lombaert IM, Wierenga PK, Kok T, Kampinga HH, deHaan G, Coppes RP. Mobilization of bone marrow stem cells by granulocyte colony-stimulating factor ameliorates radiation-induced damage to salivary glands. Clin Cancer Res. 2006;12(6):1804–12.
61. Xu J, Wang D, Liu D, Fan Z, Zhang H, Liu O, et al. Allogeneic mesenchymal stem cell treatment alleviates experimental and clinical Sjogren syndrome. Blood. 2012;120(15):3142–51.
62. Tran SD, Sumita Y, Khalili S. Bone marrow-derived cells: a potential approach for the treatment of xerostomia. Int J Biochem Cell Biol. 2011;43(1):5–9.
63. Tran SD, Liu Y, Xia D, Maria OM, Khalili S, Wang RW, et al. Paracrine effects of bone marrow soup restore organ function, regeneration, and repair in salivary glands damaged by irradiation. PLoS One. 2013;8(4):e61632.
64. Lombaert IM, Brunsting JF, Wierenga PK, Kampinga HH, de Haan G, Coppes RP. Cytokine treatment improves parenchymal and vascular damage of salivary glands after irradiation. Clin Cancer Res. 2008;14(23):7741–50.

65. Takahashi K, Yamanaka S. Induction of pluripotent stem cells from mouse embryonic and adult fibroblast cultures by defined factors. Cell. 2006;126(4):663–76.
66. Kawakami M, Ishikawa H, Tachibana T, Tanaka A, Mataga I. Functional transplantation of salivary gland cells differentiated from mouse early ES cells in vitro. Hum Cell. 2013; 26(2):80–90.
67. Vissink A, van Luijk P, Langendijk J, Coppes R. Current ideas to reduce or salvage radiation damage to salivary glands. Oral Dis. 2014. doi 10.1111/odi. 12222 epub ahead.
68. Lombaert IM, Knox SM, Hoffman MP. Salivary gland progenitor cell biology provides a rationale for therapeutic salivary gland regeneration. Oral Dis. 2011;17(5):445–9.
69. Pringle S, Nanduri LS, Marianne Z, Ronald O, Coppes RP. Isolation of mouse salivary gland stem cells. J Vis Exp. 2011;(48). pii: 2484. doi(48):10.3791/2484.
70. Feng J, van der Zwaag M, Stokman MA, van Os R, Coppes RP. Isolation and characterization of human salivary gland cells for stem cell transplantation to reduce radiation-induced hyposalivation. Radiother Oncol. 2009;92(3):466–71.
71. Nanduri LS, Lombaert IM, van der Zwaag M, Faber H, Brunsting JF, van Os RP, et al. Salisphere derived c-Kit cell transplantation restores tissue homeostasis in irradiated salivary gland. Radiother Oncol. 2013;13:240.
72. Nanduri LS, Maimets M, Pringle SA, van der Zwaag M, van Os RP, Coppes RP. Regeneration of irradiated salivary glands with stem cell marker expressing cells. Radiother Oncol. 2011;99(3):367–72.
73. Palmon A, David R, Neumann Y, Stiubea-Cohen R, Krief G, Aframian DJ. High-efficiency immunomagnetic isolation of solid tissue-originated integrin-expressing adult stem cells. Methods. 2012;56(2):305–9.
74. Beetz I, Schilstra C, Burlage FR, Koken PW, Doornaert P, Bijl HP, et al. Development of NTCP models for head and neck cancer patients treated with three-dimensional conformal radiotherapy for xerostomia and sticky saliva: the role of dosimetric and clinical factors. Radiother Oncol. 2012;105(1):86–93.
75. van de Water TA. Potential benefits of intensity-modulated proton therapy in head and neck cancer. PhD thesis, ed. Groningen: University of Groningen; 2013.
76. Jereczek-Fossa BA, Orecchia R. Radiotherapy-induced mandibular bone complications. Cancer Treat Rev. 2002;28(1):65–74.
77. Nguyen NP, Frank C, Moltz CC, Vos P, Smith HJ, Karlsson U, et al. Impact of dysphagia on quality of life after treatment of head-and-neck cancer. Int J Radiat Oncol Biol Phys. 2005;61(3):772–8.
78. Vissink A, Mitchell JB, Baum BJ, Limesand KH, Jensen SB, Fox PC, et al. Clinical management of salivary gland hypofunction and xerostomia in head-and-neck cancer patients: successes and barriers. Int J Radiat Oncol Biol Phys. 2010;78(4):983–91.
79. Humphrey SP, Williamson RT. A review of saliva: normal composition, flow, and function. J Prosthet Dent. 2001;85(2):162–9.
80. van Nieuw Amerongen A, Veerman ECI, Vissink A. Samenstelling en eigenschappen van speeksel: van dun-vloeibare tot viskeuze mondvloeistof. In: Speeksel, speekselklieren en mondgezondheid. 2nd ed. Houten: Bohn Stafleu Van Loghum bv; 2008. p. 37–51.
81. Cooper JS, Fu K, Marks J, Silverman S. Late effects of radiation therapy in the head and neck region. Int J Radiat Oncol Biol Phys. 1995;31(5):1141–64.
82. Eisbruch A, Ship JA, Dawson LA, Kim HM, Bradford CR, Terrell JE, et al. Salivary gland sparing and improved target irradiation by conformal and intensity modulated irradiation of head and neck cancer. World J Surg. 2003;27(7):832–7.
83. Kam MK, Leung SF, Zee B, Chau RM, Suen JJ, Mo F, et al. Prospective randomized study of intensity-modulated radiotherapy on salivary gland function in early-stage nasopharyngeal carcinoma patients. J Clin Oncol. 2007;25(31):4873–9.
84. Pow EH, Kwong DL, McMillan AS, Wong MC, Sham JS, Leung LH, et al. Xerostomia and quality of life after intensity-modulated radiotherapy vs. conventional radiotherapy for early-stage nasopharyngeal carcinoma: initial report on a randomized controlled clinical trial. Int J Radiat Oncol Biol Phys. 2006;66(4):981–91.

85. Slater JD, Yonemoto LT, Mantik DW, Bush DA, Preston W, Grove RI et al. Proton radiation for treatment of cancer of the oropharynx: Early experience at Loma Linda University Medical Center using a concomitant boost technique. Int J Radiat Oncol Biol Phys. 2005;62(2):494–500.
86. Tokuuye K, Akine Y, Kagei K, Hata M, Hashimoto T, Mizumoto T, et al. Proton therapy for head and neck malignancies at Tsukuba. Strahlenther Onkol. 2004;180(2):96–101.
87. Brada M, Pijls-Johannesma M, De Ruysscher D. Current clinical evidence for proton therapy. Cancer J. 2009;15(4):319–24.
88. Chan AW, Liebsch NJ. Proton radiation therapy for head and neck cancer. J Surg Oncol. 2008;97(8):697–700.
89. Schulz-Ertner D. The clinical experience with particle therapy in adults. Cancer J. 2009;15(4): 306–11.
90. van de Water TA, Lomax AJ, Bijl HP, Schilstra C, Hug EB, Langendijk JA. Using a reduced spot size for intensity-modulated proton therapy potentially improves salivary gland-sparing in oropharyngeal cancer. Int J Radiat Oncol Biol Phys. 2012;82(2):e313–9.
91. van de Water TA, Lomax AJ, Bijl HP, de Jong ME, Schilstra C, Hug EB, et al. Potential benefits of scanned intensity-modulated proton therapy versus advanced photon therapy with regard to sparing of the salivary glands in oropharyngeal cancer. Int J Radiat Oncol Biol Phys. 2011;79(4):1216–24.
92. van de Water TA, Bijl HP, Schilstra C, Pijls-Johannesma M, Langendijk JA. The potential benefit of radiotherapy with protons in head and neck cancer with respect to normal tissue sparing: a systematic review of literature. Oncologist. 2011;16(3):366–77.
93. Liu X, Su Y, Jha N, Hong M, Mai H, Fan W, et al. Submandibular salivary gland transfer for the prevention of radiation-induced xerostomia in patients with nasopharyngeal carcinoma: 5-year outcomes. Head Neck. 2010;33(3):389–95.
94. Saarilahti K, Kouri M, Collan J, Kangasmaki A, Atula T, Joensuu H, et al. Sparing of the submandibular glands by intensity modulated radiotherapy in the treatment of head and neck cancer. Radiother Oncol. 2006;78(3):270–5.

# Index

**A**
Acupuncture, SGD management, 61
Adult stem cells, 201–203
Afferent signalling, MISGD, 39–40
*Aggregatibacter actinomycetemcomitans,* 87, 89, 96
Alpha-2 adrenoceptor (α2Ad) agonists
  activation, 44–45
  central signalling, 43–44
Alzheimer's disease (AD), 19–20
American College of Rheumatology (ACR), 13
American-European classification criteria, Sjögren's syndrome, 9, 10
Amifostine, 198
Amphetamine, 44
Amyloidosis, 16
Anorexia nervosa, 23
Antimuscarinic effect, 42
Arc therapies, 161
Artificial salivas
  acidic pH, 170
  advantage, 181
  bioactives, 169
  carboxymethylcellulose/xanthan gum, 169
  composition, 169–170
  deficiency, 165
  efficacy, 168
  elasticity, 170, 171
  food proteins, 171
  intraoral lubrication and hydration, 167–168
  and natural salivas, physical properties, 170, 171
  randomised controlled trial, 166
  surface tension, 168
  usage, 167
  viscosity, 165
Autoimmune diseases
  amyloidosis, 16
  autoimmune hepatitis, 16
  chronic inflammatory bowel diseases, 15–16
  chronic inflammatory connective tissue diseases, 9–14
  endocrine diseases, 17–18
  neurological diseases, 18–20
  primary biliary cirrhosis, 16
  primary sclerosing cholangitis, 16
  sarcoidosis, 14
Autoimmune hepatitis (AIH), 16

**B**
Battery-type approaches
  Challacombe scale, 107
  item content, 106
  summated rating scale, 108–111
  visual analogue scale, 107–108
Bell's palsy, 19
BMS. *See* Burning mouth syndrome (BMS)
Bother 1 xerostomia index (BI1), 130, 131
Bother 5 xerostomia index (BI5), 129–131
Bulimia nervosa, 23
Burning mouth syndrome (BMS), 20

**C**
*Candida albicans,* 86–87, 90, 94, 95
Carbonic anhydrase VI, 74
Cell models of oral mucosa, 168
Cerebral palsy syndromes, 18
Cevimeline, MIX treatment, 46
Challacombe scale, 4, 107
Chewing gum
  and lozenges, 177
  and saliva substitutes, 46–47
  SGD management, 59
  side effects, 59
  sugar-free, 96, 123, 181–182


G. Carpenter (ed.), *Dry Mouth: A Clinical Guide on Causes, Effects and Treatments*, DOI 10.1007/978-3-642-55154-3

Clinical oral dryness score (CODS)
features, 121–123
mild dryness, 123, 124
moderate dryness, 124
mucosal dryness, 121–123
mucosal wetness, 125, 127, 128
*vs.* salivary flow, 125, 126
sensitivity, 128
severe dryness, 124
CNS trauma, 18
CODS. *See* Clinical oral dryness score (CODS)
Coeliac disease, 15–16
Crohn's disease (CD), 15
Cuckoo spit, 171–172
Cystic fibrosis (CF), 22
Cytomegalovirus (CMV), 21

**D**
Dehydration, 23, 76
Dental caries
mutans streptococci, 92–93
occurrence, 91
prediction models, 91–92
saliva, 92
Dental panoramic radiographs, 140
Dental plaque
development, 84
intensive care units *vs.* healthy controls, 91
low pH, 91, 92
microbial composition, 84
Diabetes mellitus (DM), 17
Dietary intake, 75
chewing and swallowing process, 70, 72
healthy eating index, 71
oral pain and discomfort, 70, 72
salivary secretion, 70–73
Digital subtraction fluoroscopy, 138
Draining method, 8

**E**
Eating disorders
anorexia nervosa, 23
bulimia nervosa, 24
Ectodermal dysplasia (ED), 22
Efferent signalling, MISGD
dual parasympathetic/sympathetic nerve stimulation experiments, 40
muscarinic acetylcholine receptors, 41–42
tricyclic antidepressants, 42
Embryonic stem (ES) cells, 201–202
Endoscopy, 142
Epidemic parotitis, 21
Epstein-Barr virus (EBV), 21
European League Against Rheumatism (EULAR) classification criteria, 13
External beam radiotherapy, HNC, 148

**F**
Focus scoring system, 10

**G**
Genetic and developmental diseases, oral dryness, 22
Gingivitis, 96

**H**
Head and neck cancer (HNC)
external beam radiotherapy, 148
PG-sparing IMRT, 153, 154
photon-proton techniques, 206
prophylactic pilocarpine administration, 196
radiotherapy, 195–196, 204–205
Hepatitis C virus (HCV), 21
Human immunodeficiency virus (HIV), 20–21
Hyposalivation
aging, 176
dehydration, 23
description, 8
oral symptoms, 129
signs, 120
Sjögren's syndrome, 9

**I**
Induced pluripotent stem (iPS) cells, 201, 202
Infectious diseases, oral dryness
hepatitis C virus, 21
human immunodeficiency virus, 20–21
In silico planning comparative (ISPC) studies, 206–207
Intensity-modulated radiation therapy (IMRT)
concave and convex shape, 152
description, 151–152
dose escalation, 153
HNC treatment, 153
national and international experience, 157–158
oral mucosa (*see* Oral mucosa (OM)-sparing IMRT)
principle, 151–152
quality of life, 196
Intraoral radiographs, 140

**L**
Labial salivary gland biopsy, 16
*Lactobacillus* species
  anterior sites, 93
  dental caries, 93
  intestinal flora, 94
  pH level, 94, 95
  posterior sites, 93–94

**M**
Magnetic resonance imaging (MRI), salivary gland study, 141–142
Mastication
  aging, 188
  definition, 190
  gustatory stimuli, 176
  oral food processing, 190–191
  resistance training, 189
Medication-induced dry mouth
  description, 35
  xerogenic drugs, 34
Medication-induced salivary gland hypofunction (MISGD)
  afferent signalling, 39–40
  age groups, 39
  central interruption of reflex signalling, 42–45
  definition, 35, 37
  efferent signalling
    dual parasympathetic/sympathetic nerve stimulation experiments, 40
    muscarinic acetylcholine receptors, 41–42
    tricyclic antidepressants, 42
  salivary reflex, 37, 38
  UWMS flow rate, 37
Medication-induced xerostomia (MIX)
  assessment, 35
  description, 35
  dose and duration, 36
  selective serotonin reuptake inhibitors, 36
  serotonin and noradrenaline reuptake inhibitors, 36, 37
  severity, 36
  treatment
    drug substitution, 45–46
    gum chewing and saliva substitutes, 46–47
    pharmacological stimulation, 46
Mesenchymal stem cells (MSCs), 200–201
MISGD. *See* Medication-induced salivary gland hypofunction (MISGD)
MIX. *See* Medication-induced xerostomia (MIX)
Mixed connective tissue disease (MCTD), 14
Molecular pharming, 172
MUC5B, 84, 179
Mucosa-associated lymphoid tissue (MALT) lymphoma diagnosis, 137
Mucosal dryness and CODS, 121–123
Mucosal wetness and CODS, 125, 127, 128
Multi-item approaches, xerostomia measurement. *See* Battery-type approaches
Mumps. *See* Epidemic parotitis
Muscarinic acetylcholine receptors (mAchRs), 41–42

**N**
National Cancer Institute Common Terminology Criteria for Adverse Events (CTCAE), 56, 57
Nerve-mediated reflex, 39
Neurological disorders
  Alzheimer's disease, 19–20
  Bell's palsy, 19
  cerebral palsy, 18
  CNS trauma, 18
  Parkinson's disease, 19
Nonprescriptive sialogogues
  chewing gum and lozenges, 177
  complaints and side effects, 181
  MUC5B, 179
  mucin gum, 180
  oral cavity lubrication, 179
  organic acids, 180
  patients' preferences on products, 180, 181
  saliva stimulation, 178–179
  taste stimulus, 178
Normosalivators, 182

**O**
Obstructive salivary gland disease, 135, 136
Oral Balance® gel, 62
Oral disease severity scoring systems, 120–121
Oral dryness
  artificial saliva uasge, 96–97
  autoimmune diseases (*see* Autoimmune diseases)
  dietary intake, 70, 71
  prevalence, 69–70
Oral microbiome
  hyposalivation, 85
  and saliva
    antimicrobial activity, 84
    microbial attachment, 84
    nutrient availability, 83–84
    survival, 83

Oral microflora
artificial saliva, 96–97
hyposalivation due to medication, 89–91
primary Sjögren's syndrome, 88–89
radiation-induced hyposalivation, 85
buccal mucosa, 86
dorsum of the tongue, 86
gingival crevice region, 87
supragingival plaque, 87, 88
vestibulum in molar region, 86
xerostomia treatment, 96
Oral mucosal infections, 94–95
Oral mucosa (OM)-sparing IMRT, 159–160. *See also* Intensity-modulated radiation therapy (IMRT)
Oral taste buds, 73–74
Organic acids, SGD management, 59
Organs at risk (OARs), 204
Oropharyngeal carcinoma, 2D-RT treatment, 151, 152

**P**
Parasympathomimetics, MIX treatment, 46
Parkinson's disease (PD), 19
Parotid gland (PG)
dose-response relationship and radiation tolerance, 150–151
normal tissue complication probability curves, 150, 151
radiotherapy analysis, 150
Parotid gland (PG)-sparing IMRT. *See also* Intensity-modulated radiation therapy (IMRT)
EORTC QOL HN35 dry mouth subscale score, 153–155
HNC treatment, 153, 154
LENT-SOMA subjective xerostomia, 153, 155
local disease control, 160
non-nasopharyngeal carcinoma patients, 153, 154, 156
PARSPORT trial, 153
randomised controlled trials
*vs.* conventional 2D radiotherapy, 153–156
*vs.* 3D-CRT, 156
salivary gland dysfunction, 54
Particle therapies, 161
Periodontitis, 96
Pharmacological mechanisms
centrally acting xerogenic drugs, 44
peripherally acting xerogenic drugs, 41
Pilocarpine
MIX treatment, 46
SGD management, 60
Plain radiographs, salivary glands, 140–141
Polypharmacy, 176
*Porphyromonas gingivalis,* 87, 89, 96
Prader-Willi syndrome (PWS), 22–23
Primary biliary cirrhosis (PBC), 16
Primary sclerosing cholangitis (PSC), 16
Probiotics, 94
Progenitor cells, 199, 200
Protein-energy malnutrition (PEM), 76–77
Proton therapy
advanced scanned technique, 207
Bragg peak, 205, 206
depth dose profiles, photons *vs.* proton, 205, 206
in silico planning comparative studies, 206–207
PWS. *See* Prader-Willi syndrome (PWS)

**R**
Radiation-induced hyposalivation
gene therapy, 197–198
prevention, 198–199
proton therapy, 205–207
radioprotectors, 198–199
stem cell therapy, 201–205
stimulation of regeneration
basic fibroblast growth factor, 200
mesenchymal stem cells, 200–201
progenitor cells, 199, 200
roscovitine, 200
Wnt/β-catenin, 200
Rheumatoid arthritis (RA)
onset, 12–13
salivary gland enlargement, 13
symptoms, 13
Roscovitine, 200

**S**
Saliva Orthana®, 62
Salivary bicarbonate, 74
Salivary gland dysfunction (SGD). *See also* Salivary gland hypofunction (SGH); Xerostomia
cancer patients
avoiding acidic and sugar-sweetened drinks/foods/medication, 63
avoiding xerostomic medication, 63
causes, 53
clinical features, 54
complications, 54, 55

drug treatment, 58
fluoridated toothpaste, 63
maintaining oral hygiene, 62
National Cancer Institute CTCAE, 56, 57
parotid-sparing intensity-modulated radiotherapy, 54
prevention, 58
regular dental review, 63
saliva stimulants, 58–61
saliva substitutes, 61–62
definition, 51
Salivary gland hypofunction (SGH), 103
clinical features, 54
definition, 51
presence/absence, 125, 127
prevalence, 52
signs, 56
Salivary glands
imaging modalities, 133
endoscopy, 142
MRI examination, 141–142
plain radiographs, 140–141
scintigraphy, 142
sialography, 137–140
ultrasonography, 134–137
radiotherapy
human studies, 149–150
IMRT (*see* Intensity-modulated radiation therapy (IMRT))
preclinical data, 149
response to radiation, 196–197
Salivary secretion, 3, 178
alpha-2 adrenoceptor agonists, 43, 44
autonomic nerve-mediated signals, 40
bite/occlusal force, 187–188
chewing and swallowing process, 72, 73
cytostatic drugs, 82
dietary intake, 70–73
gland size, 184, 186
muscarinic acetylcholine receptor activation, 41
number of natural teeth, 186–187
nutritional status
dehydration, 76
malnutrition and micronutrients deficiency, 76–77
oral pain and discomfort, 72
regular chewing, 183–186
resting rate, 3
tricyclic antidepressants, 42
Saliva stimulants
acupuncture, 61
chewing gum, 59
organic acids, 59
parasympathomimetic drugs, 60–61
Saliva substitutes
artificial saliva, 61–62
water, 61
Sarcoidosis, 14
Scintigraphy, 142
Scleroderma, 14
Semi-quantitative clinical score, 121
SGD. *See* Salivary gland dysfunction (SGD)
Sialography
MRI, 141
salivary glands, 137–140
Single-item approaches, xerostomia measurement, 104–106
16 S ribosomal RNA sequencing, 82
Sjögren's syndrome (SS)
American-European classification criteria, 9, 10
autoantibodies, 11
cytokines, 12
labial and parotid biopsies, 11
labial salivary gland specimens, 9, 10
lymphocytic infiltrates, 10
occurrence, 9
oral microflora, primary, 88–89
paraffin chewing-stimulated whole saliva flow rate, 12
prevalence, 9
salivary gland enlargement, 12
scintigraphy, 142
sialochemical analyses, 12
sialography, 138, 140
sialometry, 11
unstimulated whole saliva flow rate, 11–12
South Australian Dental Longitudinal Study (SADLS), 109
SS. *See* Sjögren's syndrome (SS)
Stem cell therapy
adult stem cells, 201–203
embryonic stem cells, 201–202
good manufacturing practice regulations, 204
induced pluripotent stem cells, 201, 202
proton therapy (see Proton therapy)
salisphere-derived cells, 203
tissue stem cells, 201, 202
*Streptococcus mutans,* 84, 89, 91
Submandibular gland (SG)-sparing IMRT, 158–160
Sugar-free chewing gum
advantages, 181–182
description, 96
Summated rating scale, 108–111

Summated Xerostomia Inventory (SXI), 110–111
Systemic lupus erythematosus (SLE)
 characterisation, 13
 onset, 13
 oral symptoms, 13
Systemic sclerosis, 14

**T**
Taste alteration, 75–76
Taste sensation, 74
$^{99m}$Technetium-pertechnetate, 142
Tempol, 198
3D conformal radiotherapy (3D-CRT), 151, 153, 156, 159
Thyroiditis, 18
Tiotropium, 41–42
Tramadol, 45
Tricyclic antidepressants (TCAs), 36, 42
2D radiotherapy (2D-RT), 151, 152
Type 1 and 2 diabetes, 17

**U**
Ulcerative colitis (UC), 15
Ultrasonography
 advantage, 137
 principle, 134–135
 salivary glands
  ductal obstruction, 135, 136
  hyperechoic, 135
  Sjogren's syndrome, 136, 137
Unstimulated saliva
 flow in oral cavity, 182, 183
 masticatory function
  masticatory muscles and dentition, 188–190
  oral food processing, 190–191
 salivary secretion
  bite/occlusal force, 187–188
  body position, 184
  circadian rhythm, 184
  circannual rhythm, 184
  exposure to light, 184
  gland size, 184, 186
  hydration level, 184
  number of natural teeth, 186–187
  previous stimulation, 184
  regular chewing, 183–186
 *vs.* stimulated saliva, 182
 taste perception, 182–183
Unstimulated whole saliva flow rate (UWSFR), 8, 11, 54, 70–71

**V**
Venlafaxine, 44–45
Ventilator-associated pneumonia, 91
Visual analogue scale (VAS), 107–108

**W**
Wnt/β-catenin, 200

**X**
Xerostomia, 4
 assessment, 120
 cancer patients, 55
 causes, 82
 chemotherapy, 53
 clinical features, 54, 56
 definition, 51, 103
 dehydration, 23
 description, 8
 head and neck region, radiotherapy, 52
 oral-health-related quality of life, 112
 oral symptoms, 129
 pathophysiology, 54
 prevalence, 8, 51, 52
 radioactive iodine, 52
 subjective measurement
  conceptual model, 104
  multi-item approaches, 106–111
  reliability, 104
  self-report, 104
  single-item approaches, 104–106
  validity, 104
 ventilator-associated pneumonia, 91
Xerostomia Inventory (XI)
 description, 108–109
 development, 109–110
 original and short-form versions, 108, 109
 SXI, 110–111
 validity, 110